The Evolution of Orthopaedic Surgery

The Evolution of Orthopaedic Surgery

Edited by

Leslie Klenerman

MB BCH, ChM(Wits), FRCS(Ed), FRCS(Eng)
Emeritus Professor of Orthopaedic and Accident Surgery
University of Liverpool
Liverpool, UK

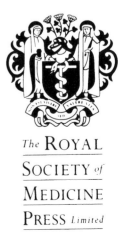

The ROYAL
SOCIETY *of*
MEDICINE
PRESS *Limited*

© 2002 Royal Society of Medicine Press Ltd
1 Wimpole Street, London W1G 0AE
207 Westminster Road, Lake IL 60045 USA
www.rsmpress.co.uk

British Library Cataloguing in Publication Data
A catalogue record for this book is available from the British
Library

ISBN: 185 315 4695

Typeset by Saxon Graphics Ltd, Derby

Printed and bound in Great Britain by
Marston Book Services Limited, Oxford

Contents

List of Contributors

Peter Abernethy MB, ChB, FRCS(Ed)
Consultant Orthopaedic Surgeon
Princess Margaret Rose Orthopaedic Hospital
Edinburgh, UK

Nicholas Barton FRCS
Emeritus Consultant Orthopaedic and Hand
Surgeon
University Hospital and Harlow Wood
Orthopaedic Hospital
Nottinghamshire, UK

Charles M. Court-Brown MD FRCS (Ed) Orth
Professor of Orthopaedics
Royal Infirmary of Edinburgh,
Edinburgh, UK

John Dove FRCS
Consultant Spinal Surgeon
Director
Stoke-on-Trent Spinal Services
North Staffordshire Hospital
Stoke-on-Trent, UK

John Fixsen M.Chir, FRCS
Formerly Consultant Orthopaedic Surgeon
Great Ormond Street Hospital for Sick Children
And The Royal Hospital of St Bartholomew's
London, UK

Robert W. Jackson OC MD MS(Tor) FRCSC FRCS
(Ed) FRCS (UK)
Professor
Baylor University Medical Center,
Department of Orthopedics,
Dallas
USA

Leslie Klenerman MB BCH, ChM(Wits), FRCS(Ed),
FRCS(Eng)
Emeritus Professor of Orthopaedic and Accident
Surgery
University of Liverpool
Liverpool, UK

Henry Mankin MD, FRCS(Hon)
Senior Surgeon Orthopaedic Oncology
Massachusetts General Hospital
Edith M. Ashley Professor of Orthopaedic Surgery
Harvard Medical School
USA

Dane A. Miller PhD
President and Chief
Executive Officer
Biomet, Inc.
USA

J. J. O'Connor
Professor
The Oxford Engineering Centre,
Nuffield Orthopaedic Centre,
Headington,
Oxford, UK

Peter Renton DMRD, FRCR
Consultant Radiologist,
Royal National Orthopaedic Hospital and
University College London Hospitals,
Honorary Senior Lecturer
University College London UK

Kingsley Peter Robinson MS, FRCS, FRCS Ed
Consultant Surgeon (retired)
Advisor in Amputee Management
Douglas Bader Unit,
Queen Mary's Hospital,
Roehampton, UK
And
Visiting Professor to Biomedical Department
School of Mechanical and Materials Engineering
University of Surrey
Guildford, UK

Neil Rushton MD FRCS
Consultant Orthopaedic Surgeon
Orthopaedic Research Unit
Addenbrooke's Hospital
Cambridge

Foreword

It is little more than a generation since orthopaedic surgery began its astounding and near exponential ascent from relative obscurity under the dominance of general surgery to itself become a major influence. How much longer will the interests of specialisation within it, allow it to remain united before it too falls victim to the fragmentation that destroyed the supremacy of its erstwhile master. In my view no more than another generation. It is timely that Professor Leslie Klenerman and his able team have set themselves the task of reviewing the remarkable evolution of the surgical speciality that has contributed more to the alleviation of man's suffering than any other. Our speciality has come along way since the two Greek words for 'straight' and 'child' were joined by Nicholas Andry in 1741 to describe his work; even further than the third century BC when Hippocrates first pronounced on articulations and the treatment of fractures. This is a fascinating story. It is of lonely visionaries and practical men who in harmony with advances in science, often in fields quite alien to medicine, had the courage to innovate and initiate such major advances as bone and joint replacement, the internal fixation of fractures and more recently arthroscopic surgery, the precursor of modern endoscopic surgery. Orthopaedic surgeons should be fascinated by this book. We all know bits of the jigsaw that is our heritage, but here we have a comprehensive perspective. Only time will tell if Professor Henry J. Mankin's forecasts are fulfilled but no one better could have been chosen to fill the role of oracle for the final chapter.

Sir Rodney Sweetnam

Preface

The arrival of the new millennium is the ideal time to review the origins and evolution of orthopaedic surgery and to look forward to its future. My plan was to start from the first use of the work 'orthopaedic' and trace its development into the surgical speciality with all the branches that we now recognise. The rapid expansion of the subject over the past fifty years has made it impossible for one person to cover the whole field. I have been extremely fortunate to have gathered a group of experts who have expressed their enthusiasm in the chapters they have written. The different interests and perspectives of these authors emphasise the diversity of disciplines now included in the field of orthopaedic surgery.

- I could not have started this project without the generous financial support of DePuy and Howmedica in advance of publication and without the help of Peter Richardson of the Royal Society of Medicine Press.
- In addition to the contributors of the various chapters, I thank John Kirkup, Tom Smith and Colin Dagnall for their friendly and helpful advice, and my wife Naomi and son Paul for their patience and constructive criticism.
- We stand on the shoulders of giants and I hope that the young orthopaedic surgeons of today who are now so technically skilled and well trained will be able to appreciate how the science and art of their speciality has evolved.

Leslie Klenerman
Sept, 2001

1

Setting the scene – the start of orthopaedic surgery

Leslie Klenerman

Surgery changed more in the nineteenth century than in the previous two millennia. The nineteenth and twentieth centuries were the age of revolutions. Industrialisation transformed the environment. Everyday life was affected by technology, steam engines and printing presses, steamships, railways, electricity, powered flight and telecommunications. In Europe and North America there was a large increase in population especially in major industrial cities, which besides producing wealth were riddled with poverty and disease (Porter 1997).

For centuries technology had played little part in the practice of medicine. Practical procedures were carried out by surgeons who were considered a lesser breed of medical practitioner. After the Industrial Revolution science and technology came together. Technology became more firmly based in science and science began to depend more on new technology. The introduction of the stethoscope by René Théophile Hyacinthe Laënnec in 1816 made possible the examination of the heart and lungs. The pioneering work of Antoni van Leeuwenhoek (1632–1723) on the microscope was belatedly taken up by pathologists more than a century later. With the improvements that followed the production of good achromatic lenses by Joseph Jackson Lister (1786–1869), Lord Lister's father, German histologists were able to show that all living organisms were made up of very small units of cells not visible to the naked eye. In disease there might be disorders of these cellular elements (Booth 1993). By 1858 Rudolf Virchow (1821–1902) in his great work *Die Cellularpathologie* demonstrated an entirely new concept of human disease. The microscope also enabled Louis Pasteur (1822–95) and Robert Koch (1843–1910) to establish the science of bacteriology. Physiology became to be regarded as one of the natural sciences based on physics and chemistry. Amongst its great contributors were François Magendie in Bordeaux, Johannes Muller in Berlin and Claude Bernard in Paris.

It is of interest to note that the word 'scientist' had been introduced by William Whewell, a Cambridge don, in 1837 and it replaced the term 'natural philosopher'.

BIRTH OF ORTHOPAEDIC SURGERY

Fractures and dislocations formed a separate topic in surgical texts from the time of Hippocrates in the fourth to fifth century BC until this century.

Orthopaedic surgery became a recognised part of operative treatment in the mid-nineteenth century at about the same time as ophthalmology. From time immemorial there had been bonesetters. Their art was handed down in families by word of mouth from one generation to another and the secrets of the art were unpublished. At first the surgical approach was limited to subcutaneous operations because of the dangers of sepsis. It was only possible to progress with the introduction of antiseptics and anaesthesia. X-rays provided a further boost and by the end of the nineteenth century orthopaedic surgery was a recognised branch of general surgery. The role of the general surgeon predominated in fracture work until the mid-twentieth century. By then orthopaedic surgery was well established, but fragmentation into regional subspecialities only became obvious from the 1970s onwards.

In 1741 Nicholas Andry (1658–1742) published *L'Orthopédie, ou l'art de prévenir et de corriger dans les enfants, les difformités du Corps*' in Paris on the art of preventing deformities in children. The work was anonymously translated into English as *Orthopaedia, or the Art of Correcting and Preventing Deformities in Children* (London, 1743) in two volumes (Andry 1743). Andry wrote, 'I have found it of two Greek words, e.g. straight, free from deformity and a child. Out of these two words I have compounded that of Orthopaedia, to express in one term, the Design I propose, which is to teach the different methods of preventing and correcting the Deformities of Children.' Andry had grasped the role of muscles as 'body moulders' (Arthur 1919). He regarded the body of a growing child as plastic. Deformities could be prevented and cured by exercises. Thus orthopaedic surgery began with orthopaedic medicine. The word has been firmly attached to the speciality despite the use of similar words such as 'orthomorphic' by Jacques Delpech in 1828 and 'orthopraxy' by Heather-Bigg in 1865, 'to make it straight' as a designation for the mechanical therapeutics of deformity (Kirkup 1993).

The earliest recorded institute for the treatment of skeletal deformities was the hospital at Orbe in Switzerland established in 1780 by another physician, Jean André Venel (1740–91) of Geneva. According to Bick (1948) it was equipped with an elaborate armamentarium of apparatus modified and adapted for individual cases. Venel used plaster casts made on admission as a visual record of his patient's deformities.

If the author of *L'Orthopaedia* is a landmark, the man who produced *De L'Orthomorphie* also merits serious attention. In 1812 Jacques Delpech (1777–1832) was appointed Professor of Surgery in the University of Montpellier. Two years later, when the French army withdrew from Spain after defeat by the Duke of Wellington, he was involved in the treatment of hundreds of wounded men. Convinced that the admission of air to wounds interfered with healing, he felt certain that if air could be excluded a wound should heal by first intention. In 1816 Delpech modified open tendo achillis tentotomy by operating through two small incisions 1 inch in length on either side of the tendon. Unfortunately the wound became infected and took months to heal and Delpech did not repeat the procedure (Kirkup 1991). In *De l'Orthomorphie* he described his methods of treatment. He originated the concept that deformities are the result of unbalanced muscle action.

Robert Chessher of Hinckley in Leicestershire (1750–1831) was a contemporary of Venel. His stepfather was a surgeon and soon after his father's death Chessher took over his practice where he had originally been apprenticed. Chessher later supplemented his medical education as a house surgeon at the Middlesex Hospital. He remained in Hinckley for the rest of his life and specialised in the correction of deformities. He was not a cutting surgeon, but made ingenious devices for the correction of deformities. He had a workshop in his house with seven or eight employees to help him. He did not publish any papers and his undoubted fame is based on records of his local reputation. Amongst his achievements was a design for a double inclined plane for treatment of femoral shaft fractures that maintained

flexion of the hip and knee. According to Roger Austin's biography of Chessher (1981), he also produced the most refined apparatus for the correction of spinal deformity before the Milwaukee brace and was the first British 'orthopaedist'.

Percivall Pott (1714–85) of London was a surgeon at St Bartholomew's Hospital from 1744 to 1787 having, in his own words, 'served it as man and boy for half a century'. He held his appointment as full surgeon until he was seventy-five 'as there were no tiresome regulations about retiring age' (Gask 1936). On a frosty morning he was riding down the Old Kent Road and was thrown from his horse and sustained a compound fracture of his leg. The bone involved was the tibia. Fortunately Pott avoided an amputation, a common treatment for this type of injury at the time. He had to lie up for a long time and made good use of his enforced leisure by writing. It was then that he wrote his book on ruptures which was his favourite subject. In 1768 his treatise *Fractures and Dislocations* appeared and the treatment he proposed became the standard around the country. One of the most important points he made was the need for immediate reduction of the fracture and that relaxation of the muscles was necessary to allow the proper setting of the bones in alignment. Pott also described what he believed to be the most frequent type of ankle fracture. The fracture is well above the tibiofibular syndesmosis, which appears to be intact despite rupture of the medial ligament and displacement of the talus laterally. Today the term 'Pott's fracture' of the ankle is a generic term for fracture dislocations around the ankle. Another important work dealt with curvature of the spine and lower limb palsy. He was the first to describe what is now known as 'Pott's Disease of the Spine'.

John Hunter (1728–93), born fourteen years after Pott, justly attained greater fame than Pott not because he was a better operator or could give a better opinion in a difficult case, but because he was a born researcher. Hunter was at heart a natural scientist. Pott devoted himself to the study and care of human disease. His early training in anatomy was the key to his attainments (Gask 1936). Hunter was interested in the growth and repair of bone. He was convinced that there were two processes involved in growth, one of deposition and the other of absorption. To Hunter is owed the first clear conception of the formation of a sequestrum and involucrum.

Hunter, recognising the inevitability of sepsis and complications of elective operations, wrote: 'The last part of surgery, namely operations, is a reflection on the healing art; it is a tacit acknowledgement of the insufficiency of surgery. It is like an armed savage who attempts to get that by force which a civilised man would get by stratagem.'

William John Little (1810–94) is very likely to have suffered childhood poliomyelitis because he developed a deformed foot from the age of two, which resulted in a typical equinovarus deformity with growth (Fig. 1.1). In 1828, when he began his medical studies at the London Hospital, he was intent on finding a cure for his foot problem. He was interested in the work of Delpech who had divided the Achilles tendon subcutaneously for treatment of clubfoot. He approached Delpech in order to have this operation, but was told to wait because of the danger of sepsis. Little hoped to become a surgeon at the London Hospital. After two years of lack of progress he resolved to become a licentiate of the College of Physicians of London instead and devote himself to medicine. He was required to spend two years at a university. He chose to go to Berlin where he was drawn by the growing fame of Johannes Muller, the founder of scientific medicine in Germany. Little also visited George Frederick Louis Stromeyer (1804–76) in Hanover who was using very fine knives and truly subcutaneous tenotomy for the correction of clubfoot. Little had his own foot successfully operated upon in 1836 by Stromeyer. Stromeyer employed the term 'operative orthopadik' (orthopaedic operation) in 1838 and as his methods rapidly spread the adjective 'orthopaedic' became synonymous with surgical treatment of deformity (Kirkup 1991). When he had recovered, Little stayed in Hanover and was given numerous opportunities to see how to perform the operation. He returned to England in 1837 and performed the procedure on 20 February of that year. According to Keith (1919) he not only cut the Achilles tendon as Stromeyer had done, but also the tendons of the tibialis posterior and flexor hallucis longus. In 1838, with the help of relatives and friends, he set up the Infirmary for the Cure of Club Foot and other Contractions (see Chapter 10). This name was soon changed to Orthopaedic Institution and was a precursor of the Royal National Orthopaedic Hospital (Cholmeley 1985). Keith acclaims Little as the pioneer of orthopaedic surgery in Britain. In 1840 he was appointed assistant physician at the London Hospital and later a full physician. His interest in deformities persisted and led to his recognition of infantile spastic paralysis or Little's disease, nowadays familiar as cerebral palsy. In his *On the Nature and Treatment of Deformities of the Human Frame*, a record of a course of lectures published in 1853, Little stated that 'Orthopaedy is something better than a mere mechanical art; whilst employing its therapeutic resources, many of whom are mechanical, the mind is also interested in other problems that have hitherto been incompletely solved.'

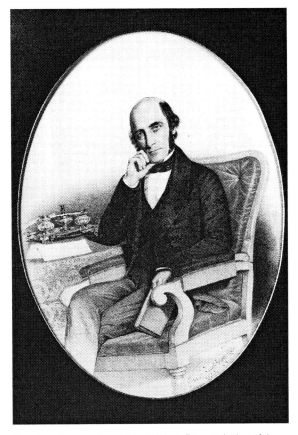

Fig. 1.1 William John Little in 1854. By permission of the Welcome Institute Library, London

At this stage, the scope of all elective orthopaedic surgery was severely restricted due to lack of anaesthesia and control of sepsis.

On 16 October 1846, Henry Jacob Bigelow (1818–90), a surgeon at the Massachusetts General Hospital, arranged for W. T. G. Morton, a dentist, to help Dr J. C. Warren, Chief of Surgery, with an operation to excise a tumour of the neck by giving ether to relieve the patient's pain (Fig. 1.2). Soon after this first demonstration in Boston, ether was used in many hospitals throughout the world. Robert Liston did an above-knee amputation at the University College Hospital London on 21 December of the same year. The next day ether anaesthesia was tried in Paris, on 23 January 1847 in Berne, on 28 January in Vienna, on 6 February in Berlin and on 8 March in The Hague (Tröhler 1993). Probably no medical discovery has ever been more rapidly adapted to clinical practice than anaesthesia. Bigelot wrote the first professional paper on anaesthesia, 'Insensibility during surgical operations by inhalation', in the *Boston Medical and Surgical Journal* in November 1846. He published a small volume *Manual of Orthopedic Surgery* in 1845, the first important work on the subject in the United States. He was also involved in work on the hip joint where his name is linked with the 'Y'-shaped ligament. He wrote about its importance in the reduction of acute dislocations in *The Mechanism of Dislocation and Fracture of the Hip with the Reduction of the Dislocations* (Peltier 1993). In addition, his name was also attached to a lithotrite and bladder evacuator.

FURTHER DEVELOPMENTS – CONTROL OF PAIN

The term 'anaesthesia' was introduced by Oliver Wendell Holmes (1809–94), Professor of Anatomy at Harvard University, who wrote to Morton five weeks after the first demonstration of anaesthesia in Boston to suggest the loss of consciousness produced by ether

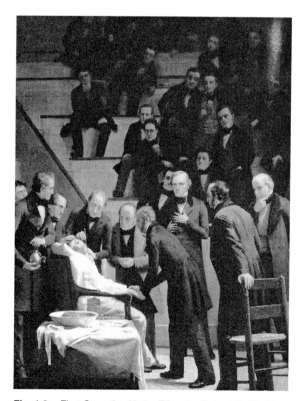

Fig. 1.2 *First Operation Under Ether*, by Robert C. Hinckley (1893), a somewhat romanticised reconstruction of the first successful public demonstration of surgical anaesthesia at the Massachusetts General Hospital on 16 October 1846. By permission of The Boston Medical Library in the Francis A. Countway Library of Medicine, Boston, Massachusetts

should be called 'anaesthesia' (Singer et al 1962). Sir John Bland Sutton describes how in his early days as a surgeon the induction of anaesthesia with ether or chloroform for an examination or operation was a rough and ready procedure. Struggling with a strong man during the administration of ether was often distressing and unpleasant. 'Occasionally the surgeons and other helpers received kicks and blows as in a scrimmage' (Sutton 1930).

The term 'local anaesthesia' was first used by James Young Simpson in a paper published in *The Lancet* in 1848 which contains an appreciation of the benefits of local as opposed to general anaesthesia that remains valid today (Wildsmith 1985). The development and use of cocaine as a local anaesthetic agent was mainly the work of Carl Koller. When Koller was house surgeon at the Vienna General Hospital his friend Sigmund Freud was studying the possibility of curing patients addicted to morphine by treating them with cocaine. Koller noticed that after he had injected a weak solution of cocaine into the eye of a frog, the eye became insensitive to pain. The use of cocaine in the eye was widely used after Koller's report to an Ophthalmological Congress in Heidelberg in Germany in 1884. Subsequently cocaine was also injected in solution into the tissues and became extensively used in dentistry and general surgery. William S. Halsted of The Johns Hopkins Hospital injected cocaine into nerve trunks and produced conduction anaesthesia in peripheral regions. Besides the nerves of the face and jaws he was the first to apply the same principles to anaesthesia at other sites (brachial plexus block, posterior tibial block, pudendal nerve block, etc.). It was late 1884 or 1885 that Halsted and his colleagues quite innocently became addicted to cocaine and Halsted's career was seriously affected from then onwards. Cocaine is far from being an ideal local anaesthetic drug and this fact was rapidly appreciated. As a result substitutes were synthesised, although no really satisfactory agent was available until 1904 when Einhorn produced procaine (Editorial 1984).

RISE OF ANTISEPSIS

In 1865, Joseph Lister (1827–1912) was working at the Glasgow Royal Infirmary when his attention was drawn to the work and writings of Louis Pasteur. The papers he read dealt with fermentation and putrefaction, and he realised their relevance to suppuration and wound infection. Putrefaction was caused by the growth of minute microscopical beings carried by dust floating in the air. The air was the only vehicle that conveyed the germ of putrefaction to the wound. Successful treatment of the wound could be achieved by purifying the air. Lister chose the carbolic spray to prevent contamination of the wound. The principles of anti-sepsis were strict attention to technique to prevent the access of organisms to the wound. Infection was not a normal stage of wound healing as many had come to accept. The outcome of the wound was the responsi-bility of the surgeon. Lister's spray was not very effective, but he and other surgeons of the time operated without gloves, caps or masks. The spray may have helped reduce contamination from the hair and hands, and droplet infection from the throat. The importance of Lister's work lay in the application of Pasteur's discoveries. Lister discarded the spray in 1887. William Halsted introduced rubber gloves at The Johns Hopkins Hospital in 1889. The Goodyear Rubber Company made two pairs with gauntlets for his scrub nurse whose hands were allergic to the corrosive sublimate hand rinse. She became Mrs Halsted not long afterwards (Wangensteen & Wangensteen 1978). It was later recog-nised that gloves also protected the patient. Johann Mickulicz-Radecki first advocated gauze masks in 1897 following the discovery by his colleague, a bacteriologist named Carl Flugge, that even during quiet speech droplets were sprayed into the air. Pasteur had by 1874 suggested immersing instruments in boiling water, passing them through a flame and rapidly cooling them before operation. Gradually, heat superseded chemical methods for the preparation of instruments, dressings and operative clothing for operations.

Robert Koch (1843–1910) of Klausthal, Hanover, conceived the experimental basis for the germ theory of wound infection by showing the value of culture and identification of bacteria. Microbiologists built early steam sterilisers. By 1883 the autoclave devised to provide moist heat under pressure was available in many bacteriological laboratories. By the end of the nine-teenth century gone were the days when a surgeon operated in a black frock coat, caked with blood, with the patient on a wooden table, the room barely lit and with sawdust on the floor.

It is interesting to note the gradual increase in the number of surgical operations performed. At St Bartholomew's Hospital, probably the largest hospital at that time, in 1865 there were 397 surgical beds. The average number of operations during the preceding five years was 370 of which seventy-eight were amputations. In 1912 there were 3561 operations of which only twenty-five were amputations (Godlee 1924).

Lister's dresser, William Macewen (1848–1924) of Glasgow perfected linear osteotomy of the distal femur for correction of deformities due to rickets and used the antiseptic technique he learned from his chief (Macewen 1878). He devised a special instrument for cutting bone that was bevelled on both sides of the cutting edge and which he called an osteotome. He also published his *The Growth of Bone* in 1912, which is a classic basic study. Macewen also demonstrated the practicality of bone grafts.

Another pupil of Lister, Thomas Annandale of Edinburgh, reported in the *British Medical Journal* of April 1885 how he had explored the knee of a thirty-year-old miner whose movements were restricted by something slipping in the knee. The patient complained of acute pain and the joint frequently locked in the flexed position. At operation the meniscus was found detached anteriorly and displaced backwards by ½ inch. Anandale drew the cartilage forwards with forceps and held it there with three chromic catgut sutures passed through it and the fascia and periosteum covering the margin of the tibia. The result achieved was 'perfect movement in the joint' and no stiffness or locking. This operation was superseded by menis-cectomy by the end of the nineteenth century. With the development of arthroscopy reattachment of the meniscus again has a place.

William Arbuthnot Lane (1856–1943) was one of the earliest surgeons to operate on fractures and use internal fixation. In his *The Operative Treatment of Fractures* first published in 1905 (Lane 1914), his words are still relevant to modern surgeons:

Apart from manual dexterity and skill the whole secret of success in these operations depends on the most rigid asepsis. The very moderate degree of cleanliness that is adopted in operations generally will not suffice when a large quantity of metal is left in a wound. To guarantee success in the performance of these operations the surgeon must not touch the interior of the wound, even with his gloved hand, as gloves are frequently punctured, especially if it be necessary to use a moderate amount of force on their introduction into the wound, when they may have been in contact with the skin for some time and may render the wound septic. All swabs intro-duced into the wound should be held in long forceps and should not be handled in any way.

To make this effective he had the artery and dissecting forceps he used lengthened from 6 to 8 inches and only then was he assured that if these instruments were used in a deep wound the fingers that held them could not touch the wound edge. He excluded contami-nation from the patient's skin by pinning a towel to the edges of the wound.

Lane was a pioneer, but his plates were poor and only fixed in one cortex. His approach was supported by Berkeley Moynihan who, in his lecture on 'The Ritual of a Surgical Operation' on 14 May 1926 (Moynihan 1920), stated that 'every operation in surgery is an experiment in bacteriology' and that the success of the experiment in respect of the patient depended not only on the skill, but also on the care exercised by the surgeon in the ritual of the operation.

According to Rocyn Jones (1958) the dozen or so years from 1870 were a productive period for orthopaedic surgery. Sir James Paget gave an exhaustive and complete description of a bone disease that produced deformities which he called osteitis deformans (still recognised as Paget's disease of bone of unknown origin). In 1875 Hugh Owen Thomas (1834–91), the first medically qualified practitioner from a family of bonesetters, published his monograph on *Diseases of the Hip, Knee and Ankle Joint*. His main treatment for diseased, that is tuberculous, joints was 'enforced, uninterrupted and prolonged rest'. His long splint for the knee was adapted for treatment of femoral fractures during the First World War of 1914–18 and drastically reduced the mortality rate of open fractures from 60 to 25%.

Robert Jones (1851–1933), Thomas' nephew, who had worked and trained with his uncle and was a passionate disciple, started using arthrodesis of the knee and ankle for stabilisation of the flail joints of poliomyelitis (Fig. 1.3). By 1894 he was able to report on fifteen patients.

Jones and Thomas were amongst the few surgeons who were interested in improving the management of fractures. They emphasised accurate repositioning of the bones and the restoration of true alignment by traction and manipulation. Jones organised a successful casualty service for the men working on the Manchester Ship Canal which was built between 1888 and 1893.

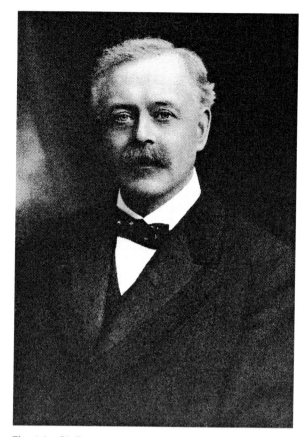

Fig. 1.3 Sir Robert Jones. By permission of the Welcome Institute Library, London

ESTABLISHING THE SPECIALTY

A group of surgeons led by Robert Jones and Alfred Tubby gathered at the Holborn Restaurant in London on 3 November 1894 and formed the British Orthopaedic Society. There were thirty-one members, thirteen from London and eighteen from the provinces. They were mostly general surgeons who were practising some orthopaedics (Waugh 1993). This was at a time when only two of the five members of the newly formed Royal National Orthopaedic Hospital confined themselves to orthopaedic surgery. Unfortunately, the society ceased to function after four years. One of the possible reasons for failure was that most members were general surgeons and not fully committed to orthopaedic surgery. The American Orthopaedic Association, founded in 1887, was the first nationally affiliated group of orthopaedic surgeons. The British Orthopaedic Association was founded in 1918. Its German counterpart was set up in 1901 and an international society,

the Société International de Chirurgie Orthopedique, in 1929, and Trauma was added to the title in 1936 at the suggestion of Vittorio Putti. In the USA the first specialist hospital called the Boston Orthopaedic Institution was set up in the city two blocks from the Massachusetts General Hospital by John Ball Brown at the same time as Little started his hospital for the treatment of club feet in London. Brown's son, Buckmaster, was an orthopaedic surgeon and was the first to limit his work to the speciality. By 1882 a Professor of Orthopaedic Surgery, Lewis Sayre, had been appointed to Bellevue Medical College, New York. The situation in Britain was very different and it was not until 1937 that Girdlestone was appointed as the first Professor of Orthopaedic Surgery at the University of Oxford. It is likely this prolonged delay was due to the power of general surgeons.

Other pioneers were Edward Hickley Bradford (1848–1926) in the USA. He was appointed as the first John Bell and Buckminster Brown Professor at Harvard

Medical School. Albert Hoffa (1859–1907) in Germany developed the operation of open reduction of a congenital dislocation of the hip, and Alessandro Codivilla (1851–1913) in Italy was Professor at the University of Bologna and Director of the Institute Rizzoli. He laid down principles for tendon transfer including tibialis posterior through the interosseous membrane for drop foot and used direct skeletal traction for bone lengthening or securing alignment (Peltier 1993).

On 28 December 1895 W. C. Röntgen, a physicist of Würzburg, announced the discovery of X-rays. A German lady, Mrs Wimpfheimer, who worked as a volunteer in Robert Jones's Sunday Clinic in Liverpool on receiving the *Frankfurter Zeitung* newspaper containing an article which described Röntgen's discovery translated the article for Jones. At the time Jones had a boy with a pellet in his wrist which could not be found by probing. Jones asked Oliver Lodge FRS, Professor of Physics at the University of Liverpool if he could help with the new X-rays. On 7 February 1896 the boy was brought to Lodge's laboratory and after a prolonged exposure of about 2 hours a radiograph was produced which showed the pellet in the third carpometacarpal joint (Jones & Lodge 1896). A link between radiology and orthopaedic surgery was forged (see Chapter 8).

In the First World War the establishment of British military hospitals with the appointment of Sir Robert Jones as Inspector of Military Orthopaedics was an indication of the potential of orthopaedic surgery to prevent crippling from skeletal injuries and help with restoration of manpower for battlefield or factory. The military orthopaedic surgeon could use his skill on his return to civilian life for the treatment of injuries caused by accidents.

The first link of fractures with an orthopaedic department in Britain was introduced by Harry Platt when he established a fracture clinic at Ancoates Hospital in Manchester in 1913. This was followed by another in Liverpool run by Reginald Watson-Jones.

Ernest William Hey Groves (1872–1944) is a good example to show how the work of orthopaedic and general surgeons overlapped. He was excluded from being a foundation member of the British Orthopaedic Association as he was not considered eligible because of his activities in general surgery. Nevertheless, he introduced a number of important orthopaedic procedures, such as intramedullary nailing of fractures, repair of what he called the crucial ligaments of the knee and replacement of the arthritic femoral head by an ivory prosthesis. His *Synopsis of Surgery* was first published in 1908 and there were eleven editions. His other text-

books included *Modern Methods of Treating Fractures* and *Surgical Operations*. He produced a primer on *Gunshot Injuries of Bones* in 1915 in which he described a method of treatment with transfixion pins incorporated into a splint, a very early external fixator (Waugh 1993). His broad approach was shown by the fact that he was President of the British Orthopaedic Association in 1928–29 and then became President of the Association of Surgeons (General Surgeons) for the next two years. According to Waugh, no other surgeon has done this except Robert Jones.

Three major developments had an important effect on orthopaedic practice in the first part of the twentieth century. There was the discovery of vitamin D and the elimination of nutritional rickets, the development of antibacterial drugs notably penicillin and streptomycin, and the introduction of the Salk and Sabin vaccines for the prevention of poliomyelitis and the discovery of blood groups.

In 1918 Edward Mellanby found that rickets could be prevented by a variety of substances rich in vitamin A, such as butter, cod liver oil and animal fats. At first this effect was attributed to vitamin A, but Hopkins in England and McCollum in the USA invented methods of destroying vitamin A and yet the cod liver oil retained its power to prevent rickets. There was another factor at work and it was called vitamin D.

Rickets had become a very common disease of one and two year olds in Northern industrial cities in Europe and the USA by 1900. The problem of growing up in Victorian industrial cities was that the smoke from burning coal absorbed most of the vitamin D-promoting ultraviolet rays and that direct solar irradiation was limited in slums with high buildings and narrow streets. Although vitamin D by mouth is a cure, rickets should perhaps be classified as a disease due to air pollution rather than as a nutritional problem (Carpenter 1993).

The beginning of antibacterial agents came with the work by Gerhard Domagk working for the I. G. Farbenindustrie in Elberfeld, Germany, in the 1930s. His introduction of the sulphonamides was a definite advance. Sulphapyridine proved to be the most potent and broad spectrum and helped save the life of Winston Churchill when he contracted pneumonia in North Africa in December 1943. Other sulphonamides widely prescribed were sulphadimidine and sulphamethazole.

The discovery of penicillin by Alexander Fleming in 1929 and its biochemical concentration by Howard W. Florey and Ernst B. Chain in Oxford in 1941 was a striking achievement which led to the control of bone infection and markedly improved the outlook of those with compound fractures. This antibacterial weapon was soon followed by another when streptomycin was found by Selman Waksman in 1943 and provided a powerful weapon against tuberculosis. Other antibiotics such as oxytetracycline followed in the 1940s. It is interesting to note that in an Editorial in the *British Journal of Bone and Joint Surgery* in 1951, a combination of sulphadiazine and penicillin was recommended as the primary treatment of acute osteomyelitis. Some of the current problems are a result of the success of antibiotics and their development of resistant organisms which are difficult to treat.

Karl Landsteiner's (1883–1943) pioneering studies of blood groups won him a Nobel Prize in 1930. Transfusions did not become a routine hospital procedure until the establishment of blood banks shortly before the Second World War. Nowadays blood transfusion is an integral part of major surgical operations (McFarland 1950).

Jonas Salk and collaborators at Pittsburgh University in 1956 produced an inactivated polio vaccine in which the virus had been treated by formaldehyde and was given by injection. Oral polio vaccine was developed with an attenuated virus by Albert Sabin. The World Health Organisation had hoped to eradicate poliomyelitis by 2000, just as has been possible with smallpox. Whether poliomyelitis can be completely eradicated in the near future, its incidence has markedly declined in the Western world, so much so that many young surgeons nowadays are unfamiliar with its associated paralytic. The common deformities that occur and their treatment were a major component of routine orthopaedic practice until the mid-twentieth century.

The history of orthopaedic surgery is one of progressive evolution. Surgery developed in parallel with the technological advances of the day. For the first forty years orthopaedic surgery was concerned with the correction of congenital and paralytic deformities by splinting, manipulation and tenotomy. From *c.*1880 the adoption of antisepsis allowed a bolder attack first by joint excision and osteotomy and later by open operations. Stabilisation of joints was achieved by tendon transplantation, arthrodesis or both. The open-air conservative treatment of skeletal tuberculosis with bone graft surgery as a refinement became part of orthopaedic practice just as an interest in trauma developed as a direct result of the First World War (Rocyn Jones 1958).

By the mid-twentieth century with the decline of poliomyelitis it was possible to focus on the major problems of arthritis and develop the regional subspecialities. Whereas orthopaedic surgery had started with an interest in children, with improved social conditions the problems of the elderly have become an ever-

increasing load. The practice of surgery is now scientific rather than merely empirical and has entered the era of joint replacement, arthroscopic and less invasive surgery.

Progress is difficult to forecast. It is of interest to read 'The Editorial of 2000 AD' by Professor Bryan McFarland of the University of Liverpool written in 1950 in the *Journal of Bone and Joint Surgery*. He thought tuberculosis of bones and joints would have disappeared. Metastases from malignant disease would no longer be a problem following discovery of a cure for malignant disease. The horrors of rheumatoid disease would have gone along with congenital and familial disorders. As will be discussed in the following Chapters these disorders are still unfortunately with us, but methods of treatment are improving all of the time.

REFERENCES

Andry N 1743 Orthopaedia. London; facsimile reproduction of the first English edn. Philadelphia, J P Lippincott 1961

Annandale T 1885 An operation for displaced semilunar cartilage. Br Med J: 779

Austin R T 1981 Robert Chessher of Hinckley 1750–1831 First English Orthopaedist. Leicestershire County Council Libraries and Information Service, Leicester

Bick E M 1948 Source Book of Orthopaedics. Williams & Wilkins, Baltimore

Bigelow H J 1845 Manual of Orthopedic Surgery. William D Tickner, Boston

Bigelow H J 1846 Insensibility during surgical operations by inhalation. Boston Med Surg J 45: 309–317

Booth C C 1993 Clinical research. In: Bynum W F, Porter R (eds) Companion Encyclopaedia of the History of Medicine, vol. 1. Routledge, London

Carpenter K 1993 Nutritional diseases. In: Bynum W F, Porter P (eds) Companion Encyclopaedia of the History of Medicine. Routledge, London, Ch 2, p 479

Cholmeley J A 1985 History of the Royal National Orthopaedic Hospital. Chapman & Hall, London

Editorial 1984 Br J Anaesth 56: 937–939

Gask G 1936 Percivall Pott. In: Sir D'Arcy Power (ed) British Masters of Medicine. Medical Press, London

Godlee R J 1924 Lord Lister. Clarendon, Oxford, p 122

Groves E W H 1908 Synopsis of Surgery. Bristol, John Wright & Sons

Groves E W H 1916 Modern Methods of Treating Fractures. Bristol, John Wright & Sons

Groves E W H 1919 Surgical Operations. London, Henry Frowde: Hodder & Stoughton

Groves E W H 1915 Gunshot Injuries of Bones. London. Henry Frowde: Hodder & Stoughton

Jones R, Lodge O 1896 The discovery of a bullet lost in the wrist by means of Röntgen rays. Lancet i: 477

Keith A 1919 Menders of the Maimed. Oxford University Press, Oxford

Kirkup J 1991 Subcutaneous tenotomy gives birth to orthopaedic surgery. Foot 2: 107–108

Kirkup J 1993 Orthopaedy, orthopaedics or 'orthosurgery'. Br Orthop News, p 7

Lane W A 1914 The Operative Treatment of Fractures, 2nd edn. The Medical Rutheday Co. Ltd, London

Lister J 1867 On the antiseptic principles in the practice of surgery. Lancet

Little W J 1853 On the Nature and Treatment of Deformities of the Human Frame. Longman Green, London

Macewen W 1878 Antiseptic osteotomy for genu valgus, genu varus and other osseous deformities. Lancet ii: 911–1914

Macewen W 1912 The Growth of Bone, Glasgow, James Maiklehose

McFarland B 1950 The Editorial of 2000 AD. J Bone Joint Surg 32B: 459–460

Moynihan B G A 1920 The ritual of a surgical operation. Br J Surg 8: 27–35

Peltier L F 1993 Orthopaedics: A History and Iconography. Norman, San Francisco

Porter R 1997 The Greatest Benefit to Mankind. HarperCollins, London

Rocyn Jones A A 1958 Review of Orthopaedic Surgery in Britain. J Bone Joint Surg 38B: 27–45

Singer C, Ashworth Underwood E, 1962 A Short History of Medicine. Clarendon, Oxford, p 351

Sutton, J B 1930 The Story of a Surgeon. Methuen, London, p 69

Thomas H O 1875 Diseases of the Hip, Knee and Ankle Joint, Liverpool. T Dobb & Co

Tröhler V 1993 Surgery (modern). In: Bynum W F, Porter R (eds) Companion Encyclopaedia of the History of Medicine, vol. 2. Routledge, London

Wangensteen O H, Wangensteen S O 1978 The Rise of Surgery. Wm Dawson & Sons, Folkestone

Waugh W A 1993 History of the British Orthopaedic Association. Bath Press, Bath

Wildsmith J A W 1985 Origins of local anaesthesia. J Roy Soc Med 78: 6–7

SECTION 1:

Major Advances in the Twentieth Century

2

Arthroplasty of the hip

Leslie Klenerman

This chapter is written from the point of view of a clinician and is intended to be complementary to Chapter 7, on biomaterials, and Chapter 15, the view from the implant industry.

Total hip replacement is one of the major advances of the twentieth century, not only in orthopaedic surgery, but also in medicine as a whole. It has been estimated that one million patients have hip replacements annually and many different implants are used (Soderman 2000). In terms of improvement of the quality of life, it surpasses coronary artery bypass operations and renal transplants (Williams 1985). A long line of bold and innovative surgeons has contributed to its development. The most significant advances were introduced by John Charnley (1911–82), working in his unit at Wrightington Hospital, near Wigan in Lancashire (Fig. 2.1). His major contributions were the principle of low friction, the fixation of the components to bone with acrylic cement and the ultraclean air-operating theatre. They were of fundamental importance and made total hip replacement a viable operation. These developments started in the 1950s and early 1960s at a time when tuberculosis was coming under control and poliomyelitis was dying out. With this large clinical burden removed, orthopaedic surgeons could concentrate on chronic degenerative diseases. This chapter is divided into three parts: the era before Charnley, the Charnley era and the era after Charnley.

THE ERA BEFORE CHARNLEY

Anthony White performed the first recorded arthroplasty at the Westminster Hospital, London, in April 1822. He divided the femur 2 inches below the greater trochanter and removed the upper end of the bone and produced a mobile joint (Rang 2000).

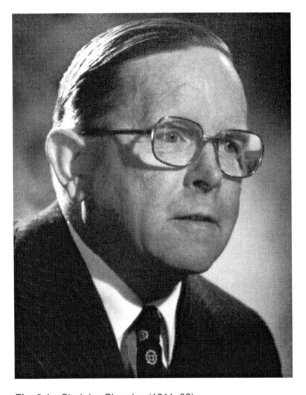

Fig. 2.1 Sir John Charnley (1911–82)

John Rhea Barton performed a different operation designed to produce a stable mobile hip on a patient with bilateral stiff hips at the Pennsylvania Hospital, Philadelphia, on 22 November 1826. The operation, a subtrochanteric osteotomy of the femur, took 7 minutes. Early movement from three weeks produced a painless pseudarthrosis (Barton 1827). According to Barton (1837), 'The patient enjoyed the use of his joint for six years during which period he pursued a business (trunk making) with great industry, earning for himself a comfortable subsistence and a small annual surplus. Pecuniary losses sunk him into a state of despondency and desperation, followed by habits of intemperance. The artificial joint gradually became more and more rigid, and finally all motion ceased in the part.'

The earliest arthroplasties were performed to produce movement in ankylosed joints. The joint surfaces were refashioned and neighbouring soft tissue or a foreign material was interposed to prevent fusion and allow movement. In the 1880s, Ollier in Lyon used muscle. In 1902, Robert Jones successfully reconstructed a hip using gold foil (Jones 1923). J. B. Murphy in Chicago published results of sixteen interpositional arthroplasties in 1913 using a pedicle flap of fat and fascia (Murphy 1913). R. Whitman described a reconstructive procedure in which the head and neck of the femur were excised and the greater trochanter transplanted to a lower level (Whitman 1924). It was originally devised for un-united fractures, particularly for those cases in which the neck of the femur had absorbed or worn away, and later used for osteoarthritic hips.

Themistocles Gluck in Germany (see Chapter 12), who had ideas well in advance of his time, replaced the hip joint with ivory components. Nickel-plated screws were used for fixation with a primitive cement of pumice powder, plaster of Paris and glue.

The surgical options for the treatment of an osteoarthritic hip in the well-known textbook *Orthopaedic Surgery* by Jones and Lovett (1923) were few. The choices were cheilectomy (i.e. trimming of bony irregularities around the joint), arthrodesis, an upper femoral pseudarthrosis without dislocation of the femoral head and neck, and an interpositional arthroplasty, as described by Murphy. It is interesting to note that Baer of The Johns Hopkins University, who in 1926 reported on one hundred cases of interposition arthroplasty with chromicised submucosa of pig's bladder, considered a good result to be an ability to flex their hip at least 25° (Baer 1926). The joint had to be painless and stable on weight bearing.

Marius Smith-Petersen, who worked at the Massachusetts General Hospital in 1923, used a glass cup to cover the reshaped head of the femur as a variant of the interpositional arthroplasty. The glass mould sometimes broke. He tried a variety of other materials such as Pyrex and Bakelite, until eventually settling on a cobalt chrome alloy (Smith-Petersen 1948). By 1947, he had operated on more than five hundred hips. Otto Aufranc, who worked with Smith-Petersen, described the results of one thousand cases of mould arthroplasty in 1957, and recorded an 82% success rate. Margaret

Shepherd, at the British Orthopaedic Association in 1954, noted that among surgeons in the UK, 54% had poor results at five years. In 1961, Charnley in his classic paper 'Arthroplasty of the hip, a new operation', wrote that 'Smith-Petersen repeatedly emphasised that the moving parts should be made to fit loosely together; in no sense therefore, could the arrangement at the finish of this operation be regarded as a mechanically stable ball-and-socket. In the course of time the spaces between the cup and femoral head and the cup and the acetabulum become filled with fibrocartilaginous material and the hip can thus become stable; but unfortunately the peri-articular soft tissues often become thick and stiff, and mobility is lost.'

E. W. Hey Groves of Bristol in 1926, in a Bradshaw Lecture at the Royal College of Surgeons, described how he had used an ivory prosthesis to replace the head of an osteoarthritic hip with a peg passing down the length of the femoral neck. In 1938, Philip Wiles of The Middlesex Hospital, London (see Chapter 7), inserted an acetabulum and femoral head of stainless steel with the two parts ground to fit accurately into the acetabulum of a cat. The acetabulum was prevented from rotating by screws and a bolt passing through the neck of the femur secured the femoral head. The animal experiments were promising and the operation was performed six times on patients severely crippled by what was then called Still's disease (juvenile chronic arthritis) (Fig. 2.2). Follow up was difficult because of the intervention of the Second World War (1939–45). All patients previously bedridden could now walk. One, who had bilateral operations, was seen in 1951. She had about 20° flexion in each hip, could walk a little and operate a mechanically propelled chair (Wiles 1958).

In 1946, the Judet brothers in Paris used a prosthesis with an acrylic head and stem that penetrated the trochanteric region as an improvement on Whitman's technique (Judet & Judet 1950). Because of severe wear, the acrylic was subsequently substituted by a cobalt chrome alloy. It was the squeak of a Judet prosthesis that stimulated Charnley to investigate friction and lubrication in normal joints. He suspected that the loosening of the femoral prosthesis was related to the degree of frictional resistance developing between it and the acetabular floor. When the squeak stopped, it was not because lubrication improved, but rather because the prosthesis had loosened. This resulted in experimental work where he showed that the extraordinary low coefficient of friction (in an animal) joint ($\mu = 0.013$) was better than a skate sliding over ice ($\mu = 0.03$). This result led to the concept of a low-friction arthroplasty (Waugh 1990).

Austin Moore of Columbia, South Carolina, in collaboration with Dr Harold Bohlman of Baltimore,

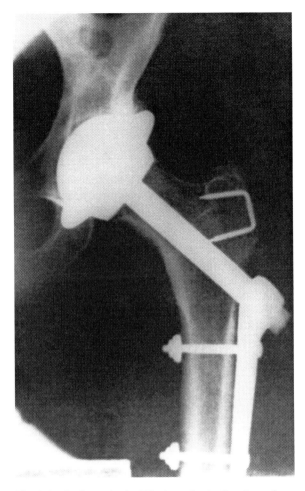

Fig. 2.2 Radiograph of a Wiles' prosthesis. Courtesy of Professor Robert Owen

inserted the first vitallium prosthesis to replace the upper portion of a femur in 1943. Following the introduction of the Judet prosthesis, Moore was not impressed with its anchoring stem and continued to search for an appliance that was more compatible with normal weight bearing. As a result, the Moore prosthesis was developed, which was inserted into the medullary cavity and had the correct angle for the femoral neck. The stem was fenestrated to allow bone ingrowth to lock the prosthesis in position and to reduce weight. A posterior approach to the hip was developed so that the prosthesis could be inserted more easily (Moore 1957). Initially known as the Southern Approach, it remains a standard means of access to the hip. F. R. Thompson of New York in 1953 developed an intramedullary prosthesis with a more curved solid stem

(Thompson 1954). Both implants remain in use today, relatively unchanged.

Kenneth McKee of Norwich was an innovative and gifted surgeon who kept the idea of a total hip replacement alive during the 1950s when arthrodesis was popular and Charnley was advocating the difficult central dislocation technique of hip fusion. In 1951, McKee, at the British Orthopaedic Association, demonstrated a hip joint that he had used on patients with an arthrodesis on one side and serious disease on the other. After visiting Thompson in New York, he adopted the Thompson femoral stem to articulate with a chrome cobalt cloverleaf socket. He used acrylic cement for fixation of the components after 1960 following its introduction by Charnley. It was McKee's design of total hip replacement that was first used clinically in North America (Amstutz & Clarke 1991) (Fig. 2.3).

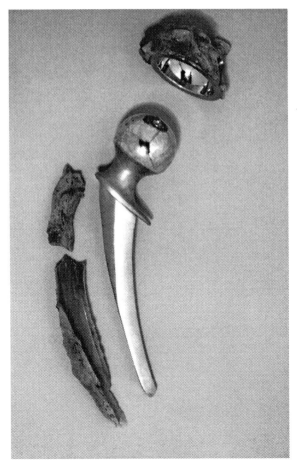

Fig. 2.3 McKee prosthesis, after removal with some surrounding cement

THE CHARNLEY ERA

Charnley's experiments on animal joints had suggested that an artificial joint could not be adequately lubricated by body fluids and he began looking for a 'slippery substance' suitable for the socket of a total hip replacement. He was introduced to polytetrafluoroethylene (PTFE), which was known in industry as Teflon or Fluon. PTFE is white and semi-translucent, looking rather like articular cartilage and can be cut with a knife. In the first instance, he devised a lining of the acetabulum with a thin shell of the plastic and for covering the femoral head, which he reshaped, using a hollow cup of the same material. The blood supply to the femoral head was affected as had occurred with Smith-Petersen's cup arthroplasty. Charnley then moved to a more radical solution. He excised and discarded the head of the femur and replaced it with a Moore's prosthesis and combined it with a PTFE socket inserted into the acetabulum.

On the advice of engineers, he gradually reduced the diameter of the femoral head to 22.25 mm to reduce frictional torque and allow a thicker socket to be used to protect against wear (Fig. 2.4). Charnley began to use dental acrylic cement to fix the prosthesis in the femur but not at this stage the socket.

During 1962, it became clear that PTFE was not a suitable material for hip replacement. This was not so much because of low resistance to wear as because of the tissue reaction caused by the wear debris. This conclusion followed the results of about three hundred operations over three to four years. Charnley came to terms with this disaster. He felt he owed a debt to his patients and did all the sometimes-difficult revision operations himself. The choice of an alternative plastic came about due to the persistence of Charnley's technician, Harry Craven, who tried out a plastic material that had been made in Germany for use in gears in the weaving trade in Lancashire, England. This was ultrahigh molecular weight polyethylene (UHMWPE). When shown the material, Charnley dug his thumbnail into it and walked out of the laboratory telling Craven that he was wasting his time. Craven, however, tested the material in the wear-testing machine and found that after three weeks it had not worn as much as PTFE did in 24 hours (Waugh 1990). UHMWPE has remained the material of choice for metal-on-plastic total hip replacements since then, despite efforts to find a better alternative, a fascinating example of serendipity.

Charnley experimented on himself and wrote a letter to *The Lancet* published on 28 December 1963. He had two specimens of PTFE injected subcutaneously into his thigh and one of high-density polyethylene prepared in finely divided form. At first, there was a systemic reaction to the PTFE for 24 hours, followed by tenderness and redness of the skin underlying the two PTFE specimens. After nine months, the two PTFE specimens were clearly palpable as nodules, and were about twice the size of the original implant. The high-density polyethylene could not be readily detected by palpation. He concluded that there were good grounds that high-density polyethylene did not produce a tissue reaction when implanted in a finely divided state.

In the late 1950s, Dr Dennis Smith, a dental materials scientist, introduced Charnley to the use of self-curing polymethymetacrylate (PMMA) to anchor

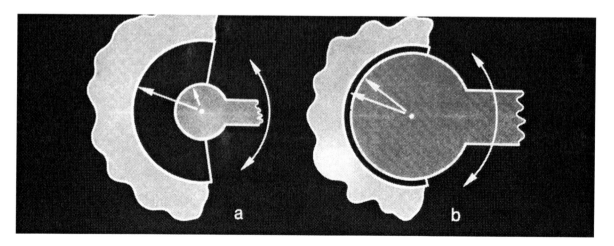

Fig. 2.4 Concept of the low-friction arthroplasty. (a) Thick socket–small femoral head with the difference in radii favouring the socket remaining stationary; (b) this is not so with only a slight difference in radii; from Charnley (1961), fig. 1.1a, b. By courtesy of *The Lancet*

prostheses to bone. PMMA cures quickly without the addition of heat and has a modulus that falls between cancellous and cortical bone. For many years, the use of this substance had been established in neurosurgery. An acrylic cranioplasty had first been performed in 1941 (Cabanela et al 1972).

Before Charnley's report in 1960, there had been tentative use of this material in joint replacements. In Scandinavia in 1941, attempts had been made to improve the fixation of a Judet prosthesis, and in New York in 1953, Haboush reported using cold-curing acrylic cement in connection with metal prostheses with an intramedullary stem. The reason for the failures encountered was probably because it was not used in sufficiently large quantities and not placed accurately (Charnley 1970). Success depended on ramming the cement down the medullary canal of the femur for the full length of the stem of the prosthesis. Charnley's first report (1960) noted that the 'grouting' in which the stem was embedded was needed only to resist compression. The cement was not a glue so that fixation was by interlocking and not by adhesion (Charnley 1960) (Fig. 2.5).

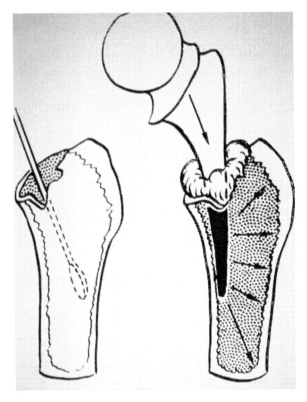

Fig. 2.5 The first picture of the insertion of cement. Courtesy of *The British Journal of Bone and Joint Surgery*

The combination of a cemented metal stem and a cemented high-density polyethylene socket revolutionised the concept of total joint replacement, and joints of similar type were developed worldwide. Maurice Mueller of Bern introduced a curved stem with a 32-mm head, calling it the Charnley–Mueller prosthesis. There were numerous other variations such as the Harris and Aufranc Turner prosthesis, which blended the features of the McKee and Charnley designs of femoral component (Amstutz & Clarke 1991).

In 1978, Ling, Lee and Thornett described their experience with a total hip replacement using a collarless stem (Ling et al 1978). Over two thousand of these prostheses had been inserted since 1970. It was considered after critical analysis that a collar was not necessary for the fixation of prostheses. The presence of a collar was thought to interfere with the satisfactory achievement of a complete cement mantle for the prosthetic stem. One particular advantage was a limited capacity for self-tightening of the implant under load. There was no radiological evidence of absorption of the calcar in the films taken after five years. These results have been maintained at a long-term follow up at an average of thirteen years (Fowler et al 1988).

Charnley reported his first long-term results following abandonment of Teflon in 1972 (Charnley 1972a, b). The follow-up period was four to seven years. The late mechanical failure was 1.3% in 210 cases. With regard to pain and the ability to walk, the grading was excellent in 90% with 10% being good. The sepsis rate was 3.8% and because of this, he devised an enclosure within the main theatre into which filtered air could be passed. This was about seven feet square and seven feet high, and was nicknamed the 'greenhouse'. Later, Charnley contacted F. W. Howarth, whose family firm had built air filtration systems since 1854. Howarth designed a permanent downflow enclosure. Charnley also always wore double gloves. A cloth hood completely invested the head and mouth, but was separate from the gown and a suction tube near the mouth and nose evacuated expired air (Waugh 1990). Charnley's sepsis rate fell to 1% following the introduction of an ultraclean environment (Charnley & Eftakar 1969). A Medical Research Council trial that compared the use of ultraclean air systems of theatre ventilation with a standard theatre with a positive pressure air supply has shown that there were substantially fewer cases of deep sepsis among patients operated on in the ultraclean theatre than in a control series. The rate was further reduced by the use of prophylactic antibiotics (Lidwell et al 1982) (Fig. 2.6).

Of the various complications of total hip replacement, there is no doubt that infection is the most serious. It

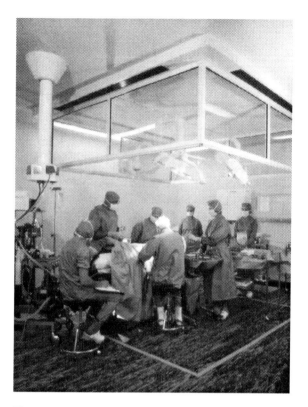

Fig. 2.6 A modern, ultraclean air theatre

arises either at the time of the operation by contamination or via the blood stream. There is little doubt that the airborne route is responsible for the major proportion of wound infections and consequent sepsis (Burke 1963). The presence of foreign material increases the likelihood of infection by relatively few bacteria (Elek & Conen 1957) and the species involved are often those thought to have negligible pathogenic potential, e.g. *Staphylococus epidermidis* or *Propionibacterium*. In the presence of a joint replacement, infection can present either as an acute superficial infection, which may eventually become deep, or as a subacute process after as long as six months. Bacteria adherent to methylmethacrylate have a remarkably higher resistance to antibiotics than bacteria on metals (Naylor et al 1990). The ability of bacteria to adhere to cement is inhibited by antibiotics within it. Bacteria that adhere to implants can encase themselves in a hydrated matrix of polysaccharide and protein and form a slimy layer known as a biofilm. These infections usually persist until the colonised surface is surgically removed (Stewart & Custerton 2001).

Thus, once the diagnosis of an infected hip replacement has been made, an 'exchange arthroplasty'

is indicated. The crucial part of the operation is an extensive wound debridement, so that the wound looks fresh and uncontaminated before the new prosthesis is inserted. Two methods are available. In the two-part exchange operation, after removal of the prosthesis and cement with a thorough debridement, a temporary spacer is inserted for six weeks of intensive chemotherapy appropriate for the organisms identified. A one-stage operation in which the infected prosthesis is removed and replaced with a new one is preferred by some.

If exchange arthroplasty is not possible, then the only effective procedure available is the removal of both components of the hip replacement, leaving a pseudarthrosis. Girdlestone first introduced this procedure in 1943 for the management of sepsis in the hip joint. With the eradication of tuberculosis and effective antibiotics, the numbers of these operations decreased. It has now been reintroduced as a salvage procedure for the total hip replacement and was the only solution available until Bucholz et al (1981) suggested re-implantation of the prosthesis with antibiotic impregnated cement.

It is only a salvage procedure. The gain is the elimination of sepsis, but the disadvantages include instability and weakness, shortening and the permanent need of a stick.

Total hip replacement is, on the whole, a very successful operation. For most implants, the revision rate is about 10% at ten years (Murray et al 1995). Revision operations cost more and do not give as good a functional result or last as long as a primary replacement. In 1995, Murray and colleagues in Oxford identified sixty-two different primary total hip replacements available on the market in the UK and found that there was little or no scientific evidence that the newer more expensive implants were better than the established designs.

In 2000, there was a report from Wrightington Hospital, where Charnley did all his pioneering work on the hip, with a twenty- to thirty-year follow up (Wroblewski et al 2000). There had obviously been modifications of the components of the prosthetic hips over the years. Of patients, 94% considered the operation to be a success. Of them, 82% were free of pain and 12% had occasional discomfort. The main long-term problem was wear and loosening of the ultrahigh molecular weight polyethylene cup, which increased with time. It was considered not possible to determine whether the process of loosening had a mechanical or biological basis.

It is interesting to compare this report from a specialised hip unit with that of one health region in the

UK where the surgery was by a variety of surgeons under fifty-six consultants in eighteen National Health hospitals and six private hospitals. There were 1198 primary total Charnley hip replacements and the outcome was assessed at five years. The rate of aseptic loosening was 2.3%, of deep infection 1.4% and of revision 3.2%. Radiological assessment revealed gross loosening that had not been previously recognised in a further 5.2%. The combined failure rate was nearly 9%, which is higher than those published from specialist centres but is probably representative of the normal state of affairs (Fender et al 1999).

THE ERA AFTER CHARNLEY

Charnley's work has been continued at Wrightington. Long-term problems have been identified as wear of the UHMWPE, which has led to the use of ceramic femoral heads and proximal strain shielding of the femur that has resulted in the change of the design of the femoral stem (the C Stem) (Fig. 2.7). This stem has a triple taper based on experimental work that allows effective load transfer from the stem to the proximal femur (B. M. Wroblewski, personal communication 2001).

This period has also seen a proliferation of prostheses, attempts to improve fixation by the introduction of hydroxyapatite and porous-coated implants to reduce wear by the use of ceramics, to restore bone stock by allografts and allograft impaction grafting for revision procedures and the reintroduction of metal-on-metal prostheses to prevent osteolysis and loosening, which are the main causes of failure of implants. Experiments have been made in vitro to increase cross-linking in UHMWP to improve resistance to wear (Muratoglu et al 2001). However, in vivo assessment of new prostheses takes a long time, a short-term follow up is for five years, an intermediate for five to ten, and in the long-term ten years or longer. The persistent problem of postoperative deep vein thrombosis, its morbidity and mortality, has received considerable attention.

Use of hydroxyapatite

Bony apposition to a metal surface can be improved by a coating of osteo-inductive material such as hydroxyapatite. The thickness of the coating of hydroxyapatite is important. Thin coatings of 50 µm or less, applications to roughened or porous-coated surfaces and preferably a fully resorbable coating are recommended. In 1985, Ronald Furlong in London implanted the first hydroxyapatite-coated prosthesis. The prosthesis had been coated by means of a technique developed by

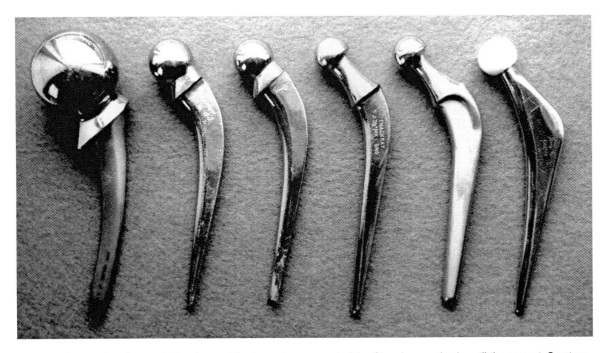

Fig. 2.7 Progressive changes in the shape of the femoral component of the Charnley prosthesis until the present. Courtesy of Professor B. M. Wroblewski

Johannes-Frederick Osborne, a maxillofacial surgeon who was a pioneer in the field (Maquelet 1996).

A recent report (McNally et al 2000) on the clinical and radiological outcome of one hundred consecutive total hip replacements in eighty-six patients with hydroxyapatite-coated femoral components indicated very successful results. Radiographs showed no translucent lines around any femoral component and there were no signs of impending failure. The authors suggested that the hydroxyapatite coating gave a satisfactory prosthesis–bone interface preferable to any other system. Apatite-coated implants can form a chemical bond with a strength comparable with cortical bone (Geesink et al 1988). It has been reported that two-thirds of the hydroxyapatite coating is resorbed within sixteen weeks and replaced by bone. The solid bonding of the prosthesis to bone may impede the transport of wear debris and prevent proximal osteopaenia and distal granulomas. Scarlett's results are supported by similar findings in a study from The Netherlands (Geesink & Hoefnagels 1995) and by a group from Norway (Rokkum et al 1999).

Ceramics

A ceramic is defined as a material that is neither metal nor organic. The ceramics familiar to orthopaedic surgeons are aluminium oxide, zirconium oxide, tricalcium phosphate and pyrolytic carbon. They are hard and brittle materials formed and are stable at high temperatures. They are biologically inert (Skinner 1996). Ceramics were the earliest structurally modified inorganic materials to be produced by man. Early tests of ceramic heads against UHMWPE were favourable compared to a metal head and have been supported by a ten-year follow up (Wroblewski et al 1999). There have been no complications and a very low rate of penetration of only 0.02 mm after two years. There has been no change in the mean rate of wear over the last five years. The authors from Charnley's old unit at Wrightington suggested that the use of ceramic heads to reduce polyethylene debris is likely to be the next logical stage in the development of the low-friction arthroplasty.

Thromboprophylaxis after total hip replacement

Venous thromboembolism remains a frequent complication despite modern surgical and anaesthetic techniques and the incidence has not changed very much since the time of Charnley. The incidence is still 50%, with 20% developing proximal obstruction (Heit 1996). Charnley was interested in the subject and thought that research should be directed towards clinical trials rather than towards sophisticated methods of detecting thrombosis not detected clinically (Charnley 1972a, b).

A paper from Bristol assessed the work of twelve teams at one centre on the results for 1162 consecutive total hip replacements carried out in 1990 and 1991 in which pharmacological prophylaxis was not routinely used. The mortality rate from pulmonary embolism was 0.34%, the total thromboembolic morbidity rate was 3.4% and the overall mortality rate at 90 days due to all causes was 1.3%. The authors concluded that the results would justify prophylaxis if it did not produce its own morbidity (Warwick et al 1995).

The published assessments of risk of death from pulmonary embolism vary from 0.1 to 1%. The two main methods of current prophylaxis are anticoagulants, low molecular weight heparin (LMWH) and mechanical means of reducing stasis. In a meta-analysis of fifty-six trials of methods designed to prevent venous thromboembolism after total hip replacement, all treatments studied reduced the risk of deep vein thrombosis with the exception of aspirin. Only LMWH and stockings reduced the risk of pulmonary embolism (Imperiale & Speroff 1994).

In a study comparing LMWH and the use of a footpump, it was concluded that the pump was a suitable alternative to LMWH (Warwick et al 1998). There are good experimental reasons for believing that reducing stasis is as effective as countering hypercoagulability in the prevention of deep vein thrombosis. It has been shown in extensive animal experiments that stasis or hypercoagulability alone do not produce venous thrombosis but the simultaneous combination of the two does so rapidly (Wessler 1962). A major difficulty with mechanical methods is the increasing evidence that shows that many thromboemboli develop after hospitalisation. Pharmacological prophylaxis can be given for a month or longer after operation. In terms of efficiency and convenience, the evidence that modern anticoagulants prevent postoperative thromboembolism far exceeds that of other prophylactic regimens (Thomas 2000).

Replacement of bone stock

The loss of bone stock secondary to the adverse effects of particulate debris and to mechanical instability of the implant in the femur is the major challenge in revision surgery.

Although the use of allografts only became popular in the late 1960s and early 1970s (Mankin et al 1983), their first use is attributed to Lexer in 1908, who transplanted twenty-three whole joints and eleven hemijoints

(Lexer 1908). These results were published in 1925. Allografts can be cancellous bone chips impacted and supplemented by methylacrylate cement (Gie et al 1993). In fifty-six hips reviewed after 18–49 months, there were few complications and a majority of satisfactory results (Gie et al 1993). An alternative method is the use of a composite consisting of a proximal femoral allograft and a prosthesis to restore the anatomical and mechanical integrity of the upper end of the femur. The allograft has an inherent capacity to incorporate and become part of the structure of the femur. It also provides a lattice for cement. The main indication for the use of an intact allograft is a circumferential defect greater than 5 cm in length. The major disadvantages are the potential for the transmission of disease and a prolonged period for healing at the graft–host interface. A number of series have been reported with good results and a substantial improvement in clinical scores (Haddad et al 1999).

Metal-on-metal prostheses

The role of polythene wear particles in osteolysis and the failure of well-fixed implants have been described in Chapter 7.

There have been considerable efforts to reduce the number of wear particles generated from polythene components to minimise the inflammatory response and increase the longevity of the arthroplasty with renewed interest in metal-on-metal bearings, which have been shown to have ten to one hundred times lower wear than metal-on-polyethylene articulations using linear and volumetric measurements.

In 1984, Muller and Weber reintroduced metal-on-metal bearings (Metasul, Sulzer Orthopaedics, Winterthur, Switzerland) and more than one hundred thousand of these have been used in Europe with the longest follow up of eleven years. A study of one hundred and eighty Metasul Retrievals reported a sixty-fold decrease in volumetric wear compared with metal-on-polyethylene with no failures due to osteolysis (Beaule et al 2000).

In retrieved specimens (Sieber et al 1999), less osteolysis suggests that the biological response is influenced more by the size of the wear particles than by the total amount of debris. The solubility of metal wear particles could lead to an improved tissue clearing capacity and thus the reduced induction of osteolysis by metal-on-metal implants. Metal surfaces have a self-polishing capacity. Scratches are worn out by further joint movement. As the rate of wear of metal-on-metal implants is lower than that of metal-on-polyethylene, the second generation of this design may increase the

overall survival rate. Studies over many years are required to confirm this.

There is a possibility that osteolysis may arise secondary to fluid pressure as happens in the pathophysiology of osteoarthritic cysts. It has been proposed that raised intracapsular joint fluid pressures can be transmitted to periprosthetic bone and play a role in the pathophysiology of osteolysis in joint replacement (Schmalzriel et al 1997). The stem–cement interface in the presence of defects in the cement mantle provides a conduit to allow access of pressure changes, joint fluid and its contents to the endosteal surface at the site of the defect in the mantle. The stem–cement interface may become part of the effective joint space particularly following abrasive wear between the stem and the cement (R. S. M. Ling, personal communication 2000).

OUTCOMES

With the vast numbers of hip replacements done each year, outcome studies are essential for quality control. From the patient's point of view, success is relief of pain and good function. The Swedes have taken the lead in this area with the establishment of The Swedish National Total Hip Arthroplasty Register, which was started in January 1979. It has been supported by the Swedish Orthopaedic Society and the National Board of Health and Welfare. Its aims are to perform epidemiological analyses, to identify risk factors for primary and revision surgery, and to facilitate improvement of surgical technique, compare regions and maintain quality assurance. Having been in place for twenty years, it is the biggest reliable database in the world. It should encourage orthopaedic surgeons to subject all their results to long-term review so that there is up-to-date evidence for continued use of specific prostheses and the surgical performance of individuals can be compared (Soderman 2000). It has shown that the quality of technique and choice of implant are of major importance in relation to loosening. The need for improved prostheses is clear, particularly for young patients who have long-life expectancies and require reliable prostheses that will last thirty years or more (Muirhead-Allwood 1998).

THE FUTURE

Joint replacement although introduced by orthopaedic surgeons is a multidisciplinary subject. The future depends on the collaboration of bioengineers, biomaterials' scientists and statisticians to help in the accurate evaluation of the data collected. The continued progress of this vast industry is now taking place against a background of major advances of molecular medicine and the grafting of chondrocytes. These biological advances will reduce the numbers of patients requiring hip replacements. With early treatment of developmental dysplasia of the hip and the control of rheumatoid arthritis, large numbers of people may be spared degenerative disease of the hip. Improved techniques should be accompanied by increased specialisation in units, so that the primary operations are done to the highest standard and the need for revision surgery is reduced to a minimum.

REFERENCES

Amstutz H C, Clarke J C 1991 The Hip. Churchill-Livingstone, New York, p 4

Aufranc O E 1957 Constructive hip surgery with the vitallium mold. J Bone Joint Surg 49A: 237–248

Baer W S 1926 Arthroplasty of the hip. J Bone Joint Surg 8: 769–802

Barton J R 1827 On the treatment of anchylosis by the formation of artificial joints. N Am Med Surg J 3: 279–292

Barton J R 1837 A new treatment in a case of anchylosis. Am J Med Sci 21: 332–340

Beaule P E, Campbell P, Mirra J, Hooper J C, Schmalzriel T P 2000 Osteolysis in a cementless second generation metal on metal hip replacement. Clin Orthop 386: 159–165

Bucholz H W, Elson R A, Engelbrecht E, Lodenkamper H, Rottger J, Siegel A 1981 Management of deep infection of total hip replacement. J Bone Joint Surg 63B: 342–353

Burke J F 1963 Identification of the sources of staphylococci contaminating the surgical wound during operation. Ann Surg 158: 287–290

Cabanela M E, Coventry M B, Macarty C S, Miller W E 1972 The fate of patients with methyl methacrylate cranioplasty. J Bone Joint Surg 54A: 278–281

Charnley J 1960 Anchorage of the femoral head prosthesis to the shaft of the bone. J Bone Joint Surg 42B: 28–29

Charnley J 1961 Arthroplasty of the hip, a new operation. Lancet i: 1129–1132

Charnley J 1963 Tissue reactions to polytetrafluoroethylene [letter]. Lancet ii: 1379

Charnley J 1970 The position of prosthesis in living bones. In: Simpson D C (ed) Modern Trends in Biomechanics. Butterworths, London, p 73

Charnley J 1972a Prophylaxis of postoperative embolism (letter). Lancet ii: 134–135

Charnley J 1972b The long term results of low friction arthroplasty of the hip performed as a primary intervention. J Bone Joint Surg 54B: 61–76

Charnley J, Eftakar N 1969 Postoperative infection in total prosthetic replacement arthroplasty of the hip joint. Br J Surg 51: 202–205

Elek S D, Conen P E 1957 The virulence of staphylococcus pyogenes for man; a study of the problems of wound infection. Br J Exp Pathol 38: 573–586

Fender D, Harper W M, Gregg P J 1999 Outcome of Charnley total hip replacement across a single health region in England. J Bone Joint Surg 81B: 577–581

Fowler J L, Gie G A, Lee A J C, Ling R S M 1988 Experience with the Exeter total hip replacement. Orthop Clin N Am 19: 477–489

Geesink R G T, de Groot K, Klein C P A T 1988 Bonding of bone to apatite coated implants. J Bone Joint Surg 70B: 17–22

Geesink R G T, Hoefnagels N H M 1995 Six-year results of hydroxyapatite coated total hip replacements. J Bone Joint Surg 77B: 534–547

Gie G A, Linder L, Ling R S, Simon J P, Slooff T J J, Timperley A J 1993 Impacted cancellous allografts and cement for revision total hip replacement. J Bone Joint Surg 75B: 14–21

Girdlestone G B 1943 Acute pyogenic arthritis of the hip. Lancet i: 419–421

Haddad F S, Garbuz D S, Masri B A, Duncan C P, Hutchison C R, Gross A E 1999 Femoral bone loss in patients managed with revision hip replacement:results of circumferential allograft replacement. J Bone Joint Surg 81A: 420–436

Heit J A 1996 Thrombophlebitis. In: Morrey B E (ed) Reconstructive Surgery of the Joints, 2nd edn. Churchill Livingstone, New York, p 72

Hey Groves E W 1927 Some contributions to the reconstructive surgery of the hip. Br J Surg 14: 486–517

Imperiale T F, Speroff T 1994 A meta-analysis of methods to prevent venous thromboembolism after total hip replacement:a prospective randomized trial. J Am Med Assoc 271: 1780–1785

Jones R 1923 Orthopaedic Surgery. Jones Sir R, Lovett R W (eds) Henry Frowds and Hodder & Stoughton, London, p 101

Judet J, Judet R 1950 The use of an artificial femoral head for arthroplasty of the hip joint. J Bone Joint Surg 32B: 166–173

Lexer E 1908 Substitution of whole or half joints from freshly amputated extremities by free plastic operations. Surg Gyn Obstet 6: 601–607

Lexer E 1925 Joint transplantations and arthroplasty. Surg Gyn Obstet 40: 782–809

Lidwell O M, Lowburg E J, Whyte W, Blowers R, Stanley S J, Lowe D 1982 Effect of ultraclean air in operating rooms on deep repairs in the joint after total hip or knee replacement: a randomized study. Br Med Journal 285: 10–14

Ling R S M, Lee A J C, Thornett C E E 1978 The collarless intramedullary stem. J Bone Joint Surg 60B: 137

Mankin H J, Doppelt S, Tomford W 1983 Clinical experience with allograft implantation. The first ten years. Clin Orth 174: 69–86

Maquelet P 1996 Foreword. In: Furlong R (ed) Hydroxyapatite Ceramic: Proceedings of a Two Day Symposium Furlong Research Foundation, London

McNally S A, Shepperd J A, Mann C V, Walezak J P 2000 The results at nine to twelve years of the use of a hydroxyapetite-coated femoral stem. J Bone Joint Surg 82B: 378–382

Muirhead-Allwood S K 1998 Editorial. Br Med J 316: 644

Moore A T 1957 The self-locking metal hip prosthesis. J Bone Joint Surg 39A: 811–827

Moore A T, Bohlman H R 1943 Metal hip joint; a case report. J Bone Joint Surg 25: 688–692

Muratoglu O K, Bragdon C R, O'Connor D C, Justy M, Harris W R 2001 A novel method of cross-linking ultra-high molecular weight polyethylene to improve wear, reduce oxidation and retain mechanical properties. J Arthrop 16: 149–160

Murphy J B 1913 Arthroplasty. Ann Surg 57: 593–647

Murray D W, Carr A J, Bulstrode 1995 Which primary total hip replacement? J Bone Joint Surg 77B: 520–527

Naylor P T, Myvrik Q N, Gristina A G 1990 Antibiotic resistance of biomaterial-adherent coagulase negative and positive staphylococci. Clin Orth 261: 126–133

Rang M 2000 The Story of Orthopaedics. W B Saunders, Philadelphia, p322

Rokkum M, Brandt M, Byek K, Hetland K R, Wange S 1999 Polyethylene wear, osteolysis and acetabular loosening with an HA-coated hip prosthesis. J Bone Joint Surg 81B: 582–589

Schmalzriel T P, Akizuki K H, Fedenko A N, Mirra J 1997 The role of access of joint fluid to bone in periarticular osteolysis. J Bone Joint Surg 79A: 447–452

Shepherd M 1954 Review of 650 arthroplasties of the hip. J Bone Joint Surg 36B: 507

Sieber H P, Riker C B, Kottig P 1999 Analysis of 118 second-generation metal-on-metal retrieved hip implants. J Bone Joint Surg 81B: 46–50

Skinner H 1996 Ceramics. In: Morrey B E (ed) Reconstructive Surgery of the Joints. Churchill Livingstone, New York, p 53

Smith-Petersen M N 1948 Evolution of mould arthroplasty of the hip joint. J Bone Joint Surg 30B: 59–75

Soderman P 2000 On the validity of the results from the Swedish National Total Hip Arthroplasty Register. Acta Orthop Scand Suppl no. 296: 71, 4

Stewart P S, Custerton J W 2001 Antibiotic resistance of bacteria in biofilms. Lancet 358: 135–138

Thomas D P 2000 Whither thrombophylaxis after total hip replacements? J Bone Joint Surg 82B: 469–472

Thompson F R 1954 Two and a half years' experience with a vitallium hip prosthesis. J Bone Joint Surg 36A: 489–500

Warwick D, Harrison J, Glew D, Mitchelmore A, Peters T J, Donovan J 1998 Comparison of the use of a foot pump with the use of low molecular weight heparin for the prevention of deep-vein thrombosis after total hip replacement: a randomized trial. J Bone Joint Surg 80A: 1158–1166

Warwick D, Williams M H, Bannister G C 1995 Death and thromboembolic disease after total hip replacement. J Bone Joint Surg 77B: 6–10

Waugh W 1990 John Charnley: The Man and the Hip. Springer, London, p 102

Wessler S 1962 Thrombosis in the presence of vascular stasis. Am J Med 33: 648–666

Whitman R 1924 The reconstruction operation for arthritis deformans of the hip joint. Ann Surg 80: 779–785

Wiles P 1958 The surgery of the osteo-arthritic hip. Br J Surg 45: 488–497

Williams A 1985 Economics of coronary artery bypass grafting. Br Med J 291: 325–326

Wroblewski B M, Fleming P A, Siney P A 2000 Charnley low frictional torque arthroplasty of the hip 20–30 year results. J Bone Joint Surg 82B: 378–382

Wroblewski B M, Siney P D, Fleming P A 1999 Low-friction arthroplasty of the hip using alumina ceramic and cross-linked polyethylene. J Bone Joint Surg 81B: 54–55

3

History of knee arthroplasty

Peter Abernethy

That men do not learn very much from the lessons of history is the most important of all the lessons that history has to teach.

(Aldous Huxley)

Epidemiological studies show a greater incidence of arthritis affecting the knee than the hip, but despite this at the beginning of the twenty-first century three hundred thousand total knee replacements and five hundred thousand total hip replacements are implanted annually world wide. What are the reasons for this apparent surgical paradox?

It is not explained by arthritis of the knee being tolerated better by the patient and as a consequence less demanding of surgery nor by the frequency with which hip fractures are treated by total hip replacement.

The development of knee replacement has been slower and more obtuse than that of the hip. The reasons for this partly relate to the fact that the first artificial knee joints were developed in an era of scientific ignorance when many of the mechanical principles of the human knee joint were still unknown. Another, but less significant, reason for its relatively tardy development related to the long-established practice of arthrodesis which afforded a means of achieving a pain-free and stable joint despite its functional limitations.

Only over the past three decades has there been an explosive increase in knee replacement surgery as increased satisfaction with the outcome has become more evident to both patient and surgeon. In the USA the frequency of knee replacement has now overtaken that of the hip, and undoubtedly this will become a global trend.

EARLY DEVELOPMENTS

In 1890 Themistocles Gluck became the first surgeon to implant an artificial knee joint. He studied first in Leipzig and then in Berlin as Von Langenbeck's last student. After a period as Professor in Bucharest he returned to Berlin as Senior Surgeon to the new Kaiser (see Chapter 12).

In a lecture to the 19th Congress of the German Surgical Society Gluck described replacements for several joints affected by tuberculosis or tumour. For the knee he devised a hinge linked to ivory stems that could be attached to bone. His choice of ivory was probably influenced by its use in dentistry at that time. Later that year, in a lecture to the Berlin Medical Society, he described the use of aseptic bone glue which he had devised to improve the mechanical fixation of the prosthesis to bone.

Even at this early stage Gluck was aware that skin closure could be compromised if the implant was too bulky and he also appreciated the important relationship between the shape and strength of implants. He is also credited with introducing the term 'arthroplasty' in 1902.

Despite these various and important contributions Gluck's work seems to have been largely disregarded during the subsequent development of knee replacement. Perhaps this is not surprising when one considers that at the height of his career he was severely criticised by his former teacher E. Von Bergmann who claimed that he was 'a discredit to German science to be combatted by every means'. No doubt such criticism was prompted by the fact that all Gluck's joint replacements rapidly became septic. Without adequate means of dealing with infection the potential of such surgery must have appeared extremely limited. Bearing in mind the circumstances, it is difficult not to have some sympathy with Von Bergmann's view.

The lack of control of infection was clearly an important factor influencing the progress of development and Gluck's extraordinary surgical vision lay dormant for the next sixty years.

In the late nineteenth century surgical interest focused on attempts to mobilise stiff joints which were usually the end result of infection or trauma. It is interesting that osteoarthritis and rheumatoid arthritis were not regarded as major indications for this type of surgery because they were seldom considered to be the cause of stiff joints. The literature from this time does not even discuss the question of pain relief which was to become the major indication for surgery only in the second half of the twentieth century.

In 1861 Ferguson of King's College Hospital in London performed excisional joint surgery on a bedbound patient following trauma to her knee. He removed two slices of bone from the tibia in addition to scooping out a quantity of dead bone. The patient's recovery was described as 'for a time rather sluggish'. Ultimately she 'was able to attend to her household duties and could run upstairs or jump off a chair as if she had had no disease and no operation'. From this description it appears that the patient had an excellent result which would be the envy of the modern arthroplasty surgeon. Pleased with this outcome, Ferguson claimed that he had put an end to the 'factious opposition of persons who knew nothing on the subject and yet declared that no good result could be obtained unless anchylosis occurred'. He re-operated on this patient five years later 'for disease in the locality of the new joint but quite unconnected with it'. There was suppuration in the upper part of the leg. Even in the absence of implanted foreign material the vagaries of bone infection were clearly a major problem for the surgeon.

Ferguson's early result was exceptional and in order to improve the general results Verneuil in 1866 interposed soft tissue between the resected bone ends. In 1885 Foederl used membranes from ovarian cysts and pigs bladders, and skin was first used in 1902 by the indefatigable Gluck.

Joint instability also proved to be a limiting factor to the success of this type of surgery. Murphy of Chicago made the most significant contribution to interpositional arthroplasty for it was he who recognised that whilst movement was important, the need to have a stable and supportive knee joint was also essential. In 1905 he introduced fascia lata first as a pedicle and then as a free flap to address this problem. Over the following thirty years or so there was considerable interest in modifying these excisional techniques directed mainly to improving stability. In 1926 Putti shaped the ends of the bone. Campbell in 1928 and Albi in 1933 further modified the bone resection.

Various reports on the results of excision arthroplasty were published and it was clear that in general they were not as good as Ferguson's published case. In 1918 Henderson collected 117 cases from the USA with poor results in sixty-four cases. In the same year Baer reported on twenty-eight interpositional arthroplasties using animal membrane of which fifteen had a good result. It is interesting to note that in this series a good result was defined as one with at least 25° of movement.

In 1923 Hey Groves of Bristol managed to collect only eighteen cases of excision arthroplasty done over the previous five years. These were drawn from his own practice and that of several English colleagues. Ten of these patients had poor results. There was little widespread enthusiasm for the operation and Hey Groves himself expressed concern over the value of the procedure. Later in 1937 Courvoisier reported on twenty-three cases from France collected over 11 years of whom seventeen had good results. Although the operation continued to be practiced it was done in very small numbers.

RESURGENCE OF METAL INTERPOSITIONAL SURGERY

It was not surprising that there was continuing interest in metal interposition as a possible means of reducing adhesions and improving the quality of these results. Any interpositional material needed to be inert and sufficiently strong.

Following its introduction into dentistry in 1933 Vitallium was found to be well tolerated by the tissues. Smith-Petersen of Boston subsequently used it as a successful interpositional material in the hip. Inspired by this Boyd devised the first Vitallium mould for the knee in 1938. He assisted Willis-Campbell of Memphis to implant it in three cases without success and its use was abandoned thereafter.

In 1939 Smith-Petersen implanted a modified knee mould and his technique was continued by the group at the Massachusetts General Hospital. In 1958 Aufranc and Jones reported a series of fourteen cases in which three different designs of shell were used, the most favoured being an 'anchor-like' device with the stem inserted into the femur and the crossbars hollowed to fit the condyles. Of these cases, only three were reported as good and three went on to arthrodesis.

The poor results of femoral moulds related mainly to the replacement of only one surface of the knee joint. Nevertheless it did prove to be a significant stage in the development of knee replacement because these devices were used subsequently as prototypes for contemporary condylar prostheses.

The indications for arthroplasty remained relatively few; most surgeons preferred arthrodesis which gave a painless and stable joint. Arthrodesis remained the operation of choice until the mid-twentieth century with excision arthroplasty restricted to those with bilateral knee ankylosis or with a stiff knee and stiff ipsilateral hip.

The concept of isolated tibial plateau substitution was first introduced by McKeever in 1952. His was an all metal device keyed into the tibial bone. In the same year this concept was modified by Jansen in Denmark who used acrylic discs and in 1959 Macintosh of Toronto modified Jansen's work using unkeyed metal discs of varying thickness. These allowed the surgeon to adjust alignment and to tighten up the slack ligaments by using an insert of appropriate thickness. At the time they afforded a means of achieving significant pain relief even though they again only addressed one of the affected articular surfaces. Their inability to relieve pain completely and their tendency to dislocate served to stimulate the need for a knee prosthesis which would resolve these important issues.

RESURGENCE OF THE HINGED JOINT

The quest for mobility led Jean and Robert Judet to implant the first hinged knee arthroplasty in 1947, but this acrylic joint quickly failed. In 1949 d'Intignano had more short-term success with a similar device and in 1953 D'Aubigne and Walldius introduced their hinged prostheses.

In his dissertation of 1957 Walldius collated the results derived from twenty-four different papers written between 1914 and 1953 relating to 896 excision arthroplasty procedures. Using the limited criteriae available only 46% were graded as successful. He contrasted these results with those he had achieved at the Karolinska Institute in Stockholm using his new acrylic and steel hinged device with 63 mm-long intramedullary stems which he had implanted in thirty-two knees, twenty-nine of which were affected by rheumatoid arthritis, two by osteoarthritis and one by post-traumatic arthritis. This was one of the earliest reports where pain relief appears to have been a major indication for surgery.

Within an average follow up period of five years good results were achieved in 75%, which meant that the patient was satisfied with the operation and in addition had no pain, good mobility and stability. The average range of postoperative movement was 84° but only eighteen patients could walk indoors without support. Nevertheless, after the unpredictable outcome of excision arthroplasty, these results were a remarkable achievement.

Some aspects of his surgery are worthy of comparison with contemporary practice. A longitudinal skin incision now regarded as the standard surgical approach for knee replacement was rejected by him after three cases because it did not give sufficient exposure of the tibial metaphysis to allow bone resection with a saw. Soft tissue mobilisation and release to allow the superb exposure using this approach were not appreciated at that time. The collateral ligaments were divided because they were not necessary for stability. Their possible role in the attenuation of forces across the joint went unrecognised. Such important soft tissue concepts were not raised as surgical issues until twenty years later.

Walldius resected 10–15 mm of bone from the tibia and 23–28 mm from the femur creating a large extension gap of 33–43 mm as opposed to about 20 mm by present-day standards, demonstrating that the principle of bone preservation was yet to be established.

His postoperative regimen involved immobilisation of the knee in a plaster cylinder for three weeks. Walking with a variety of aids was delayed for six to eight weeks and the average hospital stay for patients was two months and twenty-two days. He attested to the need for the patient to have a strong determination to cooperate and this requirement is still as important today. Contemporary management with early postoperative movement combined with more effective pain control has led to today's hospital administrator anticipating an average patient stay of between three and seven days following knee arthroplasty.

In 1953 Shiers in the UK introduced a hinge that was thinner and less bulky but still required resection of 36 mm of bone. In 1954 he stated that 'few surgeons would ever see 50 cases requiring knee replacement let alone operate on them even over a 5 year period'. This mid-century forecast of total knee replacement was wildly inaccurate. Such a statement is an excellent example of how the indications for an operative procedure are radically modified by its success. By the end of the century knee replacement had become one of the most commonly performed orthopaedic procedures.

In 1954 Jackson-Burrows in London devised a hinge, the use of which was continued by Lettin as the Stanmore Hinge. This remained in continuous use for over thirty years proving to be one of the more successful devices of its kind.

In 1970 a group of French surgeons developed the Guepar hinge (an acronym for Le Groupe L'Utilisation et le Etude des Prostheses Articulaires). This was less bulky, aligned in valgus and had a posteriorly set hinge to allow more flexion. There was also an anterior flange to allow patellar replacement. This prosthesis enjoyed considerable popularity world wide until the complications of patellar instability, prosthetic loosening and infection became increasingly evident.

In the 1970s there was a divergence of opinion and direction in the design and mechanics of knee prostheses. Although hinged devices had been reduced in size since their introduction, there was still general concern about their bulk which was known to increase infection. Furthermore, bone encroachment by the stems exposed the medullary canals to sepsis which often resulted in massive bone loss.

Concern also extended to their lack of intrinsic rotation and of adduction and abduction. Their constraint increased the transfer of force to the bone–cement interface regarded as a major factor in the loosening of the components.

This led to a variety of metal on plastic hinged joints some incorporating ingenious modifications designed to impart rotary function in order to reduce the forces acting on the bone–cement interface.

This latter concept allowed rigidity in extension and some degree of rotation in flexion. In Britain knees of this type were introduced by Sheehan (1971) and Attenborough (1973) and in the USA by Mathews and Kaufer (1973) and Murray (1974). Many of these rotational hinges still did not address the mechanical demands placed upon them and were withdrawn from routine practice within a few years.

Similar hinged devices were developed in Europe where they enjoyed much more success. Engelbrecht of Hamburg felt that hinged devices had been prematurely abandoned by others. He argued that some of the reported poor results related to metal-on-metal designs with anterior axles and that their failure had been more a function of poor design rather than pure rigidity.

The use of linked devices continued to be used by Blauth, Engelbrecht, Gschwend and others. Between 1985 and 1990 of 3193 knee replacements implanted at the Endo clinic in Hamburg, 60% were rotating hinge knees and 13% were rigid hinges. This type of practice was at odds with the majority of surgeons world wide who by then had discarded hinged knees for routine use in favour of condylar prostheses.

EMERGENCE OF A SCIENTIFIC APPROACH

In 1960 an event of enormous significance occurred when Charnley reported on his cemented hip prosthesis. This acted as the prime catalyst to the development of a more acceptable total knee replacement.

For the first time it appeared that three of the biggest problems in joint replacement had been resolved, at least in the short-term. One was the discovery of acceptable interpositional materials which surgeons had pursued for over half a century, the second was a method of fixing

them to bone and the third was the knowledge that implantation of a prosthesis could be achieved with a low rate of infection. A further admirable aspect of his work was the manner in which the general release of his operation was tightly controlled. This was a salutary omission in the development of knee arthroplasty.

In 1967 James Morrison, a doctoral student with Professor John Paul at Strathclyde University in Glasgow, produced his PhD thesis on 'Forces transmitted by the human knee joint during activities'. The realisation of the magnitude of these forces was to have a profound influence in demonstrating the need for a more scientific rather than a pure clinical approach to total knee replacement.

Morrison's work was combined with important studies by Frankel and Burstein (1971), Lamoreaux (1971), Huson (1973), Kettlekamp (1973), Menschik (1974) and Goodfellow and O'Connor (1977) on the kinematics (the study of the motion of one body over another) of the knee. This led to the definition of the axes, direction and control of movements of the knee and to the all essential successful development of knee arthroplasty.

CONDYLAR PROSTHESES

Gunston, a Canadian working with Sir John Charnley in Wrightington, developed the concept that knee arthroplasty should simulate the normal joint as closely as possible. In 1968 he implanted the first cemented metal on polyethylene knee joint. This was a four-part prosthesis with narrow femoral runners each 10 mm wide. The collateral and cruciate ligaments were preserved. Difficulty was encountered aligning the four components and in combination with the narrow runners this led to excessive polyethylene wear (Gunston 1971).

Gunston's major concern had been directed towards establishing the kinematics of the joint at the expense of achieving adequate fixation. Subsequently the device was modified and the operative instrumentation improved to allow better alignment of the components. Despite modifications by Bryan and Peterson at the Mayo Clinic, Newton in Manchester and Cavendish in Liverpool, it did not achieve long-term success.

With the increasing realisation that it was no longer appropriate for surgeons to attempt to develop joint prostheses in isolation, a multidisciplinary approach to the problem was adopted. These groups incorporated the experience of clinicians, bioengineers and material scientists and they have remained an essential and integral part of further major developments in the field.

In 1969 Freeman of the London Hospital implanted his first cemented arthroplasty which he described as a stemmed version of the Massachusetts General

Hospital shell in combination with two polyethylene hemi-arthroplasties of the McIntosh type. The cruciate ligaments were preserved. Lack of success quickly led him and Swanson of Imperial College Engineering Department to modify the design and later the same year Freeman implanted the first two-part cemented condylar prosthesis. The femoral component had a single radius of curvature and articulated with a matching dished tibial component. The cruciate ligaments were sacrificed. This 'roller in a trough' was stabilised by tight collateral ligaments and capsule which prevented the femur from moving 'uphill' either anteriorly or posteriorly.

A multicentre trial started in 1970 and problems were encountered because the tibial insert was too small to distribute the load and there was also no lateral constraint. Lack of knowledge of how to achieve correct axial alignment and how to restore tension to the ligaments combined to produce problems with instability. It did however demonstrate that total knee replacement was possible without the cruciate ligaments.

In 1971 Insall and Ranawat, surgeons at the Hospital for Special Surgery in New York, began a very productive liaison with Walker, a bioengineer. This first resulted in the development of both a unicondylar and a three-part Duocondylar prosthesis with cruciate retention. Disappointed by early sinkage of the components they went on to develop the Total Condylar prosthesis in 1974 (Insall et al 1979).

This device was strongly influenced by Freeman's earlier design. It consisted of two parts. The all plastic tibia had a short stem and was dished with a central ridge allowing some lateral constraint. The femoral component had a fixed radius of curvature with an extended anterior flange for optional patellar resurfacing. The cruciate ligaments were sacrificed and movement of the femur occurred within the conforming tibial dish. Motion was determined solely by the geometry of the prosthesis. Stability was achieved by tightening up the collateral ligaments by the use of an appropriately thick insert. Initially only one femoral component and three tibial inserts of different thickness were available. This sparcity of components sometimes led to difficulty in achieving stability especially in flexion. There was also early dissatisfaction with the achieved range of movement of 90°.

The introduction of the Total Condylar prosthesis proved to be a very successful design and was a landmark development. Insall's group ascribed its improved outcome to better operative technique, improved fixation and the ability to resurface the patella. This prosthesis is still regarded by some as the contemporary gold standard (Insall et al 1976, 1982).

GREAT CRUCIATE DEBATE

In 1971 the posterior cruciate-retaining Geometric prosthesis was introduced by a multicentre group led by Mark Coventry of the Mayo Clinic. It proved very useful but failed relatively early mainly because of inbuilt constraint and poor tibial fixation. In 1972 Waugh and Marmor introduced their four-part cruciate condylar prosthesis but the problem of correctly implanting four different components led to difficulties. It was to prove of more value as a unicompartmental device.

Retention of the anterior cruciate ligament created a tibial plateau design problem and furthermore it was often absent or attenuated in advanced arthritis. Those who argued in favour of cruciate retention generally addressed their arguments to the isolated posterior cruciate ligament claiming that it attenuated major shearing stresses across the joint and also allowed retention of a degree of proprioception. Most importantly it was considered the essential structure in initiating posterior movement or roll back of the femoral component across the tibia during flexion and by so doing improved the range of knee flexion.

This 'biological' concept was thought to reproduce natural knee kinematics, but it was soon realised that if roll back did occur in combination with a posteriorly dished tibial surface there was a risk of impingement between the femoral component and the back of the tibial component. Insall referred to this as 'kinematic conflict' (Fig. 3.1) and it led to the use of flat plastic inserts in cruciate-preserving designs. Stability was achieved by the ligaments alone and constraint by design was minimised.

Several prostheses were designed in this way. One of the most popular was the two-part Kinematic knee introduced in Boston in 1978 by Walker, Sledge and Ewald. The Press Fit Condylar (PFC) prosthesis developed by Scott and Thornhill and the Genesis knee by Rand at the Mayo Clinic were similar widely used designs. The curved femoral surface of these devices articulated against a flat tibial surface reducing constraint, but the low contact area between the two generated high stresses.

In 1978 Insall and Burstein produced the first posterior stabilised knee joint by modifying a more constrained version of the Total Condylar devised earlier by Insall and Walker. A central spine on the tibial component engaged with a transverse cam on the femoral component at 70° of flexion. This arrangement conferred anteroposterior stability and guided the femur mechanically across the tibia to produce roll back (Fig. 3.2). Immediate concern was voiced about the degree of constraint within this system. However the resultant vector of forces was directed along the line of

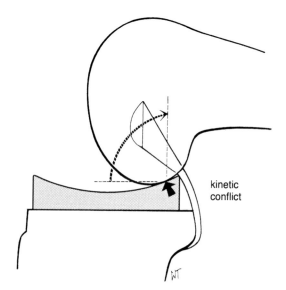

Fig. 3.1 Kinematic conflict occurs if concepts are mismatched. In this case the posterior cruciate ligament is preserved, using a dished tibial component. Impingement occurs posteriorly with flexion; from Insall et al (1993)

the tibial spine explaining why the increased constraint of the arthroplasty did not invoke increased loosening.

As it became possible to conserve, sacrifice or substitute for the posterior cruciate ligament arguments developed about which was preferable and these continue today. Contemporary outcome studies of prostheses employing these various techniques show no significant difference between them either in terms of longevity or function. No evidence has accumulated to suggest that the increased constraint present in the cruciate-sacrificing devices has given rise to increased rates of loosening nor that the preservation of the cruciate ligament has improved the function of the knee.

On a more scientific basis work by Goodfellow and O'Connor in 1977 confirmed that the cruciate ligaments worked together as a four-bar linkage system and when one was sacrificed this mechanism became ineffective. Recent fluoroscopic studies by Stiehl and Komistek and others have demonstrated that the isolated posterior cruciate ligament does not function in a predictable way and sometimes produces 'roll forward' rather than 'roll back'.

The initial arguments about the need to preserve the cruciate ligament are much less convincing now than when initially suggested almost thirty years ago.

SOFT TISSUE PATHOLOGY

In 1977 Freeman et al first drew attention to the fact that the soft tissue pathology around an arthritic joint

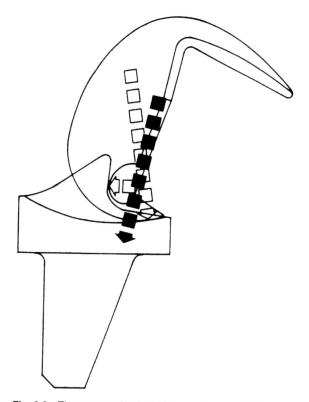

Fig. 3.2 The cam mechanism of the posterior stabilised knee stimulates the function of the posterior cruciate ligament and causes a roll back of the femur on the tibia with flexion. The resulting vector of forces passes distally through the fixation peg; from Insall et al (1982)

was of great importance. As a result of erosion of the articular cartilage the ligaments are relatively lengthened and slack. The use of a spacer in the form of a total knee replacement could be used to jack out the stretched ligaments and restore their normal length (Fig. 3.3).

In the event of one of these structures being contracted Insall in 1979 described an extensive soft tissue release of the contracted ligament on the concave side of the joint. In the case of a fixed varus deformity release of the soft tissues from the upper medial tibial metaphysis was necessary (Fig. 3.4) whilst a sequential lateral soft tissue release was described for a fixed valgus deformity.

Initial fears that surgical release of the soft tissues in this manner may create instability were unfounded and it came as a revelation to many surgeons that such extensive soft tissue surgery enabled them to restore soft tissue balance around the knee whilst also maintaining stability of the joint.

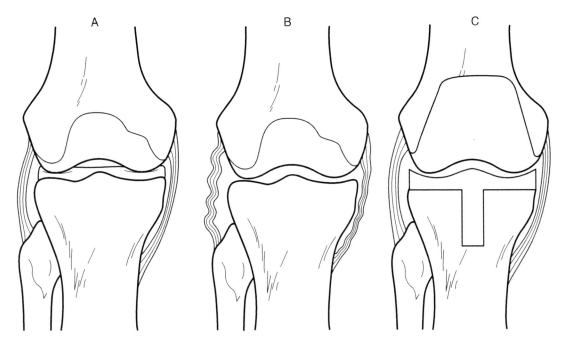

Fig. 3.3 (A) Normal joint. (B) Symmetrical erosion of the articular cartilage, laxity of both ligaments. (C) Spacer effect of knee prosthesis with restoration of ligament length

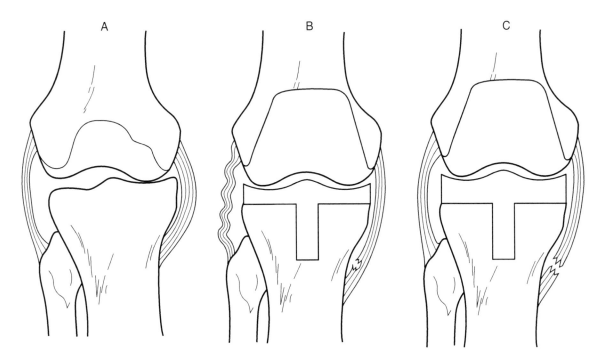

Fig. 3.4 (A) Varus deformity with contracted medial ligament and lengthening lateral ligament. (B) Knee remains unbalanced because the medial structures were incompletely released and the lateral ligament remains lax. (C) The medial structures are adequately released allowing insertion of a thicker spacer to tense the slack lateral ligament

ACHIEVING OPTIMAL ALIGNMENT

In 1972 Lanz and Wachsmuth introduced the concept of the mechanical axis of the limb. This was defined as a line connecting the centre of the hip to the centre of the ankle which normally intersects the intermediate one-third of the knee (Fig. 3.5). This was not the line of weightbearing

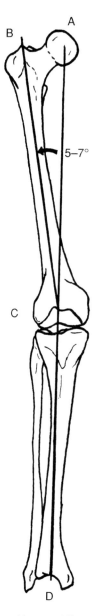

Fig. 3.5 When alignment is normal the mechanical axis (ACD) passes through the intermediate one-third of the knee. The upper limb of the anatomical axis (BC) subtends an angle 5–7° at the knee. The distal limb (CD) is common to both axis.

but represented ideal leg alignment ensuring optimal distribution of loading across the knee. The literature has attested to the importance of the restoration of optimal axial alignment in relation to longevity of the prosthesis.

In most patients the mechanical axis was found to subtend 5–7° with the line of the femoral shaft (anatomical axis). The operative introduction of femoral intramedullary rods linked to an appropriate jig allowed the surgeon to cut the distal femur at this measured angle. In combination with a 90° cut on the proximal tibia optimal limb, alignment could be restored by this so-called 'classical technique'.

The alternative 'anatomic technique' acknowledged the normal varus inclination of the tibia and achieved optimal alignment by cutting the tibia in 3° of varus and balancing this with a more valgus cut of 10° on the femur. There was little leeway for error and even 5° of tibial varus was recognised as a significant factor in increasing the risk of failure. Most surgeons adhered to the classical technique finding it technically easier and more accurate to cut at 90° to the axis of the tibia (Fig. 3.6).

The restoration of a stable knee in both extension and flexion and an optimally aligned limb with balanced soft tissues around the joint allowed the surgeon to deal with severe knee deformities using unlinked condylar replacements. It also obviated the obligatory use of hinged devices to address such problems.

Increasing emphasis on the technique of implantation led to the adoption of a greater degree of surgical sophistication with the development of a plethora of instruments designed to assist the surgeon to achieve optimal bone cuts, soft tissue balance and optimal alignment.

It became recognised that implanting the femoral component in 3° external rotation not only allowed femoral adjustment to the normal 3° varus slope of the tibia, but it also reduced the 'quadriceps angle' allowing better tracking of the extensor mechanism.

Two basic sequences of bone resection emerged. The 'gap technique', which depended upon the creation of equal bone gaps in flexion and extension, and the 'measured bone resection technique'. The essential difference between them related to the method by which external rotation of the femoral component was achieved and also of determining the thickness of the posterior condylar cuts.

EVALUATION OF TOTAL KNEE REPLACEMENT

It became increasingly evident that it was impossible to compare the results of different knee replacements without the application of standardised knee function rating systems before and after surgery. These evolved to

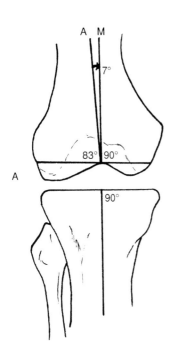
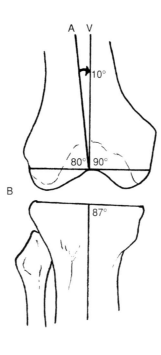

Fig. 3.6 (A) Classical technique of bone resection: 7° distal femoral cut, 90° proximal tibial cut. Joint line perpendicular to mechanical axis. (B) Anatomical technique of bone resection: 10° distal femoral cut, 3° varus proximal tibial cut. Joint line perpendicular to vertical axis.

separate the function of the knee itself from the overall function of the patient, which could be influenced by factors remote from the knee.

In 1982 Tew and Waugh described a method of analysing the results which made it possible to estimate the annual failure rate and to predict the proportion of implants that would survive successfully for a given number of years.

Whilst it is now clear that the result of knee replacement is highly dependent on technique, comparative analyses have afforded an opportunity of establishing criteriae against which individual prostheses could be matched before being accepted into widespread practice. It is hoped that such evidence based comparison will help both clinician and manager to select the best prosthesis from the enormous number available on the market.

Further progress has been made in establishing the value of the procedure with the introduction of outcome studies. These allow a subjective contribution by the patient in addition to standard objective assessments and have confirmed the symptomatic, functional and economic value of the operation even in the very elderly.

PROBLEM OF POLYETHYLENE WEAR

Evidence that the biological response to wear debris could cause osteolysis and loosening gave grounds for concern about failure of total knee arthroplasty due to long-term wear.

In 1992 Engh reported a disturbing incidence of wear and delamination in 51% of retrieved polyethylene inserts from posterior cruciate ligament retaining prostheses. The observed degree of change was related not only to the length of time for which the inserts had been implanted, but also to the lack of congruence between the articulating surfaces which generated stresses in polyethylene known to exceed its yield strength (Fig. 3.7).

The use of thin or heat-pressed polyethylene was also recognised as a cause of wear despite the fact that as early as 1976 Marmor had pointed out that 6 mm plastic inserts were insufficiently thick and had abandoned their use at that time. Later Bartel confirmed that the contact stresses within polyethylene increased as the thickness decreased and that they increased exponentially for thicknesses less than 6 mm.

The resurgence of thin polyethylene inserts had arisen as a result of a philosophy demanding more conservative resection of tibial bone in order to retain stronger bony support for the component. This overemphasised concept together with the introduction of metal backing led to a commensurate reduction in the thickness of plastic inserts.

In his 1992 Editorial for the *British Journal of Bone and Joint Surgery* Goodfellow described the adoption of minimal constraint and thin plastic as 'one step forward

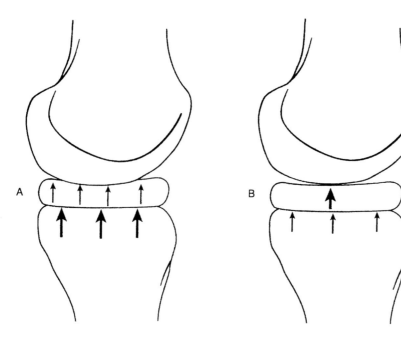

Fig. 3.7 (A) A greater contact area generates less stress in polyethylene and more at the cement interface. (B) A lesser contact area generates more stress in polyethylene and less at the cement interface

and two steps back'. Subsequently the use of thicker and more congruent inserts in PCL-retaining devices was adopted.

MOBILE BEARING KNEES

The concern about polyethylene wear and the general adoption of increased congruency encouraged the concept of mobile bearing knee replacements. In these devices the kinematics of the joint were separated into two systems. The tibial components were designed like menisci, with a flat inferior surface which slid across a flat metal tibial plate offering no constraint. At the articular surface the menisci were dished to increase congruency. Intact cruciate ligaments were an essential requisite to maintain the correct kinematics allowing the femur to move posteriorly in flexion. With a femoral component of single radius of curvature as in the Oxford unicompart-mental knee, this congruency was maintained throughout flexion. In other knees like the LCS (Low Contact Stress) design the radius of the femoral component decreased in flexion reducing the tibiofemoral contact at a time when the joint loading was maximum. However this feature also reduced the excursion of the menisci and the risk of posterior dislocation in flexion.

The LCS knee had dovetail grooves on the under-surface of the menisci which fitted reciprocal ridges on the baseplate to control the anteroposterior glide and further diminish the tendency to posterior meniscal displacement.

Recent information from combined anatomical and MRI studies confirms German studies carried out in the nineteenth century that roll back in the normal knee occurs only in the lateral compartment of the joint. The medial condyle does not translate but rotates around a fixed axis an observation which is now being addressed in some contemporary designs. It also gives credence to Stiehl's fluoroscopic findings that mobile bearing knees may also move in an unpredictable fashion.

There has been no evidence to date that mobile bearing knees generate better function or movement than fixed bearing knees. Postoperative movement is probably not determined by the type of knee prosthesis but more by the preoperative range of movement, the restoration of the joint line and size of the components.

The available ten-year results suggest that mobile bearing knees are at least as good as fixed bearing knees, but whether they will prove to be superior is speculative at present. Currently about 30% of all knee replace-ments are of the mobile bearing type.

METAL BACKING AND MODULARITY

Metal backing of the tibial component was first used clinically by Insall in 1979. In 1981 Riley, Ewald and Walker confirmed its beneficial effects using *in vivo* strain gauge analysis of tibial components showing that the bending stress on a plastic stem was ten times greater than on a metal stem. In 1982 Bartel et al using a combination of finite-element analysis and clinical studies demonstrated that the addition of a metal casing to the undersurface of the tibial component did reduce the stresses on the underlying cancellous bone.

There was some concern that stress shielding may occur as a result of bypassing the load, but this was not evident on ten-year follow up of these components.

The overall evidence has suggested that all plastic tibial components have been quite acceptable for the elderly group but that metal backing remains advantageous to the younger patient to reduce the stresses within the plastic and increase the longevity of the component. In general metal-backed components have continued to be used for all age groups despite being approximately 30% more expensive. The use of all plastic components in older patients could be an effective contribution to cost saving in a world-wide climate of financial constraint.

Metal backing also permitted the introduction of modularity with snap-in plastic inserts theoretically allowing easy exchange in the event of wear. In addition distal stem extenders, metal wedges and blocks became available principally for use in cases of revision. Knee prostheses were increasingly referred to as knee systems. They afforded the surgeon the luxury of knowing that the majority of problems of bone and ligament loss could be dealt with by making simple adjustments to the basic prosthesis.

This development may not be without consequences as there is current concern about fretting at the junctions of these components and of micromovement of the plastic insert within the metal backing possibly leading to increased wear.

FIXATION DEBATE

A further property of metal casing was the opportunity it afforded to obviate the need for tibial cement fixation by using it in either pressfit mode or with a porous coating. It was thought that this might have a particular application in younger and more active patients who were considered to be at risk of fatigue at the bone–cement interface. To be accepted any uncemented technique had to better the results of cemented arthroplasty.

The contemporary literature contains many reviews of different types of cemented condylar prosthesis demonstrating excellent long-term results with projected ten-year survival rates of 94% or more. Fewer series have detailed equally successful results following uncemented fixation.

Whiteside found that the uncemented Ortholoc knee had a survival rate equal to that of other cemented fixed bearing knees, and Beuchal presented similar results using a variety of mobile bearing joints. The best comparative clinical information available for fixed bearing devices derives from the prospective Leicester trial published in 1998 in which 139 patients were randomised to receive a cemented or uncemented Press Fit Condylar prosthesis. At five years follow up no differences were found in terms of longevity or function. The case for the routine use of the much more expensive coated devices was not supported by the results within this time scale.

Failure of uncemented devices has occurred most frequently on the tibial side persuading some surgeons to adopt a hybrid policy of cement fixation for the tibia alone. The advantages of this policy seem somewhat limited.

The excellent surgical outcome of knee prostheses led to the indications for replacement surgery being modified to include younger patients with knee pathology beyond the scope of other surgical procedures except arthrodesis.

A review from New York in 1998 by Diduch et al suggested that the outcome of cemented knee arthroplasty in the younger patient in the first eight years was at least comparable with that in older patients despite a return to significant activity levels by many of the patients. These excellent midterm results do little to strengthen the argument for uncemented replacements even in the young.

PATELLAR RESURFACING

The need to resurface the patella with polyethylene as part of a total knee arthroplasty continues to be keenly debated since the concept was introduced by Insall in 1979. In the early 1970s and 1980s reports from the USA suggested that a lack of resurfacing was responsible for residual anterior knee pain in 10–50% of cases. There was, and indeed still is, some difference of opinion on the precise significance of this as a clinical problem. Nevertheless it led the way to the addition of extended anterior femoral flanges and to the possibility of tricompartmental arthroplasty.

There was an unfortunate tendency to consider patellofemoral replacements in generic rather than specific terms. The individual design of the trochlear groove in particular and of the insert itself were fundamental to the behaviour of the patellofemoral mechanism. A significant incidence of complications was reported after patellar surfacing mainly relating to dislocation, fracture and wear. Redesign of the trochlear groove and a more anatomical patellar button with two facets helped to address some of these complications. More recently instrumentation has also been developed to optimise the amount of patellar bone which is resected.

The addition of metal backing of the patellar button, unlike the tibia, proved a generic failure because it reduced the thickness of the plastic, especially at the edges of the insert. Beyond 90° of flexion these areas are in contact with the femoral condyles and are subjected to maximum loads resulting in plastic wear and metallosis. Metal backing of the patella was consequently abandoned in most knee systems, one apparent exception being the rotating patellar mechanism of the LCS knee system.

Despite considerable revision in the design of the patellofemoral joint and modification of the surgical implantation of these inserts controlled trials have not demonstrated unequivocal evidence of an improved outcome to support the routine use of patellar resurfacing.

UNICOMPARTMENTAL REPLACEMENT

The possibility of selective compartmental replacement was based on the concept of the earlier tibial hemi-arthroplasty. It was a natural extension to attempt to replace the articular surface of the femoral condyle. Unicompartmental replacements were first introduced by Engelbrecht (1969), Insall and Walker (1972) and Marmor (1972) for use in unicompartmental osteoarthritis rather than inflammatory disease where the joint pathology is more widespread. Their subsequent evolution was accompanied by considerable disagreement. Early designs were criticised because the femoral runners were too narrow leading to excessive stresses in the polyethylene. Early failures due to the use of thin plastic combined with some unfavourable reports in the literature by Insall in 1976 and 1980 led to a reduction of enthusiasm for the procedure.

Unicompartmental prosthetic design also created difficulty for the surgeon because of the need to match up the femoral and tibial components through a full range of movement. Any malalignment led to edge loading and increased wear. For this reason they were designed with minimal congruency which unfortunately increased their potential for wear. Accelerated wear was further compounded with the Porous Coated Anatomic prosthesis in which heat-pressed polyethylene was used.

Another concern was that failure might occur as a result of the natural progression of degenerative change in the opposite compartment of the knee. Recent studies have suggested that this is not a major cause of failure.

More precisely defined indications for unicompartmental surgery to exclude those with fixed deformity, advanced disease or loss of a cruciate ligament coupled with improvements in prosthetic design have led to better results.

The results of various fixed bearing unicompartmental knee replacements have shown similar survival rates. The Swedish national multicentre series with a total of over two thousand unicompartmental joints had a projected 90% survival rate at six years. Scott et al from Boston had an 82% survival rate at ten years.

Comparison of the outcomes of unicompartmental and total knee replacement in the same patient suggested that after unicompartmental surgery the patient recovered faster and their knee felt better and had a greater range of movement.

The survivorship of these fixed bearing unicompartmental devices into the second decade has not been as good as total knee replacement and this raised some issues about the optimal age group best served by the procedure. This was compounded by some early suggestions that revising the unicompartmental prosthesis was often difficult due to the loss of bone, although the veracity of this argument is now questionable.

In 1998 the Oxford group (Murray et al) reported on the use of their medial compartment fully congruent mobile polyethylene bearing in 144 knees with a 98% ten-year survival rate comparing favourably with the best results of tricompartmental replacements.

During the period 1997–98 unicompartmental replacement represented only 1% of all knee arthroplasties carried out in the USA. Based on the potential number of patients for whom the procedure may have been appropriate, this percentage is considerably less than one would have expected if the operation was being widely used. Recent reports on its improved outcome the procedure has lead to it being more widely adopted by the international orthopaedic community.

REVISION KNEE SURGERY

Commensurate with the steadily increasing number of primary knee replacements carried out over the past twenty-five years the rate of revisional knee surgery has also increased adding to the financial and organisational demands on orthopaedic services.

Approximately 5–10% of all knee replacement operations are now revision procedures. The collective results in terms of pain relief, function and prosthetic longevity have been shown to be significantly poorer than after primary implantation. The results deteriorate with further revisional surgery. These findings have attested to the great importance for the need to optimise the result of primary replacement.

The most common mechanisms of failure of primary knee arthroplasty are mechanical or infective. Mechanical failure due to polyethylene wear may relate to its faulty production, storage, sterilization or design. Some of these factors have been modified over the years and there is now general acceptance that the technique of implantation is critical and that most failures can be ascribed to surgical errors rather than to the specific prosthesis.

Despite changes in prosthetic design, operating environments and the judicious use of antibiotics, failures still result from infection, the consequences of which are catastrophic for the patient and health economist alike. Significant predisposing factors to sepsis have been shown to include impaired wound healing, septic foci and rheumatoid arthritis.

The indications for revisional surgery have changed over the years. In the 1970s the most common reasons were for infection or loosening particularly of constrained devices. Recent reports from several North American authors showed that 50% of their revision cases were now due to complications of the extensor mechanism.

There is irrefutable evidence to show that it is axiomatic to establish the cause of failure before revisional surgery is undertaken. Without such knowledge a successful outcome is jeopardised and surgery should be avoided. The chance of an 'exploratory arthrotomy' being helpful under such circumstances is negligible and should be avoided.

In suspected infection isolation of the offending organism has been demonstrated to be essential to maximise the chance of ablating the sepsis.

Careful pre-operative planning of revision surgery has been increasingly emphasised. Selection of the optimal incision in relation to pre-existing scars in order to minimise the risk of skin necrosis is essential. Exposure has proven to be very difficult in the presence of a stiff knee with a tight extensor mechanism, leading to the introduction of additional soft tissue and bony surgery to avoid the extremely serious consequences of its disruption.

Assessment of the nature and degree of major bone loss was also shown to be critically important to allow the surgeon to ensure that the appropriate armamentarium was available at the time of surgery. Recent developments in the harvesting, storage, sterilisation and application of bone-grafting techniques combined with the availability of modular and custom-built knee systems have been major factors in allowing the implantion of knee prostheses in the absence of adequate supportive bone stock.

Contained bony defects have been dealt with effectively using morsellised autograft or allograft bone as confirmed by Whiteside and others.

Metallic wedges and blocks, or blocks of bonegraft have been used successfully to deal with uncontained bone defects depending on their size. Mankin and Gross were mainly responsible for establishing segmental allografting

as an effective method of dealing with very severe bone deficiencies resulting from tumour excision or failed joint replacement surgery. Optimal allograft fixation has been achieved by fashioning a step cut between the donor and recipient bone used in combination with a long-stemmed prosthetic component cemented into the allograft but not in the donor bone.

The comparative results of using segmental allografts as opposed to custom-built prostheses have not yet been clearly established.

Resetting the joint line to a near normal level to enhance the mechanics of the arthroplasty has been recognised as one of the principal aims of total knee replacement surgery. This has been particularly difficult to achieve in revision surgery due to bone and ligament deficiency. There was an initial tendency simply to fill an increased extension gap with a thicker tibial plastic insert resulting in a proximal shift of the joint line and the creation of a patellar baja which can limit flexion. The introduction of 5 or 10 mm-thick distal femoral metal blocks or 'add-ons' helped to address this problem to a degree by allowing the surgeon to shift the femoral component distally toward its original position.

It was also tempting for the surgeon to use a smaller femoral component to fit the diminished skeleton. The resulting reduction in prosthetic anteroposterior diameter increased the flexion gap and sometimes led to instability in flexion despite the use of stabilizer components. A larger ill-fitting femoral component was in danger of toggling and tilting increasing the risk of loosening. The introduction of modular posterior condylar metal add-ons enabled many such deficiencies to be readily filled improving the femoral fit.

Greater degrees of bone loss have demanded additional augmentation with bone graft or custom devices in order to maintain the joint line.

CONCLUSION

Whilst conceived last century, knee arthroplasty has developed essentially in the second half of the twentieth century. Its development was not a smooth, logically planned sequence first based on sound engineering and design principles followed by regulated surgical implantation. Unfortunately it was characterized by trial and error leading to frequent setbacks. It has been the actual process of developing an acceptable knee replacement which has continued to do much to teach the surgeon how the human knee works.

Major lessons have derived from the need to produce a prosthesis that not only reproduced the behaviour of the normal knee as closely as possible, but which also required minimal sacrifice of bone to allow its implantation. Its design features have demanded minimal constraint compatible with the generation of forces acceptable to its material structure. Its outcome has been highly dependent on the technique of implantation and the need to achieve periarticular soft tissue balance and an optimally aligned limb.

For most patients the present results of knee replacement are excellent, although it is prudent to bear in mind that most of the results of knee replacement surgery reported to date relate to the use of earlier nonmodular components.

Polyethylene wear has been a major determinant of prosthetic longevity. Future developments in material science, prosthetic design and a healthy recognition of previous experience may demonstrate that even further improvement in function and longevity may not necessarily be mutually exclusive.

REFERENCES

Freeman M A R, Sculco T, Todd R C 1977 The replacement of the severely damaged knee by the I.C.L.H. (Freeman–Swanson) arthroplasty. J Bone Joint Surg 59: 64

Gunston F H 1971 Polycentric knee arthroplasty. Prosthetic simulation of normal knee joint movements. J Bone Joint Surg 53: 272

Hawk A 1993 Recreating the Knee: The History of Knee Arthroplasty. Caduceus, Health Sciences Library, University of Maryland, Baltimore

Insall J N, Lachiewicz P F, Burstein A H 1982 The posterior stabilized condylar prosthesis: a modification of the total condylar design: two to four year follow up clinical experience. J Bone Joint Surg 64: 1317

Insall J N, Ranawat C S, Aglietti P, Shine J 1976 A comparison of four models of total knee replacement prostheses. J Bone Joint Surg 56: 754

Insall J N, Scott W N, Ranawat C S 1979 Total condylar knee prosthesis: a report of two hundred and twenty cases. J Bone Joint Surg 61: 173

Insall J N, Windsor, Scott W N, Kelly D, Aglietti P, 1993 Surgery of the Knee, 2nd edn. Churchill Livingstone, Edinburgh

Murray D W, Goodfellow J W, O'Connor J J 1998 The Oxford medial unicompartmental arthroplasty. A ten year survival study. J Bone Joint Surg 80: 983

Walldius B 1957 Arthroplasty of the knee joint using an endoprosthesis. Acta Orthop Scand 24 (suppl.): 19

4

Arthroscopy and arthroscopic surgery

Robert W. Jackson

There have been dramatic changes in orthopaedic surgery in the past century. Tuberculosis and poliomyelitis have virtually been eliminated, thus relegating to history many of the operations that were commonplace fifty years ago. New techniques have replaced the muscle transfers and arthrodeses that marked the old era. Arthroscopic surgery along with joint replacement and the open reduction and internal fixation of fractures are probably the most important developments that have truly revolutionised orthopaedic surgery and dramatically improved the quality of life.

HISTORY OF ARTHROSCOPY

Arthroscopy is an offshoot of cystoscopy, which had its beginning in 1806 when Bozzini invented the first endoscopic device specifically designed to look inside the bladder (National Museum for the History of Science 1973). Other notable contributors to the field of cystoscopy included Désormeaux with his 'gazogene endoscope' in 1853 (National Museum for the History of Science 1973), Leiter and Nitze in Germany who presented their cystoscope to the Vienna Medical Society in 1879, and Thomas Edison who invented the incandescent lamp in 1880. From that point cystoscopy gradually, but slowly, developed as a surgical science.

In 1910, H. C. Jacobaeus, a Swedish surgeon, developed an endoscopic device to look inside the abdomen and the thorax and became the pioneer of endoscopic surgery. He used the device to operate inside the pleural cavity by resecting adhesions under direct vision. The technique was advantageous in the pneumothorax treatment of tuberculosis, as adhesions often prevented the full collapse of a lung. The success of Jacobaeus's thoracoscope led other pioneers such as Severin Nordentoft to apply similar techniques to other body cavities.

In 1912, Nordentoft from Aarhus in Denmark, who was primarily a radiologist and radiotherapist, described an instrument that he and his brother designed that could be applied to the abdomen, the bladder and to the knee joint. His description of the anatomical structures seen within the knee, as presented in a paper given at a conference of surgeons in Berlin, leaves no doubt that Nordentoft was the first to insert an endoscopic device into the knee joint (Nordentoft 1912). His work was done on cadavers and there is no record of his having used it on living patients.

Before this recent discovery of Nordentoft's work in the German literature, it was generally considered that Professor Kenji Takagi of Tokyo University was the initial pioneer in knee endoscopy. He is reported to have applied a cystoscope to a knee joint in 1918 in an effort to identify tuberculous knees early in the disease process and thus to prevent the serious complication of ankylosis, which made squatting and kneeling ultimately impossible. This work, however, did not come to light until his first presentation on the subject in 1933 to the Japanese Orthopaedic Association.

The first clinical publication on the subject of arthroscopy is credited to Eugen Bircher from Switzerland. His paper of 1921 described the use of a Jacobaeus laparoscope in the knee joint. However, the instrument was not really suitable for the knee joint as there was a 90° side-viewing optic, and a considerable amount of dead space between the tip of the instrument and the lens. Records show that Bircher performed only seventy arthroscopy procedures, and after 1930 there is no further mention of the procedure in the reports of the hospital at which he worked (Kieser 1999). At this time Bircher was also studying the use of contrast media for arthrography, and subsequently developed the double arthrographic contrast technique in 1930.

Although it has not been directly confirmed, it is possible that Bircher and the American pioneer Michael Burman compared notes at meetings in Berlin in 1930 as Burman was doing a fellowship in Germany at that time. Burman's fellowship was in Dresden at the Institute of Pathology under Professor Schmorl, where he studied the joints of cadavers using an arthroscope. In 1933, at a meeting of the German Society of Surgery in Berlin, Bircher commented on his frustrations and why he gave up on arthroscopy and mentioned that Burman's technique might bring better results (Kieser 1999). Reinhold Wappler in New York, the founder of the company called American Cystoscope Makers Incorporate (ACMI), built the first forward oblique-viewing system for a urologist named McCarthy in 1923. Subsequently, Burman's first paper on arthroscopy, written in New York in 1931, described his experience with the 25° forward oblique-altered cystoscope produced by Wappler. However, Burman's ideas were not accepted by his colleagues and although he wrote an 'Atlas' of arthroscopy he could not find an editor or publisher. A copy of the unpublished manuscript is in the archives of the Arthroscopy Association of North America (AANA).

Special mention must also be made of Philip Kreuscher, who preceded Burman by publishing in 1925 the first paper in English. This was a plea for the early diagnosis of semilunar cartilage disease by arthroscopy in the *Illinois Medical Journal*. Unfortunately, to date, there is little information about his arthroscope or what motivated Kreuscher. It appears likely, however, that he was influenced by an associate in general surgery who was aware of the work of Jacobaeus.

Kenji Takagi presented his first paper on arthroscopy at the Japanese Orthopaedic Association annual meeting in 1933. He commented that his first efforts at arthroscopy occurred in 1918, but he waited until he had developed an effective instrument before publishing the technique. Takagi's endoscope was rebuilt from a cystoscope and had a 60° forward oblique optic.

Other European arthroscopists who published on arthroscopy were Dr R. Sommer, a trauma surgeon (1937); Dr Ernest Vaubel, a rheumatologist from Frankfurt (1938); and Dr K. H. Wilcke, a surgical intern at the University Hospital in Berlin (1939). Also of interest is the fact that Vaubel travelled from Europe in the early 1930s to do a fellowship in tissue culture at the Rockefeller Institute in New York. Apparently, he did not meet Burman, neither did he know about his work as he did not visit the Hospital for Joint Diseases. On Vaubel's return to Europe, he performed at the Leipzig University Hospital his first arthroscopies and in 1938 published a sixty-four-page monograph on arthroscopy. This is probably the first book on the topic in the world literature.

It was based on twenty-two rheumatological cases and dealt solely with the changes of synovial membranes and articular surfaces seen in rheumatoid arthritis.

When the Second World War started in 1939 all activity in this area was halted. Twenty years later, in 1959, Dr R. Suckert, using a Wolf arthroscope, reported on eighty arthroscopies at a Swiss trauma surgeon's meeting in a paper entitled 'Photo arthroscopy of the knee joint' (Suckert 1960).

Back in Japan, the 'father' of modern arthroscopy, Dr Masaki Watanabe (Fig. 4.1) was diligently working with the Takei Medical Optical Instrument manufacturers, consecutively developing the Number 19 arthroscope, the Number 21 arthroscope (which became the first production arthroscope) (Fig. 4.2), the Number 22 arthroscope (with fibre light), and the Number 24 arthroscope (the precursor to the needlescope – 1.7 mm diameter).

In 1957, Watanabe obtained a permit to travel from Japan to the SICOT (Societé Internationale de Chirurgie Orthopédique et de Traumatologie) Congress in Barcelona. He subsequently visited several centres in Europe and North America armed with a motion film on arthroscopy and the first edition of his *Atlas of Arthroscopy*, which was beautifully illustrated by an artist named Fujihashi and co-authored by Watanabe's colleagues Drs H. Ikeuchi and S. Takeda.

In the late 1950s and early 1960s, significant advances in optics and light transmission occurred. While there is some question as to the originator of fibre light, Karl Storz in 1960 produced a 'cold lamp' with the light transmitted through flexible optical fibres. It is also on record that in 1954 French optical engineers produced a bronchoscope

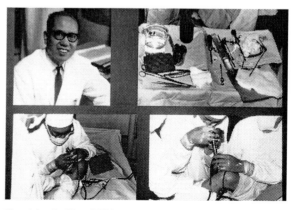

Fig. 4.1   Dr Masaki Watanabe (1921–94), the true 'father of arthroscopy'. He is shown in his office (upper left), at the back table during surgery (upper right) and during an arthroscopic procedure done in 1964 using the Number 19 arthroscope (lower)

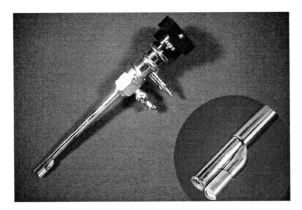

Fig. 4.2 Watanabe Number 21 arthroscope, which became the first production model. Note the offset light bulb and the straight-ahead optics, with a field of vision of 102° in saline solution and a depth of focus from 1 mm to infinity

with an external high-intensity light source that conducted the light to the tip of the bronchoscope by a quartz rod. This probably was the first external light source, but as quartz rods were difficult to work with, glass-fibre illumination became the method of choice for illuminating a field (Kieser 1999).

The rod lens system was developed by the English physicist Harold Hopkins in 1959 (Hopkins 1978). Storz recognised the importance of this system and joined forces with Hopkins in 1967 to develop some spectacular new cystoscopes that combined fibre light with the rod lens optical system. However it was several years before Storz commenced the manufacture of true arthroscopes.

REAWAKENING OF THE WESTERN WORLD

In 1964, R. W. Jackson from the University of Toronto went to Japan on a scholarship, primarily to study tissue culture techniques at the University of Tokyo. Before leaving Canada, his mentor, Dr Ian Macnab, mentioned that there was a doctor in Japan who had talked about arthroscopy in 1957 at the SICOT meeting in Barcelona, but he could not remember his name or where he was from. On his arrival Jackson tried to find the doctor who was virtually unknown, even in his own country. Eventually contact was made, and during many subsequent visits to the Tokyo Teishin Hospital to observe Watanabe and his technique of arthroscopy, Jackson learned the technique and in return tried to teach Watanabe conversational English.

On Jackson's return to Canada with a Number 21 arthroscope, which was a gift from Watanabe, he

continued the work and gave his first presentation on the subject at the inaugural meeting of the Association of Academic Surgeons, which was held in Toronto in 1967. It was also in that year that Drs Ward Casscells, Jack McGinty and John Joyce made individual trips to Toronto out of interest to learn the technique (Jackson 1987).

In 1968, Dr Leonard Peltier at the University of Kansas ordered and received directly from Japan the first Number 21 Watanabe arthroscope. However, the supply and repair of the arthroscopes was difficult. Problems frequently occurred in the early days including inadvertent autoclaving for sterilisation, which would ruin the lens seal and melt the insulation on the electrical cords. Great delays would then be encountered in trying to get replacement parts from Japan as the production of Number 21 scopes was limited to about twenty-five a month, with each lens being hand ground by technicians.

In 1969, Dr Dick O'Connor visited Watanabe and on his return worked with the Richard Wolf Corporation of Rosemont, Illinois, to develop instrumentation for arthroscopic surgery (O'Connor 1977). The Wolf diagnostic arthroscope also used fibre light and became the early standard, along with modified Storz cystoscopes, that were adapted for arthroscopy. O'Connor also developed the first operating arthroscope (Fig. 4.3).

In 1972, Dr Lanny Johnson, working with Dyonics Corporation, introduced the 'needle scope', which was a modification of Watanabe's Number 24 (Johnson 1977). In subsequent years, many arthroscopes and new instruments were introduced to the marketplace and arthroscopy rapidly changed from a diagnostic to a surgical subspecialty.

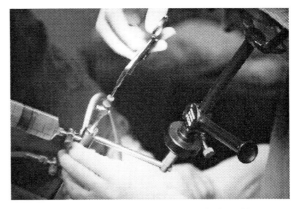

Fig. 4.3 The first operating arthroscope designed by Dr Richard O'Connor and built by the Wolf Corporation of Rosemont, Illinois. It featured an offset eyepiece and a long operating channel through which torn meniscal fragments could be resected under direct vision

ARTIFACTS

Most of the early arthroscopes were modified cystoscopes. Takagi used a Charrière Number 22 cystoscope to examine knees first. Bircher used a Jacobaeus laparoscope. Kreuscher in 1925 called his instrument an 'arthroscope', but it was most likely a small cystoscope that he used in the knee. Takagi, however, began to develop instruments especially for the knee, some as large as 7 mm in diameter, others as small as 3 mm. Originally the interior views were obtained by looking directly down a tube. Lenses were then added to magnify the scene. One of the major advances came from the Zeiss Corporation, with the invention of the Amici prism, which turned the inverted lens image right side up. As mentioned, the development of the incandescent bulb was a major breakthrough, which was soon followed by the advent of fibre light (known as cold light). The next advance was the rod lens system (Hopkins 1978). More recent advances have included zooming of the image to enlarge and focus on specific pathologies.

Most modern arthroscopes are now about 4 mm in diameter and are suitable for use in major joints, with smaller arthroscopes available for smaller joints.

The first instruments to be used for arthroscopic surgery were biopsy forceps, which permitted a patch of synovium to be selected under direct vision and removed for histological examination. In the early days, rheumatologists had a definite interest in arthroscopy, as evidenced by the work of Jason and Dixon in Britain (1968) and Robles-Gil and Katona in Mexico (1972). However, the rheumatologists' ability to progress in this field was limited as they did not have easy access to operating rooms. Also, as the science of arthroscopy expanded and the number of procedures became more complex, the potential for instrument breakage and other complications increased. Consequently, rheumatologists tended to leave even the biopsies to their surgical colleagues.

One of the important developments was the hook probe, which is now commonly used to explore the interior of a joint. Originally, crochet hooks and harpoon tips were used for this purpose, but they would catch on the tissues making it difficult to remove them. Other innovations such as flat or diamond-shaped tips at the end of probes were developed, whereby the instrument would be inserted under the meniscus and turned 90°, thus elevating the meniscus and allowing the inferior surface to be examined. Eventually the neurosurgical nerve hook was adapted as the arthroscopic probe, and this has proven to be a most useful instrument.

The first true arthroscopic surgical procedure on record was performed by Watanabe in 1957 and consisted of the removal of a synovial tumour through a separate sheath. In 1961, he removed a loose body from a joint, and in 1962 performed the first partial meniscectomy.

The concept of 'triangulation', whereby visualisation was through one portal and an operating tool was introduced through a second portal to do the surgery, was another important development (Fig. 4.4).

Miniature scissors were developed, originally with straight cutting edges but eventually with a hooked cutting tip, that would grasp the tissues and prevent them from squirting away as the scissors were closed. One early surgical tool called a 'basket' forceps was adapted from cystoscopic surgery where every bit of tissue removed from the prostate had to be preserved for histological examination. Therefore, these instruments had wire baskets in the lower jaw of the cutting mechanism to collect the tissue fragments. The basket concept, however, proved disadvantageous in arthroscopy as the wires would break and, when debriding large amounts of articular cartilage, it was a nuisance to take the arthroscope out of the joint to empty the basket after each bite. It became a common technique to let the fragments float free, then flush them out of the joint or extract them using suction from the joint at the end of the procedure. Other types of cutting forceps were developed, some with shovel noses to go underneath a meniscus, some with blunt tips, and others with tips angled to right or left or upward (Fig. 4.5). This variety of tips was necessary to reach the various lesions seen. Originally, these manual cutting tools had ring grips for thumb and finger, but it soon became obvious that the flexing of all the fingers of the hand was an ergonomically more effective method of using the instruments. Consequently handgrips were developed. Retractable knife blades, backward-cutting instruments and retrograde knives were also developed.

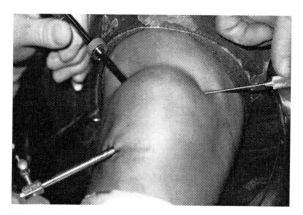

Fig. 4.4 The technique of triangulation whereby visualisation was through one portal and operative tools were introduced through a second portal

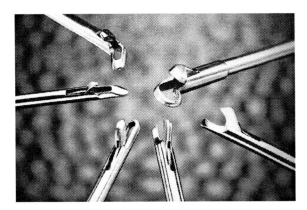

Fig. 4.5 A variety of tips of manual instruments showing hook scissors, shovelled nose basket forceps, blunt nose basket forceps and various angled tips

In the mid-1970s Dyonics Corporation developed the first rotating suction shaver. Shaving of the patella then became a fairly routine procedure. Following the shavers, burrs of various types and shapes were developed to remove osteophytes, to widen the intercondylar notch and to debride the undersurface of the acromion.

Breakage of instruments was a significant problem in the beginning and accounted for 18% of all complications in the first report on the subject of complications by the AANA (Sprague 1989). The instrument designers, however, soon solved that problem and now breakage is no longer considered a significant worry.

In recent years new energy sources have been explored. The Holmium Yag 2:1 laser, which has a small depth of penetration and can be used in saline, has become the laser of choice (Brillhart 1995). Also, more recently, heat-producing units such as bipolar radiofrequency devices capable of producing temperatures of 65°C are used to shrink collagen or ablate tissues at higher settings.

IMPROVEMENT OF TECHNIQUE

Fear of contamination was one of the early worries and sterilisation of the instrumentation was a problem as the early arthroscope could not be autoclaved. The Watanabe Number 21 arthroscope was originally sterilised in formalin vapour. Later the electrical and optical equipment was sterilised by soaking in cidex. Eventually, ethylene oxide gas sterilisation on an overnight cycle was considered the best way to sterilise this equipment. It therefore became necessary to have more than one set of instruments in the operating room to do back-to-back cases. Fear of contaminating the eyepiece was also a common early concern and sterile masks and hoods were often worn by the operating surgeons.

Eventually, television was developed and this was another major advance. The first black-and-white television images were achieved in 1968, and by 1974 live video presentations were being presented at conferences and videotapes started to appear in instructional courses. Coloured television was a further advance and by miniaturising the camera and placing some of the electronic components in a box away from the operating field cameras became small enough to be attached directly to the arthroscope. Apart from the advantage of better sterility and less chance for facial or eye contamination, television provided the opportunity for all of the operating room team to be involved in the procedure. A major level of quality control was now provided as everyone in the operating room could witness what was being done. The use of television also eliminated the necessity to kneel or crouch down to look into the suprapatellar region and soon many surgeons were operating by sitting in a comfortable position, with the television monitor at eye level. New stereotactic skills had to be developed as the surgeon was actually working off the monitor and not looking directly into the joint.

Some basic principles were involved in the arthroscopic examination of any joint. Distraction of the joint as much as possible, a good flow of physiological saline or Ringer's solution to keep the field clear and sometimes an increase in pressure produced by a pump to stop minor bleeding became the mainstays of technique. Tourniquets were used where possible, but they have proven to be less necessary as pumps were developed that controlled pressure and flow. Leg holders around the thigh enabled varus or valgus strains to be applied, thus opening the knee compartments slightly for better visualisation.

Complications did occur with infection, thromboembolism, haemarthrosis, instrument failure and vascular or neurologic injury being seen occasionally. However, the overall complication rate in a multicentre study was less than 2% (Sprague 1989).

Early concerns about infection and anaesthesia delayed the use of the technique as an outpatient procedure. Eventually, however, outpatient procedures became common as the incidence of infection was virtually nil and as local anaesthesia proved adequate in many cases. Soon, it was realised that both knees could be arthroscoped at the same sitting and under the same light general anaesthetic. Outpatient procedures soon became customary and rapidly led to arthroscopies being done in an 'office' setting, i.e. a sterile room attached to the office. Anaesthesia has ranged from general to regional to local, and has usually depended on circumstances such as the patient's apprehension and the surgeon's skill.

TEACHING OF ARTHROSCOPY

As the technique of arthroscopy became more sophisticated, it became necessary to have courses to teach the newer techniques and the concepts and principles of the science. The first instructional course at the Academy of Orthopaedic Surgeons annual meeting was given by Jackson in 1970. By the mid-1970s the AANA and several universities were holding annual courses. Skilled individuals would also arrange a faculty and hold private courses with some of the prominent teachers being: Dr Robert Metcalf in Salt Lake City, USA; Dr Theo van Rens in Nijmegen, The Netherlands; and David Dandy in Cambridge, UK.

Before the advent of television, teaching attachments enabled one student at a time to observe a procedure (Fig. 4.6) and rubber or plastic models were used to practice new stereotactic skills.

Slides of pathology, taken with 35-mm cameras, were originally used for teaching presentations. Soon videotapes became the standard for teaching. Cadaver courses became common actually to demonstrate procedures, and an expert would be televised doing a procedure on a cadaver. Then courses were arranged whereby the participants would themselves perform procedures on cadaver parts (Fig. 4.7).

Although the Japanese had an arthroscopy journal for many years, it was not until 1985 that the AANA developed its own journal called *Arthroscopy and Related Surgery*. It has grown rapidly and is now one of the major journals in the world literature. The AANA also produced a video journal that had a short life of three years in the early 1990s. The cost of production was not met by demand as everybody had their own television cameras at this stage.

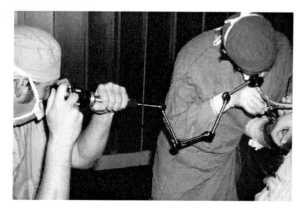

Fig. 4.6 A flexible teaching attachment made by Karl Storz with prisms at each joint enabled the student to watch the operation and take 35-mm single-lens reflex pictures of the procedure

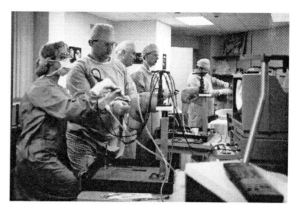

Fig. 4.7 A typical cadaver course with students practising the techniques of meniscal repair, anterior crucial ligament reconstruction, etc. on cadaver knees

In terms of the printed book, the first *Atlas of Arthroscopy* was published in 1957 by Watanabe, Ikeuchi and Takeda. The third edition of the *Atlas* is beautifully illustrated with actual photographs as well as artistic renderings. The first textbook on the subject of arthroscopy in the English language was a small monograph of 1976 by Jackson and Dandy. Since then, there has been a proliferation of books on operative arthroscopy of the ankle, shoulder, elbow, etc., each adding something to the wealth of knowledge about this new technique.

ORGANISATIONS INVOLVED IN THE DEVELOPMENT OF ARTHROSCOPY

In 1972, the first course in arthroscopy was held in Philadelphia, organised by Dr John Joyce III. In 1974, a second course was held in Philadelphia, and at that time the International Arthroscopy Association (IAA) was formed, with Dr Masaki Watanabe being elected as President, Dr Robert Jackson as Vice-President and Dr Ward Casscells as Secretary. Dr Richard O'Connor was the Treasurer and Dr John Joyce was the named President of the North American Chapter of the IAA.

The first meeting of the IAA was held in 1975 in Copenhagen in conjunction with SICOT (Societé Internationale de Chirurgie Orthopédique et de Traumatologie). It was the organising committee's thought that each country should have its own organisation, and that once every three years in conjunction with SICOT the best papers from each country would be presented. It was thought that the plan would create a type of competition, which would lead to the more rapid development of arthroscopy as a surgical specialty. The meeting in Copenhagen was exciting with about forty participants from all over the world.

One of the most memorable aspects of the meeting concerned the Treasurer, Richard O'Connor. He had been thinking for some time that gold was safer than paper money. He consequently took the dues obtained from the seventy founding members of the IAA and converted them into gold coins, which he purchased illegally. At that time the price of gold worldwide was $40.00 per ounce and was tightly controlled by the US mint. It was actually illegal to own or buy gold privately. Somehow, O'Connor managed to obtain gold from elsewhere, mostly Krugerrands from South Africa. He carried these coins in a money belt, adding many pounds to his body weight. Following the meeting, he spent two weeks in a secluded seaside villa, wrote his textbook on arthroscopy (O'Connor 1977) and then went to Zurich, Switzerland, where he opened a numbered Swiss bank account and deposited the gold. That was April 1975. Just eight months later, in December, government control over the price of gold was lifted and its price rose rapidly from $40.00 to over $300.00 per ounce. Over the next two years the value continued to rise and the IAA executive finally sold the gold at about $700.00 an ounce and made a significant profit of more than $60 000. With this money the IAA was able to hire a professional executive director who established the Association on a business-like basis and assured that membership dues were paid, meetings were properly organised and so on.

New chapters then began to develop in countries like Brazil, India and Australia. Any country that had ten or more members could become a chapter of the IAA. The second IAA meeting combined with SICOT was held in 1978 in Kyoto, Japan, where Watanabe was a magnificent host. The third meeting, with almost two hundred members in attendance, was in Rio de Janeiro in Brazil in 1981. At that meeting the first Dr John Joyce Awards were given for the best research and clinical papers. Again, the awards were a further stimulation for young people in the field of arthroscopy.

Owing to the rapid growth of the IAA, it was proposed to hold meetings more frequently and to align the organisation with the International Knee Society (IKS), which also had formed in the early 1970s. Although some arthroscopic explorations of shoulder and elbow were being done, arthroscopy at that time was primarily focused on the knee. IAA meetings, therefore, were changed and held every two years to coincide with the IKS meetings. At first the IAA meeting was held in the same place, either before or just after the IKS meeting. However, by 1984 combined meetings were arranged so that arthroscopic topics were interwoven with all knee topics.

In 1982, the American chapter of the IAA formally established itself as a separate legal entity, becoming the AANA and the annual meetings became more diverse. Shoulder problems assumed a major role in the meetings. Eventually, in 1993 the IKS, the IAA and the Sports Medicine Society were all merged into one organisation known as the International Society of Arthroscopy, Knee Surgery and Orthopaedic Sports Medicine (ISAKOS). At this point, arthroscopy was no longer considered a separate entity but generally was regarded as a useful adjunct in the management of most joint problems related to sports.

While all this activity was going on in North America, a similar amount of activity was occurring in Europe and the Far East. The European Society for Surgery of the Knee and Arthroscopy (ESSKA) was established in 1984. It served a useful purpose in bringing the European countries together in an organisation where their papers could be presented. A German-speaking Arthroscopy Association, consisting of German, Swiss and Austrian arthroscopists, was also established. The Japanese Arthroscopy Association continued to flourish, holding its own meetings, publishing a journal and reaching out to the countries of the Pacific rim.

EVOLUTION OF ARTHROSCOPIC SURGERY

In the early to mid-1980s the concept of arthroscopy changed from a purely diagnostic mode to a diagnostic and surgical mode, and in the mid-1990s this changed again to a pure surgical mode. Almost every arthroscopic procedure now performed is done to correct some pathology or abnormality within a joint. The diagnostic aspects of joint pathology have largely been taken over by non-invasive techniques such as magnetic resonance imaging (MRI). Arthrography at one time was in competition with arthroscopy for diagnostic purposes. Soon it became obvious that arthrography, even good double-contrast arthrography, did not reveal the true state of the interior of the joint as well as a visual examination.

Although Watanabe and Ikeuchi did the first recorded partial meniscectomy in 1962, O'Connor must gain credit for the promotion of partial meniscectomy as an effective treatment method. Before his efforts the standard of care for torn menisci in the Western world demanded the total removal of the torn meniscus in order to permit the peripheral tissues to recreate a new meniscus. This was the teaching of Ian Smillie. To do less than a total meniscectomy, therefore, was almost tantamount to malpractice. O'Connor, however, on seeing small flaps of meniscus, would remove only the torn fragment, even though it was removed through a small arthrotomy incision. Later, using biopsy forceps and small scissors, these fragments were removed through arthroscopy portals. The results of the early partial meniscectomies were remarkable. The reduction in recovery time from several weeks to several days was hailed by the sporting world as one of the great advances in the century. It soon became obvious that it was not the torn meniscus that had previously required six to eight weeks of rehabilitation but that it was the arthrotomy incision that took time to heal, leading to the loss of muscle strength, reaction time and endurance. The removal of the loose meniscal fragments under arthroscopic control through two or three puncture wounds enabled the professional athlete to go back on the field within a week. This ability to treat athletes was both a boon and a bane to arthroscopy. The publicity gained through the professional athletes was a tremendous aid in establishing the credibility of the technique. However, many patients with arthritic knees would expect to be cured within days and would be upset when it did not happen.

The efficacy of partial meniscectomy was not only in the lessened morbidity and the earlier return to normal activity, but also in the much-reduced incidence of complications such as infection or deep vein thrombosis. Also, the midrange studies at ten to twelve years following partial meniscectomy showed a dramatic decrease in the amount of post-traumatic osteoarthritis (Schimmer et al 1998). While not perfect, the results of partial meniscectomy have been most gratifying. Other procedures in the knee such as patella shave and chondroplasty (removing loose and scaling articular cartilage fragments) have yet to be proven by long-term follow-up studies.

As early as 1985, an AANA course advertised the teaching of arthroscopic anterior cruciate ligament (ACL) reconstruction and shoulder stabilisation. Now much emphasis is on stabilisation techniques of lax capsules by reattaching them to the glenoid, shrinking them, decompressing tight areas and so on. Lesions of the ACL are currently diagnosed in large numbers by MRI techniques and by clinical awareness, and are being treated in almost every instance by an ACL reconstruction. The end results of these aggressive approaches to restoring normal joint kinematics is yet to be proven in the long-term. However, it shows tremendous potential as in most instances the end result is a normal joint.

Degenerative arthritis is also a condition that can be helped significantly by arthroscopic procedures. The benefits of lavage or the washing out of fragments of debris from the joint have been known and commented on since Bircher's day. The ability to smooth irregular surfaces and to remove loose fragments has made this an important adjunct in the treatment of the degenerative knee (Jackson 1998). Arthroscopy will become

even more important as we move on to biological resurfacing of these knees, using methods to promote the redevelopment and growth of articular cartilage. As the general population ages, minimally invasive techniques for treating arthritis will become even more important.

As a result of all of these procedures in knees and shoulders, arthroscopy has become the most commonly performed orthopaedic procedure. At Baylor University Medical Center in Dallas, Texas, for example, a hospital of about one thousand beds, there are more than five thousand arthroscopic procedures done each year. This amounts to one-fifth of all the surgical procedures performed in all the surgical specialties.

FROM THE PAST TO THE FUTURE

The initial response to the introduction of arthroscopy into the armamentarium of the orthopaedic surgeon was one of scepticism and ridicule. Established surgeons comfortable with arthrotomies had great doubts that anyone could see or do anything through the small portals involved in arthroscopic surgery. Gradually the value of minimally invasive surgery was appreciated and resident doctors began to learn the techniques in training. Courses around the world also promoted the technique. The ingenuity of the practitioners and the support of the technical trade in making appropriate instrumentation has made a reality of the concept that 'if you can see pathology you should be able to deal with it'.

The success of arthroscopic surgery appears to have been the catalyst for a similar effort in every other surgical field. Before the obvious success of arthroscopic surgery, many surgical specialties occasionally used diagnostic endoscopes. Now virtually all surgical specialties are developing surgical procedures done under endoscopic control.

Considering the number of patients around the world that have been helped and the number of procedures that can and are being performed, it is not unreasonable to state that arthroscopic surgery has become one of the three most important surgical procedures of the last century. The other two major surgical advances would be total joint replacement, which revolutionised the treatment of degenerative arthritis, and the open reduction internal fixation of fractures, which has evolved to a science that enables most victims of trauma to return quickly to a normal life.

In the future the emphasis in arthroscopic surgery will stress tissue repair rather than resection. Arthroplasty, through the biological resurfacing of joints, is something that will probably succeed in the near future. Imaging will also improve. All of the great advances in arthroscopy have in the past come through improvements in lenses or light. It is therefore highly probable that three-dimensional imaging, perhaps even holographic images, will soon be routine. New energy sources will also be explored. Lasers are just the first of these, and different lasers, which will be smaller and more powerful with different wavelengths, will be used for specific purposes. There is tremendous unexplored energy potential in the electromagnetic spectrum.

Other advances will include robotic units, which will be devised to assist the arthroscopic surgeon, and synthetic tissues that will be developed to replace the ACL, the joint surface or the meniscus under arthroscopic control. Arthroscopy of the spine will also become a reality, and flexible endoscopes that will enable the instrument to be inserted into previously inaccessible places such as nerve root canals.

There is no question that minimally invasive surgery has changed the face of orthopaedics and surgery in general. We have come a long way in three decades. However the journey is only halfway over and the future is truly exciting.

REFERENCES

Bircher E 1921 Die arthroendoskopie. Zentralbl Chir 48: 1460–1461

Brillhart A T (ed) 1995 Arthroscopic Laser Surgery: Clinical Applications. Springer, New York

Burman M S 1931 Arthroscopy or direct visualization of joints. An experimental cadaver study. J Bone Joint Surg 13: 669–695

Hopkins H H 1978 The modern urological endoscope. In: Gow J G, Hopkins H H (eds) Handbook of Urological Endoscopy. Churchill Livingstone, Edinburgh

Jackson R W 1987 Memories of the early days of arthroscopy: 1965–1975. The formative years. Arthroscopy. J Arthroscopic Related Surg 3: 1–3

Jackson R W 1998 Osteoarthritis of the knee: arthroscopic surgery and a new classification system. Am J Knee Surg 11: 51–54

Jackson R W, Dandy D J 1976 Arthroscopy of the Knee. Gruen & Stratton, New York

Jacobaeus H C 1910 Ueber die Moeglichkeit die Zystoskopie bei Untersuchung seroeser Hoehlungen anzuwenden. Muenchen Med. Wchnschr 57: 2090–2092

Jason M I V, Dixon A S T J 1968 Arthroscopy of the knee in rheumatic diseases. Am J Rheumatoid Dis 27: 503

Johnson L L 1977 Comprehensive Arthroscopic Examination of the Knee. C V Mosby, St Louis

Kieser C 1999 Die arthroskopie zwischen Weltgeschichte und Technik. Arthroskopie 12: 111–116

Kreuscher P 1925 Semilunar cartilage disease, a plea for early recognition by means of the arthroscope and early treatment of this condition. Illinois Med J 47: 290–292

Leiter J, Nitze M 1879 Ein neue beleuchtungs und Untersuchungsmethode für die harnrohre, harnblase, und rektum. Wien Med W'schr 29: 649–662

National Museum for the History of Science 1973 From Lichleiter to Fiber Optics. Catalogue for the XVI Congress of the International Society for Urology, Amsterdam. National Museum for the History of Science, Leiden

Nordentoft S 1912 Ueber Endoskopie geschlossener Kavitäten mittels Trokarendoskops. Zentralbl Chir 39: 95–97

O'Connor R L 1977 Arthroscopy. J B Lippincott, Philadelphia

Robles-Gil J, Katona G 1972 Clinical and therapeutic usefulness of arthroscopy. Gazz Sanit 20: 16 [in Italian]

Schimmer D C, Brillhart K B, Duff C, Gling W 1998 Arthroscopic partial meniscectomy: a 12 year follow-up and a two-step evaluation of the long term course. Arthroscopy 14: 136–142

Sommer R 1937 Die endoskopie des kniegelenkes. Zentralbl Chir 64: 1692–1697

Sprague N F 1989 Complications in Arthroscopy. Raven, New York

Suckert R 1960 Die photoarthroskopie des kniegelenkes. Z Unfallmed. Berufski 53: 65–67

Takagi K 1933 Practical experiences using Takagi's arthroscope. J Jpn Orthop Assoc 8: 132 [in Japanese]

Vaubel E 1938 Die endoskopie des kniegelenkes. Zeitschrift fur Rheumaforschung 1: 210–213

Watanabe M, Takeda S, Ikeuchi H 1957 Atlas of Arthroscopy. Igaku Shoin, Tokyo

Wilke K H 1939 Die endoskopie des kniegelenks an der leiche. Bruns Beitr Klin Chir 169: 75–83

5

History of orthopaedic trauma

Charles M. Court-Brown

The management of orthopaedic trauma has always presented a challenge to surgeons. Man's desire to wage war has ensured a steady supply of musculoskeletal injuries over the years and many advances in orthopaedic trauma management have come about as a result of having to treat progressively more serious injuries caused by warfare. However, progress has also been affected by major social changes such as the Industrial Revolution and the invention of the internal combustion engine. Advances in metallurgy, anaesthesia and antibiotics have also played a significant part in altering the way that orthopaedic injuries have been treated, but it has primarily been surgical interest and ingenuity which have been the major driving forces for change over the centuries.

The pace of change has accelerated with time and it is interesting to observe that the fracture treatment advocated by Hippocrates, namely the use of stiffened bandages which were changed fairly frequently, was essentially the method taught to the Arabic surgeon Albucasis over a millennium later. He is reported to have continued with the use of stiffened bandages but to have suggested that they be maintained for a prolonged period. This form of early cast management remained unchallenged for a further 850 years when following the development of antisepsis and anaesthesia direct surgical intervention in the management of fractures became popular. In the last 150 years there has been considerable change with the development of internal and external fixation systems and an increased awareness of the importance of not only preserving life and limb, but also actually assessing patient function after treatment.

The last 250 years have also seen considerable changes in the causes of fracture and the requirements of patients. Before the Industrial Revolution all countries had rural economies. Most severe musculoskeletal injuries were caused by war and treatment was often prolonged with considerable morbidity and mortality. Increasing industrialisation and urbanisation together with the large numbers of casualties produced by the Napoleonic Wars meant that the advanced European countries had to find more effective and quicker methods of returning patients to maximal function. However, warfare continued to be the main cause of musculoskeletal injuries in these countries and in the USA until after the Second World War. The Korean and Vietnam Wars were responsible for considerable advances in the assessment and treatment of severely injured patients but since the end of the Second World War it has been the motorcar which has been mainly responsible for the need for improvement in the management of severe musculoskeletal injuries.

Road traffic accidents have resulted in the establishment of sophisticated trauma systems in the USA and some of the advanced European countries. In many countries the number of road traffic accident victims continues to rise. Recently there has been a further change in the type of patient who requires treatment for musculoskeletal injuries. Increasing affluence and leisure time has been responsible for an increase in the numbers of sports injuries that require treatment. However, the major epidemic in musculoskeletal injury that will affect the twenty-first century will not be caused by warfare, motor vehicle accidents or sport but by osteoporosis. It will be the large number of osteoporotic fractures occurring in the elderly population that will affect the health systems of most countries. Inevitably injuries related to our ability to prolong life beyond the effective life span of the skeleton will become progressively more common and many countries are reporting an annual increase in the incidence of fractures in the elderly. Osteoporotic fractures are already becoming the commonest fractures treated by orthopaedic surgeons and it is likely that the number will increase fairly rapidly.

HISTORY OF FRACTURE MANAGEMENT

The earliest references to the management of fractures are in the Edwin Smith Papyrus. This was written *c.*2800 BC and acquired by Edwin Smith the American Egyptologist in Luxor *c.*1867 (Breasted 1930). The papyrus contains forty-eight case reports of different medical conditions and the concepts of open fracture and comminution were introduced for the first time. It is interesting to observe that Case 37 consists of a fracture of the humerus and a wound over the upper arm. The author suggests that if the wound does not connect with the fracture the arm should be splinted and the wound dressed daily with grease, honey and lint. However if the wound connects with the fracture the ailment should not be treated, presumably because of the uniformly poor prognosis at that time.

The Ancient Egyptians and Ancient Chinese employed wooden splints held by stiffened bandages. This method of management is still used in different parts of the world but it was refined by Hippocrates who advocated the use of bandages stiffened with cerate, this being an ointment consisting of lard or oil mixed with wax, resin or pitch. Rigid fracture fixation was gained by increasing the number of bandages. Hippocrates used mechanical aids to reduce displaced fractures and dislocations but recommended that reduction of the fracture be delayed until the swelling had resolved (Adams 1939).

The teachings of Hippocrates dominated surgical thinking until internal and external fixation was introduced *c.*1850 AD. His bandaging methods were altered by Albucasis whose major contribution was to suggest that the stiffened bandages be left in position for a prolonged period rather than being changed frequently as advocated by Hippocrates. The Arabic School of Medicine, as represented by Albucasis, provided the link between the teachings of the Ancient Greeks and Romans and the European School of Surgery, which produced all of the advances in musculoskeletal surgery over the next eight centuries. Progress was relatively slow between 1000 and 1800 AD, although there were some notable advances made during this period, which includes the development of isometric traction by Guy de Chauliac in the fourteenth century. De Chauliac's principles were extended by Percivall Pott and Robert Chessher who developed the double inclined plane method of lower limb traction (Peltier 1990).

The most important advances that occurred between 1000 and 1800 AD were in the treatment of the soft tissue injuries associated with open fractures. Paul of Aegina (652–90), the last of the great Greco-Roman physicians, had suggested that open wounds should be treated with ointments and be allowed to suppurate. The concept of 'laudable pus' became accepted but was eventually challenged by a number of surgeons of whom Ambroise Paré (1510–90) was the most famous. He began his surgical career as a surgeon to General Montejean who commanded the army of François I of France. He followed the prevailing opinion of the day and dressed open wounds with boiling oil. Apparently the supply of oil became exhausted and Paré was forced to dress the soldiers open wounds with a paste containing oil of roses, turpentine and egg yolks. He discovered that the results were better and he abandoned the use of boiling oil. It is clear from Paré's account of the treatment of his own open tibial fracture that he understood the importance of proper wound debridement and removal of devitalised bone fragments. He also appreciated the importance of early mobilisation.

Paré's work was extended by Pierre Desault (1744–95) and his pupil Larrey (1766–1842). These surgeons also understood the importance of the management of the soft tissues in open fractures. Desault popularised the operation of wound toilet and in fact gave it the name 'debridement', which is derived from the French *débrider*, meaning to unbridle. Larrey became the chief surgeon of the French army during the Napoleonic Wars. His surgical skills were legendary. The shortened working week was not for Larrey! He is reported to have performed two hundred amputations in a day at the Battle of Borodino (1812). He is also recognised as having introduced the field ambulance service to facilitate the removal of wounded soldiers from the various Napoleonic battlefields.

Larrey would have been involved in the greatest innovation in fracture management since the time of Albucasis, the introduction of gypsum-impregnated bandages. The principle of stiffened bandages remained unchanged but the use of gypsum permitted a rigid external cast to be made thereby facilitating early mobilisation of the patient. Gypsum or plaster of Paris bandages were introduced by Mathijsen (1805–78) and by Pirogov (1810–81). Both surgeons used coarsely woven cloth into which dry plaster of Paris had been rubbed thoroughly. The bandages were moistened and then rubbed by hand until hard. They were first used in the treatment of mass casualties in the Crimean War by Pirogov and represented a major step forward in fracture management. Their use was quickly adopted throughout Europe, but it is interesting that they were not used to any extent in the American Civil War. In the USA it was Lewis Sayre and Lewis Stimson in New York and Scudder in Boston who advocated the use of plaster casts in the management of fractures.

Despite the obvious advantages of using a quick-drying cast that permitted the ambulatory treatment of fractures, there was some hesitancy about adopting this method of treatment. Hugh Owen Thomas felt that the immobilisation of a fractured limb was essentially unphysiological and he and his nephew Robert Jones advocated the use of ambulatory splints made from metal. It is difficult to discern Thomas's logic as presumably the splints immobilised the leg as much as the casts did. Eventually the Thomas splint became used mainly for transportation purposes and remains in use to this day.

The use of a mouldable material such as plaster of Paris allowed surgeons to design different types of cast. Delbet (1861–1925) introduced a functional cast with flares around the knee and ankle. This, like the later Sarmiento cast, theoretically allowed joint movement. Krause (1857–1937) introduced the concept of early weight bearing with a walking cast, but the great Austrian surgeon Lorenz Böhler (1885–1973) was a firm believer in rest. He advocated accurate reduction, using traction if necessary, followed by the application of a skin-tight cast. His clinical audit was legendary and there is little doubt that his results were good, although it must be emphasised that surgeons at that time were primarily concerned with achieving bone union rather than good long-term functional results.

The next debate about cast management of lower limb fractures concerned the role of early weight bearing. British surgeons such as Reginald Watson-Jones (1902–72) and John Charnley (1911–87) were conservative and continued with non-weight-bearing mobilisation. However Dehne (1905–83) and later A. Sarmiento (1967) strongly advocated early mobilisation and their results proved them correct. Unfortunately the literature about the use of casts and braces in the management of tibial and other fractures is now rather dated and most of it was written before the importance of assessing patient function was appreciated. Cast management remains a popular method of managing fractures of the humerus and tibia.

The other major development of the nineteenth century was the introduction of operative fracture fixation. It is recorded that Lapeyode and Sicre, surgeons from Toulouse in France, were successfully fixing open fractures *c.*1775 but the major advances were unquestionably made during the nineteenth century. The timing of the advances is not well recorded but the first book of techniques of internal fixation written by Laurent Jean Baptiste and Bérenger-Féraud in 1870 describes six methods of managing fractures (Fig. 5.1). Two were actually forms of external fixation, both having been invented by the eminent Parisian

surgeon Malgaigne (1806–65). These were the Malgaigne point designed to push the spike of a tibial fracture back into position and the Malgaigne clamp designed to reduce and fix patellar fractures. The other methods described by Bérenger-Féraud were the wiring of adjacent teeth placed through the bone near the fracture, interosseous bone suturing, cerclage wiring and enclavement. 'Enclavement' was a term given to the fashioning of the bone ends to facilitate bone interposition and thereby increase stability. Interosseous and cerclage wiring techniques are still used and it is interesting to note that Bérenger-Féraud believed that cerclage wiring was the most useful surgical technique available to him. Cerclage wiring was also used by Joseph Lister in London and Samuel Cooper to fix open patellar fractures and their technique soon became accepted and used by many surgeons.

The first bone plate was devised in 1886 by Hansmann in Hamburg, Germany (Fig. 5.2a). He employed the novel concept of inserting the screws percutaneously, presumably so that they might be removed easily. However the infection rate was not recorded and might well have been somewhat high! Plate fixation was rapidly extended and popularised by three orthopaedic surgeons of note. Albin Lambotte (1866–1956) in Belgium, William Arbuthnot Lane (1856–1943) in England and William Sherman (1880–1979) in the USA not only developed plating systems, but also undertook clinical research to improve patient management. Lambotte could reasonably lay claim to be the father of modern fracture surgery. He was a genius and was responsible for the development of a number of internal and external fixation techniques. He is probably best known for his work with external fixation, but he also developed plates, screws and staples, and obviously had clear indications for the use of these devices as well as flexible wires, cerclage wires and wire sutures in different situations. In addition, he was a master violin-maker and it is recorded that he made 182 violins. He also recorded his findings fastidiously and wrote one of the famous books of orthopaedic traumatology, *L'Intervention opératoire dans les fractures récentes et anciennes* (1907).

Lane was another great innovator. He became disenchanted with non-operative management of fractures and in 1884 advocated the use of internal fixation provided surgeons adhered strictly to aseptic surgical techniques. He wrote *The Operative Treatment of Fractures* (1905) and devised the Lane plate in 1907. Sherman also produced his own plate. He had some experience in this field as he was the surgeon for the Carnegie Steel Company. He developed a series of plates and self-tapping screws that he used in both closed and open fractures and malunions

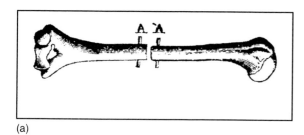

(a)

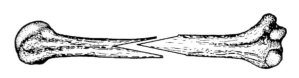

(d)

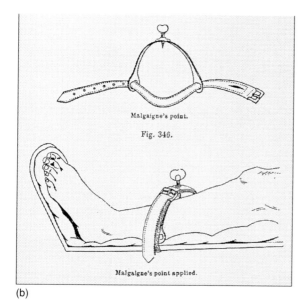

(b)

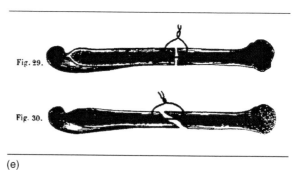

(e)

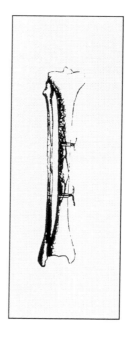

(c)

(f)

Fig. 5.1　The earliest internal fixation methods detailed by Bérenger-Féraud (1870):
(a) direct fixation by wiring 'teeth' placed through the bone, (b) Malgaigne's point, (c) Malgaigne's patellar clamp,
(d) enclavement, (e) bone suture, (f) Cerclage wiring

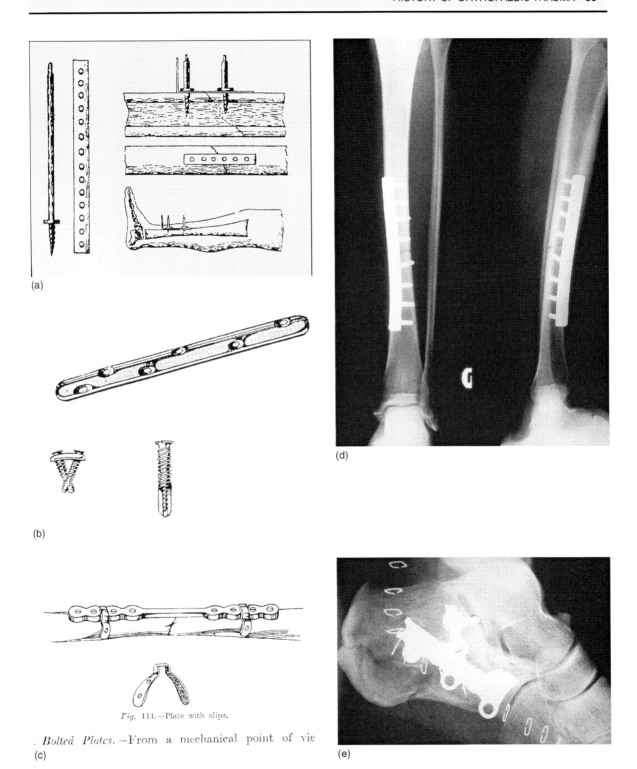

(a)

(b)

Fig. 111.—Plate with clips.

. *Bolted Plates.* —From a mechanical point of vie

(c)

(d)

(e)

Fig. 5.2 The evolution of bone plates: (a) the first bone plate designed by Hansmann in Hamburg, Germany, in 1886, (b) the curved plate devised by Lambotte, (c) plate clips for use with Lane's plates, (d) the Dynamic Compression Plate (DCP) devised by the AO group, (e) an AO calcaneal plate, which is location specific but can be cut to suit the exact shape of the bone

(Sherman 1912). Both Lane and Sherman believed in early mobilisation after plate fixation.

In the early days of bone plating there was considerable discussion about plate and screw design. Surgeons recognised that loosening of the plate was a problem and attempted to address it by devising different designs of plate and screws. Lane's screw was essentially of wood and early biomechanical testing showed that it achieved a poor hold in diaphyseal cortical bone. Ernest Hey Groves (1872–1944) of Bristol in Britain pointed out that bone was a dense homogeneous material much more like metal than wood (Hey Groves 1921). He felt that the design of bone screws should be based on the 'engineers screw' used by Lambotte. The use of a slit at the distal end of the screw to permit self-tapping was also recognised and employed at this time.

Surgeons remained concerned about the fact that all the bone screws were in the same plane if a standard plate was used. Lambotte designed a curved plate that allowed surgeons to implant the bone screws in different planes (Fig. 5.2b). It was recognised that this was biomechanically advantageous but that the greater width of the plate resulted in increased periosteal damage. Plate clips designed to minimise periosteal damage were applied to a standard Lane plate and screws were allowed to be inserted in different planes without significantly increasing the area of periosteal damage (Fig. 5.2c). A number of other methods were used to improve stability of the plate. Bolts were used with nuts placed on the opposite side of the diaphysis with a guide being devised to minimise soft tissue damage. Surgeons also experimented with plates of ivory and bone but they found that they had to be comparatively thick and clumsy to provide adequate strength. As they also required thicker bone screws their use was short lived (Hey Groves 1921).

The next major advance in plate design and technique followed the work of Robert Danis (1880–1962), Professor of Theoretical and Practical Surgery at the University of Brussels. His philosophy guided the Arbeitgemeinschaft für Osteosynthesefragen (AO) group. He believed in early rigid fracture fixation to allow immediate active mobilisation of the adjacent joints and muscles, and also in the restoration of normal osseous anatomy and in primary bone healing without callus formation. He had invented a 'coapteur' or compression plate that achieved sufficient rigidity to fulfil his criteria for successful fracture management. Danis was a visionary but it might reasonably be suggested that his main contribution was to influence Maurice Müller who together with Hans Willenegger, Robert Schneider and Martin Allgöwer formed the AO.

This group has been responsible for all of the advances in plating since 1950. It has also contributed extensively to orthopaedic research and to the dissemination of knowledge to young surgeons (Müller et al 1964). The group's first plate was the dynamic compression plate (DCP) which was so designed that the plate could move as the screws were tightened so compressing the fracture (Fig. 5.2d). The plate was more adaptable than Danis's coapteur and it remains the basic plate used throughout the world. The use of the DCP has declined in recent years as surgeons have adopted intramedullary nailing and external skeletal fixation. Dynamic compression plating became associated with a relatively high incidence of infection and non-union but it must be remembered that of all the commonly used methods of bone fixation plating is the most difficult. Indeed with hindsight the early results of bone plating can be seen to have been good. Surgeons such as Ruedi plated open tibial fractures without the benefits of plastic surgery and still achieved reasonable results (Ruedi et al 1976). In recent years the AO group has developed bone-specific plates such as those for the calcaneus, distal radius, distal femur and distal clavicle (Fig. 5.2e). All of these plates are well designed and widely used. In addition the group has detailed the use of the wave plate for non-unions and introduced the concept of minimally invasive plating.

EXTERNAL SKELETAL FIXATION

The patellar clamp of Malgaigne has already been mentioned (Fig. 5.1c). This was the first external fixation device, but it was not the first implant to be used in this manner. In 1850 in Strasbourg, France, Cucel and Rigaud had used two transcutaneous screws held by string to immobilise an olecranon fracture. There were a considerable number of external fixation devices invented in the second half of the nineteenth century but the breakthrough in external fixation came from the work of Clayton Parkhill (1860–1902) in the USA (Parkhill 1897) and Lambotte in Belgium (1907). Parkhill was an enthusiast who reported good results in eight of nine patients with tibial fractures or non-union. His device was a very simple unilateral frame that required supplementary support from a plaster cast. Lambotte's external fixation device was also unilateral (Fig. 5.3a) but it was biomechanically superior and supplementary cast fixation was not required. Lambotte enlarged the indication for the use of external fixation in fresh fractures and it was widely used for the treatment of tibial, humeral, forearm and clavicle fractures. There is no doubt that Lambotte understood the mechanics of external fixation and he achieved good results.

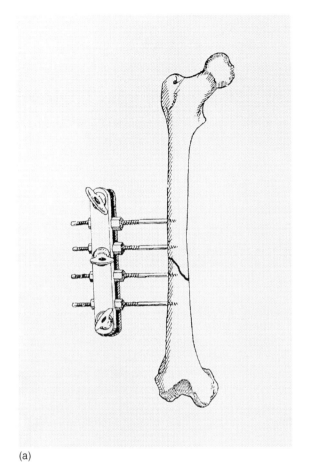

(a)

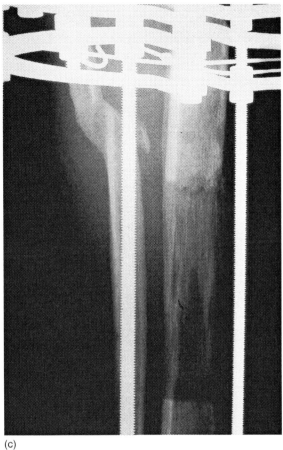

(c)

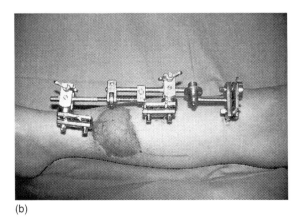

(b)

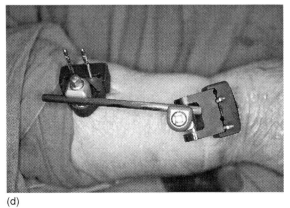

(d)

Fig. 5.3 The evolution of external skeletal fixation: (a) the original external fixator designed by Lambotte, (b) a unilateral configuration of the Hoffmann external fixator, (c) an Ilizarov frame for distraction osteogenesis, (d) a peri-articular configuration of the Hoffmann 2 external fixator used to treat a distal radial fracture

In the early nineteenth century surgeons in Britain were still influenced by the non-operative school of fracture treatment but there were two surgeons at the time who advocated the use of external fixation. Keetley (1893) used a unilateral frame and experimented with the use of transfixion pins made of different material. However it was Hey Groves who investigated external fixation in detail. He undertook a series of experiments in cats and concluded that the results were good if there was perfect anatomical reduction, the fixator was retained in place long enough to permit fracture union and the limb was kept free to allow early mobilisation (Hey Groves 1921).

External fixation was not widely used during the First World War because of the enormous number of casualties and the comparatively small number of experienced surgeons. However the technique became much more popular after the War and a number of frames were devised to facilitate fracture management. Some surgeons also adapted external fixators to allow limb lengthening. Vittorio Putti from Bologna, Italy, was very influential in this regard. In 1921 he wrote that he considered that an aligned leg length discrepancy of less than 2 inches did not require operative correction. However for more severe discrepancies he advocated the use of an external fixator which utilised a telescopic tube containing a spring. He was able to apply controlled distraction and to measure the amount of daily lengthening. He also detailed the precise method of introduction of pins and he described a 'Z'-shaped osteotomy which he created with a power saw. He reported on ten cases gaining between 3 and 4 inches in length. Putti's work essentially created a new discipline within orthopaedic surgery and led to the introduction of more sophisticated frames such as the Wagner device.

Fracture management using external fixation was popularised mainly by Raoul Hoffmann (1938) of Geneva who designed a multiplanar frame that could be applied in a variety of configurations depending on the morphology of the fracture and the surgeon's desire to have more or less rigid fixation (Fig. 5.3b). This was the first external fixation frame to be tested biomechanically (Lindahl 1965). In the USA external fixation was popularised by Conn (1931), Stader (1937) and Haynes (1939), but it was the work of Roger Anderson that has stood the test of time (Anderson & O'Neill 1944). He devised a transarticular frame for the management of distal radial fractures. In recent years distal radial frame design has improved but Anderson's general principles are still followed by many surgeons.

External fixation again fell out of favour in America after the Second World War. A study undertaken by the American Academy of Orthopaedic Surgeons (Johnson & Stovald 1950) criticised the technique and it was left to European surgeons to maintain the use of external fixation over the next twenty years. The Hoffmann device

remained popular largely because of the work of Vidal in France (Vidal et al 1970) and Burny in Belgium (Burny & Bourgois 1972). It is interesting to note that these surgeons used the same device but with a different philosophy of fracture treatment. The multiplanar Hoffmann frame permitted surgeons to make many different external fixator configurations. Vidal believed in rigid fixation and used configurations that had transfixion pins and four side bars. Burny, on the other hand, believed in flexible fixation and mainly used unilateral frames. This difference of opinion about rigidity of fracture fixation was never resolved and surgeons continue to argue about the merits of both rigid and flexible fracture fixation. A review of the literature concerning external skeletal fixation suggests that there is no advantage of one type of fixator configuration over another.

The other significant advance that occurred after the War was the evolution of the Ilizarov external frame. Gavriil Ilizarov worked in Kurgan in Russia. He was faced with a considerable number of post-War reconstructive problems and minimal resources. He developed a circular frame that consisted of a number of circular and semicircular rings held to the limb by multiple thin transfixion wires (Ilizarov 1954). His main contribution however was the discovery of distraction osteogenesis and his device is now widely used throughout the world to treat osteomyelitis, non-union, malunion and limb length discrepancies (Fig. 5.3c).

In recent years the use of external fixation to treat diaphyseal fractures has waned as intramedullary nailing has become more popular, but it remains a very popular technique for the treatment of metaphyseal fractures. With the invention of new frames (Fig. 5.3d) external fixation has become particularly popular for the treatment of distal radial fractures (McQueen 1998) and tibial plafond fractures but there are many other indications including temporary fixation in the multiply injured patient, complex diaphyseal fractures and severe pelvic fractures.

INTRAMEDULLARY NAILING

The earliest intramedullary devices were used in the nineteenth century. It is reported that in 1841 Dieffenbach was treating diaphyseal non-unions by stabilising them with ivory pegs. Other surgeons such as Heine and Bardenheur in Germany used similar techniques in the later part of the century. However Bircher in Germany used ivory pegs and clamps for the primary treatment of diaphyseal and metaphyseal fractures (Bircher 1893). The ivory diaphyseal pegs were of a simple design but the metaphyseal clamps were 'H'-shaped with one leg of the 'H' being extramedullary and the other intramedullary (Fig. 5.4a). Senn in the USA used intramedullary

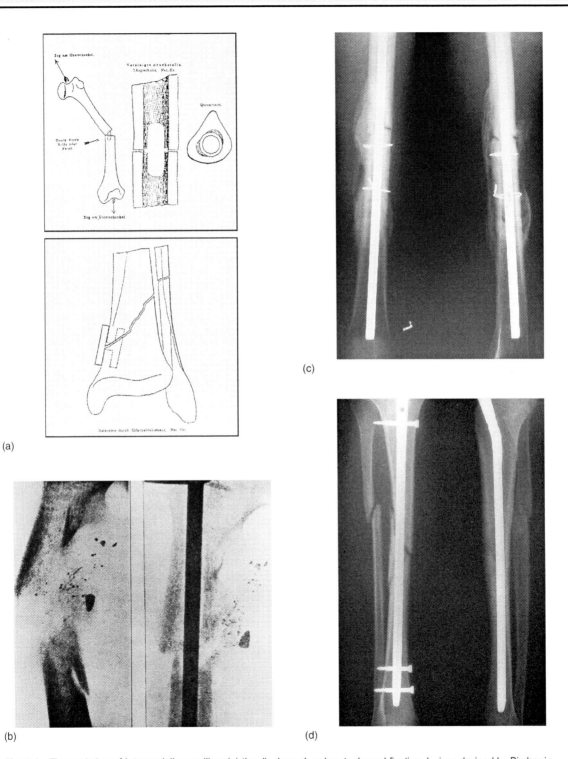

Fig. 5.4 The evolution of intramedullary nailing: (a) the diaphyseal and metaphyseal fixation devices devised by Bircher in 1893, (b) a metal intramedullary nail used by Hey Groves in 1921 to treat an open femoral fracture, (c) the original Küntscher nail used to treat a comminuted femoral diaphyseal fracture with cerclage wires stabilising the bone fragments, (d) a statically locked Grosse–Kempf intramedullary nail used to treat a tibial fracture

de-ossified animal bone cylinders instead of ivory pegs for the treatment of diaphyseal fractures but the surgical technique would have been similar (Senn 1893).

Hey Groves may have undertaken a number of studies using external fixation but he is actually best known for his work with intramedullary nailing. He used intramedullary ivory pegs to treat femoral diaphyseal fractures employing a retrograde nailing technique. He was enthusiastic about the technique and wrote that it was a straightforward procedure that could be done through a small incision with minimal periosteal damage. He felt that movement between the bone ends facilitated rapid union and was impressed that mobilisation of the joints could be instituted soon after surgery. Hey Groves carried out these operations before the First World War but by the end of the War he was using long metal nails to stabilise femoral fractures (Fig. 5.4b).

Hey Groves was an extraordinary man. He and Lane should be regarded as the principal pioneers of British orthopaedic trauma surgery. He undertook a series of experiments in cats to investigate intramedullary nailing. He used nails made of different materials and found that magnesium nails were not rigid enough to prevent malalignment. He had used magnesium because he thought that it might be absorbed by the body making nail removal unnecessary. The softness of the metal prevented it from being used clinically but Hey Groves was impressed with the periosteal reaction caused by magnesium. He also used nails made of metal coils, the rationale being that he could remove the nails merely by pulling on one end of the coil (Hey Groves 1921). Unfortunately this did not work! It would be interesting to know if Hey Groves's work influenced Gerhard Küntscher (1900–72) in any way. They did not live all that far apart and their professional activities may well have brought them into contact. Whether or not Küntscher was influenced by Hey Groves, he was undoubtedly the main force behind intramedullary nailing and his clinical research is responsible for the current popularity of intramedullary nailing throughout the world (Küntscher 1962).

Küntscher also undertook animal experiments investigating the advantages of intramedullary nailing. He felt that for successful nailing the fixation should be such that limb function was unimpaired. The incision should be as far from the fracture as possible and the fixation should enhance callus formation. Küntscher not only developed the classic cloverleaf nail with his engineer Pohl (Fig. 5.4c), but also devised the first reconstruction nail where a side arm could be placed through the nail into the femoral neck. In addition he used small flexible intramedullary nails and developed the first intramedullary saw.

Initially Küntscher was wary about reaming as he believed it would damage the endosteal surface of the bone and might cause fat embolus. However, he was clearly a pragmatist and he quickly realised the advantages of the technique. He subsequently produced the first set of intramedullary reamers. Küntscher's last invention was the 'detensornagel', a locked intramedullary nail. He designed this close to the end of his life but the device made a considerable impression on Klaus Klemm who together with Schellmann devised an interlocking nail (Klemm & Schellmann 1972). At the same time a similar nail was introduced by Ivan Kempf and Arsene Grosse in Strasbourg (Kempf et al 1978). These nails were to revolutionise the management of femoral and tibial diaphyseal fractures (Fig. 5.4d). Küntscher's work with flexible unreamed nails was advanced by Hackenthal in Germany and Ender in Austria, but outside selected centres these techniques are not in widespread use today.

It is interesting to compare the evolution of nailing in Europe and the USA. Internal metal splints had been used in America as early as 1911 by Dr Lilienthal in New York, but the technique of intramedullary nailing was popularised in America by the Rush family. J. Hack Rush and his two sons worked in Mississippi. They treated a Monteggia fracture dislocation with a Steinmann pin introduced antegrade into the olecranon (Rush & Rush 1937). Following the success of this operation they designed a set of thin flexible nails that relied on three-point fixation to gain stability. They also published a manual of their techniques (Rush 1955) and pioneered the use of closed nailing using fluoroscopy. Their techniques became widely used but as Rush nails do not provide stable fixation for all fracture types their use has declined in recent years. They influenced a generation of orthopaedic surgeons and the principle of unreamed nailing was advanced by Otto Lottes (1952) and Dana Street (1951) in the USA. Much of the credit for the widespread introduction of intramedullary nailing into America must however go to the surgeons of Harborview Medical Centre in Seattle who popularised both the technique of femoral intramedullary nailing and a system of Level 1 Trauma Centres (Winquist et al 1984).

In recent years there has been considerable debate about the role of unreamed nails and the potential disadvantages of reaming. The AO group produced a solid unreamed nail which was popularised by the Hannover group under Harald Tscherne (Krettek et al 1996). However, comparative studies have shown that there are considerable clinical advantages associated with reaming particularly when used in closed tibial and femoral fractures (Court-Brown et al 1996, Tornetta & Tiburzi 2000). In addition, Christie et al (1995) failed to show significant fat embolus problems in non-pathological long bone fractures treated by reamed intramedullary nailing. In the 1990s attention turned to investigating the treatment of the complications associated with intramedullary nailing and a considerable amount of work has been undertaken to examine exchange nailing, infection and knee pain. Surgeons have also investigated the role of nailing in upper limb fractures, but although there are some enthusiasts many surgeons prefer non-operative management or plating of the diaphyseal fractures of the humerus and forearm.

HIP FRACTURE TREATMENT

Hip pinning is essentially an intramedullary technique although many surgeons have used a side plate to supplement the intramedullary pins or screws placed into the femoral neck and head. Internal fixation of hip fractures commenced at about the beginning of the twentieth century. Before this time hip fractures had been managed non-operatively. Nicolas Senn (1844–1908) was the first surgeon to consider internal fixation of femoral neck fractures. He undertook a series of animal experiments that demonstrated that experimentally produced fractures in cats and dogs could be fixed internally with metal nails or ivory or bone pegs. A sceptical surgical profession criticised him and he did not operate on patients with proximal femoral fractures.

Other surgeons did undertake internal fixation. Lambotte used crossed metal hip pins (Fig. 5.5a) and surgeons such as Albee (1917) and Hey Groves made extensive use of bone pegs. Smith-Petersen (1917) devised a new approach to the hip joint and devised a triflanged nail which influenced surgical technique for the next fifty years. The major problem that the early surgeons encountered was the difficulty in positioning their pegs or nails correctly in the femoral neck and head. X-rays and later fluoroscopy facilitated placement of pins as did the technique of cannulated nail fixation popularised by Lorenz Böhler and others.

Once the technique of hip pinning had became accepted there was considerable debate about the optimal method of fixation. Many surgeons developed hip screw and side plate systems designed to gain maximal hold in the femoral head and to compress the subcapital fracture. Other surgeons developed multiple pin fixation systems of which the best known was the Deyerle system of hip pinning (Deyerle 1959). It is clearly the forerunner of modern cannulated screw systems (Fig. 5.5b). Both techniques persist to this day with multiple cannulated screws being popular for the treatment of subcapital fractures and hip screw systems being used for intertrochanteric fractures.

In the last decade true intramedullary fixation was introduced for the management of intertrochanteric fractures. These devices are reconstruction nails that consist of a short intramedullary nail which is distally locked by one or two screws (Fig. 5.5c). Proximal locking is obtained by passing a screw through the nail into the femoral head and neck. Trials were undertaken to compare these devices with hip screw and plate systems in intertrochanteric fractures. There appears to be little difference between the two implants and only time will tell which device becomes more popular.

The use of prosthetic replacement of the head of the femur was pioneered by Hey Groves who used an ivory prosthesis to replace the head of the femur. This prosthesis had a stem that gained stability from being positioned in the femoral neck and greater trochanter rather than in the femoral diaphysis. A similar design was used by Robert and Jean Judet from Paris who used acrylic rather than ivory. The devices were clearly poor and it was not until surgeons used metal implants for hemiarthroplasty passed into the femoral diaphysis that the operation of femoral hemiarthroplasty became popular. The two best-known devices were the Moore and Thompson prostheses designed to be used with and without bone cement. In later years surgeons have used a number of bipolar prostheses and total hip arthroplasties although the latter continue to be associated with a number of problems when used to treat subcapital fractures.

OPEN FRACTURES

The use of antiseptic solutions to clean open wounds has already been described, as has the beginning of the evolution of debridement under Desault and Larrey. The first surgeon actually to describe the operation of wound toilet or debridement in detail was Milligan (1915) who was with the British Expeditionary Force in the First World War. Later Trueta (1944) described the operation of wound excision in detail.

The problem that faced all surgeons until comparatively recently was what to do with the open wound? Primary closure was either impossible or disastrous. The only treatment was to try to keep the wound as clean as possible until it granulated or closed sufficiently to allow secondary suture. A number of techniques were devised to maintain a clean wound. The Winnett-Orr (1877–1956) method of occlusive dressing was popular. It consisted of packing the wound with Vaseline gauze and immobilising the limb in a plaster cast (Winnett-Orr 1941). The dressings were changed at infrequent intervals and the wound closed when it was possible. Alternatives to the use of the Winnett-Orr technique

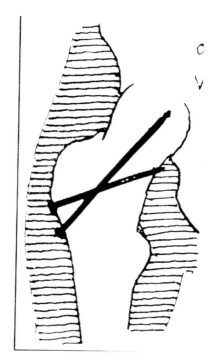

(a)

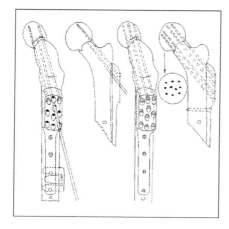

(b)

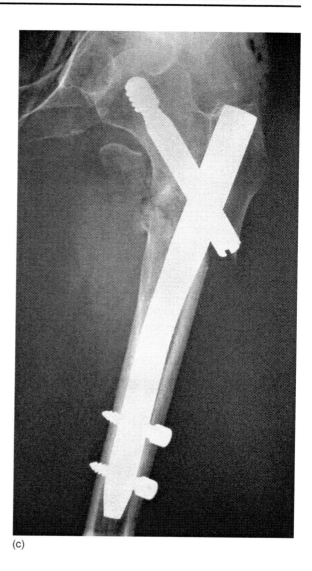

(c)

Fig. 5.5 The evolution of the management of hip fractures: (a) crossed metal pins used by Lambotte, (b) the Deyerle hip fixation system, which employs multiple pins and a guidance template, (c) a Gamma Nail. A short reconstruction nail used for intertrochanteric fractures

were the use of Dakin's solution of sodium hypochlorite and merely to expose the wound to air through a window in the plaster. Dakin's solution was popularised by Carrel who used perforated irrigation tubes placed around the wound. The fractures were reduced and immobilised in a cast and the wound irrigated every 2 hours. The wounds were therefore kept clean until they could be sutured secondarily.

Despite the fact that plastic surgery has been performed for at least 1500 years it is perhaps surprising that plastic surgical procedures for the management of open fractures have only been in widespread use for about twenty years. Rudimentary flap techniques existed in the fifteenth century but do not appear to have been used to close the open wounds that presented to the surgeons of the time. However the main purpose behind the treatment of open wounds at this time was the preservation of life and the preservation of limbs and their function was a secondary consideration. Thus surgeons such as Verdun, Ravaton and Vermale contented themselves by designing better skin flaps following amputation in an effort to improve the stump (Aldea & Shaw 1986). The first recorded human skin graft was undertaken by Sir Astley Cooper in 1817. However it was Reverdin in 1870 who demonstrated the usefulness of small split thickness skin grafts. Thiersch advocated the use of long split skin grafts in 1874 but they were not used very much until the Second World War.

The use of flaps in open fracture surgery followed the introduction of the tubed pedicle flap by Sir Harold Gilles during the First World War. These flaps were originally used to treat the chronic osteomyelitis that frequently resulted from open fractures, with considerable benefit. The methods of transferring a flap from one part of the body to another were slow and uncomfortable for the patient and the technique was not readily applicable to the management of open fractures. The two major advances that allowed flaps to be used to treat open fractures were the development of microsurgery and the understanding of the anatomy of local flaps. Microvascular surgery became popular in the 1960s and 1970s with the first successful implantation being performed in Boston in 1962 (Malt & McKhann 1964). Within the next twenty years the use of free flaps became widespread. In the 1970s and 1980s there was considerable interest in the use of local flaps to cover open wounds. These were quicker and easier to use than free flaps and were therefore associated with a lower morbidity (Erdmann et al 1997). Currently both techniques are in widespread use and it is likely that history will record that it was the evolution of flap cover in the late twentieth century that revolutionised the management of open fractures.

REFERENCES

Adams F 1939 Hippocrates: The Genuine Works of Hippocrates. Williams & Wilkins, Baltimore

Albee F H 1917 Bone Graft Surgery. W B Saunders, Philadelphia

Aldea P A, Shaw W W 1986 The evolution of the surgical management of severe lower limb trauma. Clin Plast Surg 13: 549–569

Anderson R, O'Neill G 1944 Comminuted fractures of the distal end of the radius. Surg Gynae Obstet 78: 434–440

Bérenger-Féraud L J B 1870 Traité de l'immobilisation directe des fragment osseux dans les fractures. Adrien Delahaye, Paris

Bircher H 1893 Eine neue method unmittelbarer retention bei fracturen des rohrenkochen. Ann Klin Chir 34: 410–422

Breasted J H 1930 The Edwin Smith Papyrus. University of Chicago Press, Chicago

Burny F, Bourgois R 1972 Etude biomechanique du fixateur externe de Hoffmann. Acta Orthop Belg 38: 265–279

Christie J, Robinson C M, Pell A C, McBirnie J, Burnett R 1995 Transcardiac echocardiography during invasive intramedullary procedures. J Bone Joint Surg 77B: 450–455

Conn H R 1931 The internal fixation of fractures. J Bone Joint Surg 9: 261–268

Court-Brown C M, Will E, Christie J, McQueen M M 1996 Reamed or unreamed nailing for closed tibial fractures. A prospective study in Tscherne C1 fractures. J Bone Joint Surg 78B: 580–583

Cucel L R, Rigaud R 1850 Des vis métalliques enfoncés dans les tissues des os, pour le traitement de certaines fractures. Rev Med Chir Paris 8: 115

Deyerle W M 1959 Absolute fixation with contact compression in hip fractures. Clin Orthop 13: 279–297

Erdmann M W, Court-Brown C M, Quaba A A 1997 A five year review of islanded distally bases fasciocutaneous flaps on the lower limb. Br J Plasr Surg 50: 421–427

Hansmann G 1886 Eine neue methode der fixierung der fragmentes bei komplizierten frakturen. Dtsch Ges Chir: 134–137

Haynes H H 1939 Treating fractures by skeletal fixation of the individual bone. South Med J 32: 720–724

Hey Groves E W 1921 On Modern Methods of Treating Fractures, 2nd edn. John Wright, Bristol

Hoffmann R 1938 Rotules à os pour la réduction dirigée, non sanglante, des fractures (osteotaxis). Helv Med Acta: 844–850

Ilizarov G A 1954 A new principle of osteosynthesis with the use of crossing pins and rings. In: Collected Scientific Works of the Kurgan Regional Scientific Medical Society. Kurgan Regional Medical Society, pp 145–160

Johnston H E, Stovald S L 1950 External fixation of fractures. J Bone Joint Surg 32A: 460–467

Keetley C B 1893 On the prevention of shortening and other forms of mal-union after fracture. Lancet i: 1377–1379

Kempf I, Grosse A, Laffourge D 1978 L'apport du verouillage dans l'enclouge centromédullaire des os longs. Rev Chir Orthop 64: 635

Klemm K, Schellmann W D 1972 Dynamische und statische Verriegelung des marknagels. Monatsschr Unfallheilkunde 75: 568

Krettek C, Rudolf J, Schandelmaier P, Guy P, Konemann B, Tscherne H 1996 Unreamed intramedullary nailing of femoral shaft fractures: operative technique and early clinical experience with the standard locking option. Injury 27: 233–254

Küntscher G 1962 Praxis der marknagelung. F K Schattauer, Stuttgart

Lambotte A 1907 L'intervention opératoire das les fracture récents et anciennes envisagée particulièrement au point de vue de l'ostéo-synthèse. Lamertin, Brussels

Lane W A 1905 The Operative Treatment of Fractures. The Medical Rutheday Co. Ltd, London

Lilienthal H 1911 Fracture of the femur: open operation with introduction of intramedullary splint. Ann Surg 53: 541–542

Lindahl O 1962 Rigidity of immobilisation of transverse fractures. Acta Orthop Scand 32: 237–246

Lottes J O 1952 Intramedullary fixation for fractures of the shaft of the tibia. South Med J 45: 407–414

Malt R A, McKhann C F 1964 Replantation of severed arms. J Am Med Assoc 189: 716–722

McQueen M M 1998 Redisplacable unstable fractures of the distal radius. A randomised prospective study of bridging versus non-bridging external fixation. J Bone Joint Surg 80B: 665–669

Milligan E T C 1915 The early treatment of projectile wounds by excision of the damage tissues. Br Med J 1: 1081

Müller M E, Allgöwer M, Schneider R, Willenegger H 1965 Technique of Internal Fixation of Fractures. Springer, Berlin

Parkhill C 1898 Further observations regarding the use of the bone clamp in ununited fractures, fractures with mal-union and recent fractures with a tendency to displacement. Ann Surg 27: 553–570

Peltier L F 1990 Fractures: A History and Iconography of their Treatment. Norman, San Francisco

Putti V 1921 The operative lengthening of the femur. J Am Med Assoc 77: 934–935

Ruedi T, Webb J K, Allgower M 1976 Experience with the dynamic compression plate (DCP) in 418 recent fractures of the tibial shaft. Injury 7: 252–257

Rush L V 1955 Atlas of Rush Pin Techniques. Beviron, Meridian

Rush L V, Rush H L 1937 A reconstructive operation for comminuted fractures of the upper third of the ulna. Am J Surg 38: 332–333

Sarmiento A 1967 A functional below-the-knee cast for tibial fractures. J Bone Joint Surg 49A: 855–875

Senn N 1893 A new method of direct fixation of the fragments in compound and ununited fractures. Trans Am Surg Assoc 11: 125–151

Sherman W O 1912 Vanadium steel bone plates and screws. Surg Gynae Obstet 14: 629–634

Smith-Petersen M N 1917 New approach to the hip joint. Am J Orthop 15: 592

Stader O 1937 A preliminary announcement of a new method of treating fractures. N Am Vet 18: 37–38

Street D M 1951 One hundred fractures of the femur treated by means of the diamond-shaped medullary nail. J Bone Joint Surg 33A: 659–669

Tornetta P, Tiburzi D 2000 Reamed versus nonreamed antero-grade femoral nailing. J Orthop Trauma 14: 15–19

Trueta J 1944 The Principles and Practice of War Surgery, 2nd edn. Hamish Hamilton, London

Vidal J, Rabischong P, Boneel F 1970 Étude bioméchanique du fixateur externe d'Hoffmann das les fractures de jambe. Montpelier Chir 16: 43–52

Winnett-Orr H 1941 Wound and Fractures. A Clinical Guide to Civil and Military Practice. Charles C Thomas, Springfield

Winquist R A, Hansen S T, Clawson D K 1984 Closed intramedullary nailing of femoral fractures. J Bone Joint Surg 66A: 529–539

SECTION 2:

The Scientific Background

6

Biomechanics

John J. O'Connor

The term 'biomechanics' might be interpreted strictly to mean the study of the interactions of living tissues with their mechanical environments. However, exploration of that mechanical environment is itself a significant challenge and biomechanics has come to embrace the study of the geometry and mechanics of living tissues and their mechanical properties.

That biomechanics is a thriving scientific subject may be judged from the fact that the 33rd volume of *Journal of Biomechanics* (2000) ran to 1750 pages, about 230 papers, many devoted to the musculoskeletal system. It is clearly not possible to summarise all this work in one chapter. There are textbooks that provide up-to-date reviews (Mow & Hayes 1997, Nigg & Herzog 1998). It is a subject of interest in its own right; the recent edition of Y. C. Fung's *Biomechanics: Mechanical Properties of Living Tissues* (1993) is addressed to 'students of bioengineering, physiology and mechanics'. The clinical significance of the subject is not universally acknowledged; Brand (1992) discussed the clinical usefulness or otherwise of locomotion analysis: 'not one measure of locomotion has gained wide acceptance in clinical practice (say compared to certain blood tests, imaging techniques, or pulmonary function techniques)'. The thrust of the present chapter is to review the contribution that biomechanics has made or could make to the practice of orthopaedic surgery. In the era of joint replacement, the contribution might seem enormous and fundamental, but such an assessment assumes that joint replacements are designed and implanted with a thorough understanding of how they will interact with the retained tissues, an assumption which can still be questioned.

In his Presidential Address to the British Orthopaedic Association in 1989, J. W. Goodfellow declared that 'engineering mechanics is the basic science of orthopaedic surgery'. To what extent does this assertion meet the Brand test?

ARTISTS, ANATOMISTS, SCIENTISTS

Knowledge of the geometrical arrangements of the bones, muscles and ligaments is the starting point for studies in musculoskeletal mechanics. Indeed, changes in those geometrical arrangements (kinematics) as the body changes its shape during activity are an essential topic within the mechanical analysis. Artists as well as medical scientists have long been interested in anatomy. So must the biomechanic.

The editors of *Leonardo da Vinci on the Human Body* attributed to Mundinus (1270–1326) the first attempt to consider anatomy as a study of the function as well as the structure of the human body, while the sculptor Donatello (?1386–1466) was the first artist actually to perform dissection (O'Malley & Saunders 1983). Although they concluded that Vesalius in 1538 introduced anatomically correct and naturalistic illustrations produced by artists (from the School of Titian) (Boorstin 1983) under the direction of the anatomist and carefully related to the text, it was Leonardo (1452–1519) who considered the mechanics. 'By the eventual application of his physical laws to human anatomy, Leonardo achieved a wholly unique penetration into the mechanical principles of physiology. ... Thus he reduced bones and joints to levers acting on fulcra, and muscles to lines of force acting on these levers' (Keele 1977).

Leonardo's anatomical drawings of the arms, legs, neck and trunk, produced mainly between 1508 and 1510, were based on the dissection of more than 30 bodies (Keele 1977). They showed anterior, posterior and lateral views, as in a modern engineering drawing. With the notes written beside them, they represent the earliest scientific investigations into the mechanics of the human musculoskeletal system. He distinguished between the actions of flexor, extensor, abductor, adductor and rotator muscles at the joints. He also defined the lines of action of the muscle forces and his advice to the anatomy instructor was: 'Before you form the muscles make in their place threads which should demonstrate the positions of these muscles; the ends of these [threads] should terminate at the centre of the attachments of the muscles to the bones.' It is still assumed that the resultant muscle force acts through the centroid of its attachment area.

Leonardo's drawings of the bones of the leg contain the following (O'Malley & Saunders 1983):

Note here that the tendon which takes hold of the heel **c** [tendo Achilles] raises a man on the ball of his foot **a**, the weight of the man being at the fulcrum **b** [the internal malleolus of the ankle]. And because the lever **b**–**c** enters twice into the counter-lever **b**–**a**, 400 lbs of force at **c** produces a power of 200 lbs [the weight of a man in Florentine pounds] at **a** with a man standing on one foot.

Thus, he uses the geometry of the musculoskeletal system to deduce that muscle forces are usually larger than the external loads applied through the ends of limbs because their lever arms at the joints are shorter. In his study of standing on the ball of the foot, Leonardo demonstrated that the downward compressive force on the articular surface of the ankle has to balance not only the upward thrust of the force applied to the forefoot by the ground, but also the upward pull of the force in the Achilles tendon at the other end of the lever, the first demonstration that the articular surfaces of joints have to transmit compressive forces even larger than the muscle forces, which themselves are larger than the external loads. Most recent confirmation of these deductions comes from instrumented hip replacements, which have detected hip contact forces up to 8.7 times body weight (Bergmann et al 1983).

Leonardo showed that the system of muscles stabilising the cervical spine 'holds it erect just as the ropes of a ship support its mast' (O'Malley & Saunders 1983). Lateral forces tending to bend a limb produce a combination of tensile forces in the muscles and compressive forces in the bones. Recent *in vivo* measurement with an instrumented prosthesis have confirmed this deduction and showed that the compressive force in the shaft of the prosthesis (and, therefore, in the shaft of the bone) can also be many times larger than the external loads (Lu et al 1997).

Leonardo, therefore, stated or implied the basic principles underlying musculoskeletal mechanics:

- Limbs are stabilised against lateral forces by a combination of tension in the muscles and compression in the bones.
- Muscle forces are larger than the external loads acting at the ends of limbs because their lever-arms from the centres of the joints are shorter.
- Compression forces on the articular surfaces of joints are larger than the external loads because they also have to balance the forces in the muscle and tendons spanning the joints.
- Compression forces in the long bones are larger than the external loads for the same reason.

George Stubbs (1724–1806), referred to by William Hunter as 'that excellent painter of animals', was an active anatomist, not only for artistic purposes. Unlike many anatomical artists, he suspended and drew his cadaver animals in positions of activity and carried out dissections right down to the skeleton. His drawings of the horse reflect successive dissection and definition of the muscles, the arterial system and the bones. There are several drawings of the skeleton of the horse that show all the bones – the compression-carrying elements – while the only soft tissues present are the menisci of the knee (Egerton 1976). Perhaps he perceived that the menisci transmitted compressive force between the incongruent articular surfaces of the femur and the tibia and greatly increased the effective contact areas over which those loads were transmitted. It took a further two centuries before the load-bearing function of the menisci was demonstrated (Walker & Erkman 1975, Shrive et al 1978, Maquet 1984) and for analogues of the menisci to be introduced into a knee prosthesis (Goodfellow & O'Connor 1978).

MUSCULOSKELETAL MECHANICS

Giovanni A. Borelli was one of the first experimental scientists, following Galileo Galilei (1564–1642). Part I of his *De motu animalium* was published posthumously in 1680. He gave detailed descriptions of bird flight, of the walking and running of bipeds and quadrupeds, and of the swimming of fish, bipeds and quadrupeds. He explained the differences between species and activities as consequences of the mechanics of the different anatomy. He organised extensive experiments to study muscles and the forces they transmit. Borelli confirmed Leonardo's important deductions experimentally (Borelli 1680). His experiments demonstrated that muscle forces can be many times greater than the external loads they support and that, as a consequence, the compressive forces transmitted through joints can be even larger.

He used pulleys and hanging weights to measure forces in the muscle and tendons spanning joints and explained that they obey the theory of the lever: 'The magnitude of the force of any animal muscle necessarily must be greater than the weight which the muscle raises and never smaller' (Chapter VIII) because 'the ratio of the muscular force to the resistance is always equal to the ratio of the longer distance of the resistance to the shorter distance of the muscular force from the fulcrum'. The fulcrum is the 'centre of rotation' of the joint. A muscle force passing across the centre of rotation will be unable 'either to flex the limb against resistance or even maintain the limb in its position'. In terms of increased lever-arm lengths, he explained the mechanical advantage gained by attachment of tendons 'on tuberosities in the vicinity of the joint with their direction oblique to the longitudinal axis of the bone'.

He deduced (Chapter XII) that the forces exerted by the rectus femoris and gastrocnemius of a stevedore carrying a load on his neck may be 'fifty times the supported load'. Taking the forces in the intervertebral discs as his example, he argued that the compressive forces transmitted by the articular surfaces of joints have to balance not only the downward push of the weight of the body above the joint, but also – and more importantly – the upward pull of the muscles spanning the joint.

Although it is easy to find fault with the detailed mechanics and calculations, his work having been completed before Sir Isaac Newton (1642–1727) published his *Principia* (1687), the general principles described in the 224 Propositions of Part I of *De motu animalium* have mainly stood the test of time, and, with Leonardo's conclusions, continue to form the basis for our analysis of musculoskeletal mechanics.

WOLFF'S LAW

Roesler (1987) attributed to Bourgery (1832) the first description of the architectural structure of cancellous bone. Culmann (1862) and von Meyer (1867), possibly the first engineer/clinician team, recognised that the trabecular patterns in the proximal femur could reflect the trajectories of the stresses induced under load. Roux (1895) sought to relate similar trajectories in an anky-losed knee by coating a rubber model with paraffin wax and observing the patterns of cracks that appeared when the model was loaded. He concluded that there must be some 'quantitative self-regulating mechanism' requiring a 'functional stimulus' to the cells to control the process of adaptation (Roesler 1987), a statement of the theory of functional adaptation. Wolff (1899) claimed that Roux's work gave quantitative verification of his own principle that 'Every change in the form and function of the bones, or their function alone, is followed by certain definite changes in their internal

architecture and equally definite changes in their external construction, in accordance with mathematical laws.' Not all mechanical influences are benign: excessive mechanical loading leads to fracture of bones; excessive rigidity of compression plates leads to post-union osteopenia (Bradley et al 1979).

At any point in the bone, the most general and complex state of stress can be described most simply as a set of companion principal stresses acting on three planes at right angles, with no shear stresses. In bending, the maximum principal stress is tensile, the minimum compressive, located at the convex and concave edges of the bent beam and acting on planes perpendicular to the axis of the beam. In torsion, such planes transmit shear stresses, but the tensile and compressive principal stresses act on planes at 45° to the axis. These differences between bending and torsion explain the differences between transverse and spiral fractures of the long bones.

The trajectories of the principal stresses pass normal to the planes on which they act. It is a feature of photoelasticity that the patterns of the optical fringes (technically the isostatics derived from the observed isoclinics) that appear when a birefringent material is loaded under polarised light can be made to coincide with the trajectories of the principal stresses (Fig. 6.1). There is a difficulty, though, in relating the two-dimensional radiograph images of three-dimen-sional trabecular structures to the two-dimensional photoelastic images.

Pauwels (1954a) criticised some of the details of Roux's analysis, using photoelastic models both of Roux's specimen and of a further more complete specimen. Nonetheless, he concluded that 'the cancellous architecture represents an embodiment of the stress trajectories which arise in the ankylosis when the skeleton of the limb is loaded'. Pauwels subsequently explained in similar manner the differ-ences between the trabecular architectures in the femoral necks below a normal and an ankylosed hip (Pauwels 1960).

A century after Wolff, and after a vast body of work, the precise form of the mathematical laws is not yet defined. Bertram & Swartz (1991) provided a compre-hensive and critical survey of the experimental investi-gations into the relationships between mechanical strain and bone remodelling (e.g. Lanyon & Rubin 1984). Fritton *et al* (2000) made continuous recordings of bone strains from sheep and found that strains > 1000 μ occurred only a few times a day, whereas strains < 10 μ occurred several thousand times. They concluded that 'until the mechanism of bone's mechanosensory system is fully understood, all portions of bone's strain history

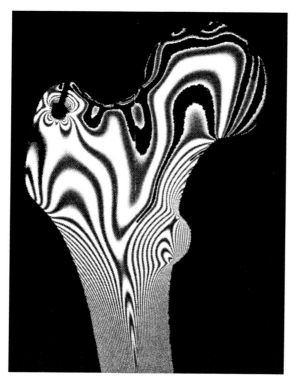

Fig. 6.1 Birefringent material loaded under polarised light

should be considered to possibly play a role in bone adaptation'. Nonetheless, postoperative radiographs of osteotomies and joint replacements appear to confirm the general truth of the proposition. There is experimental evidence that repeated micromovement can influence the rate of healing of bone fractures (Goodship & Kenwright 1985). Perhaps the most spectacular example is distraction osteogenesis, first described by Codivilla in 1905. There have been many advances in the surgical technique since then, most notably the use in 1939 of the external fixator for lengthening human legs (Abbott & Saunders 1939). Kenwright & White (1993), in reviewing virtually a century of development in this area, remarked that recent work 'supports the direct role of the mechanical stimulus of stretch, or tension, to the architecture of the osteoblast' and that 'there is an optimal strain to which newly formed bone should be subjected'.

While we await the experiments that will define the precise form of the mathematical laws of function adaptation and bone remodelling, the alternative is to advance plausible hypothetical laws and see whether the consequences of those laws conform to observation. This was the approach taken by Pauwels (1948). Many subsequent attempts have been made to model

mathematically the processes of functional adaptation and the effects of the mechanical environment on tissue differentiation, recently reviewed by Carter et al (1998). Finite-element methods are now preferred to photoelasticity to determine the distributions of stress and strain throughout a bone in response to loads applied through joints and through muscle insertions. Models of remodelling allow bone density to increase in regions of high strain and to decrease in regions of low strain. Some of the features of natural bone architecture can thereby be reproduced. Huiskes et al (1992) used finite-element stress analysis and hypothetical remodelling laws to study stress shielding and remodelling around the stems of hip replacements. A requirement of such studies is to develop an accurate view of the day-to-day history of load transmission through the tissues as well as an accurate view of how the tissues then remodel. The models of the proximal femur most frequently used appear to predict levels of strain much higher than those measured *in vivo* (Ling et al 1996, Taylor et al 1996). However, increasing use of instrumented implants (Bergmann et al 1997) will help validate more accurate methods of load analysis and may lead to a more accurate description of functional adaptation.

ANALYSIS OF LOCOMOTION

The analysis of movement has intrigued mankind since primitive times. Borelli described level walking and explained the need for side-to-side movement of the centre of gravity of the body (Proposition CLVII) with rotations of the pelvis in the transverse plane (Table XI and Figure 12) as well as coordinated flexion/extension movements at the hip, knee and ankle (Proposition CLVIII). Quantification of these movements (Inman et al 1981, Winter 1995) and of the internal forces that initiate and maintain them had to await – indeed prompted – the development of appropriate instruments and methods of analysis, developments which still continue.

Instrumentation

Simple measures of gait – cadence, stride length, walking speed – can be based on measurements of length and time and were described by the brothers Weber and Weber (one an anatomist, the other a mathematician) in 1836. More sophisticated methods are necessary for mechanical analysis. For instance, the double-support phase of normal level walking, with both feet on the floor, lasts < 0.1 s, too fast for its accurate measurement with a stopwatch.

Marey and his student Carlet developed pneumatic pads placed within shoes and connected with tubes to a recording device carried by the subject. They could then time the phases of single and double support during walking (Marey 1873). Similar pads over the hooves of horses demonstrated that all four hooves are briefly off the ground during trotting, a phenomenon which Muybridge (1882) subsequently showed photographically. Having seen Muybridge's photographs in 1878, Marey developed first his photographic rifle and later his cinecamera to study human and animal movement (Bouisset 1992).

The cinecamera or interrupted light photography became the most popular methods for the detection of movement, although many other techniques, such as goniometry (Karpovitch et al 1960, Chao & Hoffmann 1978), and the use of accelerometers (Morris 1973), have been attempted. Cine- or videorecords of gait can readily be obtained, but if they are to be used for other than qualitative assessment, methods of analysing movement quantitatively are needed. Bernstein (1934) introduced the techniques of stereophotogrammetry to obtain three-dimensional data from groups of two-dimensional images. Very considerable labour was involved in making measurements from the successive frames of cinefilm (Bresler & Frankel 1950) so that methods of performing the data-reduction automatically were sought. Using large photodiodes to follow the movements of light-emitting diodes placed on the subject has been the basis for one type of commercial gait analysis system (Woltring 1974). Furnee (1967) is credited with the first use of the videocamera, together with the fast modern computer. The cameras record the movements of stroboscopically illuminated reflective markers placed over anatomical landmarks on the limbs and torso of the subject. Winter et al (1972) and the Strathclyde group (Jarrett et al 1974) developed camera–computer interfaces and the use of spherical reflective markers together with a method of estimating the position of the centre of the circular image of each marker seen by each camera. Active markers can be of different shapes and their separate tracks can be distinguished readily, but they require an on-board power supply. Reflective markers require no power supply but clever algorithms are needed to keep separate the tracks of individual markers, particularly when they are close together (as on the foot).

Marey (1883) and his students also developed the second ingredient of the gait laboratory – the force plate – and used it to measure the vertical and anteroposterior components of the force transmitted between the foot and the ground during a range of activities (normal and brisk walking, running, and jumping) (Bouisset 1992).

With combined information on forces and movements, they sought to calculate the mechanical work done during level walking (Marey 1885). The rectangular six-component force plates developed by the California group (Bresler & Frankel 1950) used strain-gauged pillars at each corner that allowed the measurement of the three components of the ground reaction force, the two coordinates of the point at which its line of action cut the surface of the force-plate and the spin-moment about a vertical axis. Modern force-plates follow these design principles.

The third ingredient of the gait laboratory, electromyography (EMG), was based on Luigi Galvani's (1737–98) discovery between 1786 and 1792 of muscular electricity (Clarys & Lewillie 1992). Du Bois Reymond (1849) perfected various electrical machines for detecting voluntary electrical signals from human muscles in contraction, but Duchenne de Boulogne (1855) is credited with the establishment of the modern science of EMG, having investigated the dynamics and function of most of the superficial muscles and mapped out their motor points (Clarys & Lewillie 1992). Patterns of EMG activity of the main lower limb muscles during level walking were described by the California group (University of California 1953). However, it still remains true that EMG can, at best, detect whether a muscle is active, but it cannot measure the level of its activation or the instantaneous force transmitted by the muscle (Basmajian & De Luca 1985).

Analysis

Having the three basic instruments in place is only the beginning. Ideally, the information to be extracted from the measurements includes (1) kinematic data: the angles of flexion/extension, abduction/adduction and axial rotation as well as the relative translations of the bones in three directions at each joint, and (2) kinetic data: the tensile forces transmitted by each of the muscles and ligaments and the compressive forces transmitted across the articular surfaces of the joints. Determination of these quantities requires development of appropriate mathematical models of the musculoskeletal system with which to interpret the data and which describe how the shape of the body changes during activity and how it transmits its loads.

The mathematical models should include geometrical descriptions of the body segments and the bones, incorporating the different constraints to motion imposed by different joints, the layout of the muscles and their origins and insertions of their tendons on the bones. The mass distribution and inertial properties of each body segment should be defined. These are all quantities (parameters) that differ between individuals; the ideal of customising models to individual subjects is the objective of much current work. Orthopaedic surgeons alter these parameters when performing osteotomy, leg lengthening, joint replacement, ligament reconstruction and tendon transfer. The simulation of orthopaedic surgery and its consequences can therefore be an objective of gait analysis.

Braune and Fischer, between 1889 and 1904, provided some of the data for such a mathematical model. They froze cadavers and hung them from three axes to determine the weight and position of the centre of gravity of the body as a whole and, after dissection, of each segment. They found the moments of inertia of the body and its segments by measuring periods of oscillation about linear axes. These valuable data are still available (Braune & Fischer 1985, 1988. Dempster (1955), Drillis & Contini (1966) and Contini (1972) have added to this database and a summary of their data is provided by Winter (1979).

Braune and Fischer found a living subject whose external dimensions closely fitted one of their cadaver specimens (obviating the need to sacrifice the subject after gait analysis) and dressed him in a black suit with thin incandescent light tubes flashing at regular intervals to identify the centres of the joints and the centres of gravity of the body segments. They used four cameras to photograph him during level walking (Maquet 1992), producing stick figure images. They used glass photographic plates to minimise image distortion and a travelling microscope to digitise the positions of the images on the plates, achieving a level of accuracy still competitive with the most modern gait analysis systems.

From the observed movements in three dimensions of the centre of mass of the whole body and the assumed distribution of weight, they deduced the ground reaction force transmitted between ground and foot over the gait cycle. By considering the movements of each body segment in turn, they then calculated the resultant moment of the combined muscle, ligament and articular contact forces at the joints of the foot. This has been the main method of calculation ever since, called inverse dynamics, although the first step, calculation of the ground reaction forces, can be avoided when force-plates are used to acquire the data. The information provided by Braune and Fischer was so detailed that it has been used by subsequent research workers for other purposes: Pauwels used it to calculate hip joint forces (1935b) and Maquet (1984) to calculate knee joint forces during walking. Most recently, Woltring (1987) used it to show that the instantaneous helical axis (IHA) of the knee joint moves relative to the

both the femur and tibia during walking, confirming Borelli's observation (Chapter IX) that the knee is not a simple hinge.

Outstanding problems of gait analysis

Despite intensive development of gait analysis systems both by commercial firms and in research laboratories, there are still some fundamental problems that help to restrict clinical applications of these systems.

Presentation of results

First is the sheer volume of data that can be produced. A full gait analysis report using one of the current commercial systems can contain up to 60 separate graphs, with records over a single gait cycle of the angles of flexion/extension, abduction/adduction and axial rotation at the hips, knees and ankles, as well as the resultant moments of the internal forces about three axes and the powers generated (the product of moment and angular velocity) at each joint. The report may also contain graphs of the three components of the ground reaction force under each foot over the gait cycle and EMG signals from ten muscles. The practitioner has to learn the characteristic shapes of each graph in the normal subject and recognise deviations from those shapes that are typical of various pathologies. Similar sets of graphs can be obtained for every activity, stair climbing, rising from a chair, etc. Sutherland et al (1988) demonstrated the wide variation within each graph amongst the 'normal' population, making identification of pathology even more difficult.

The problem of data presentation can be helped by the use of computer graphics and animations. Very simple animations have been created in the form of moving stick figures generated by joining together the images of the marker balls on each body segment and these can be quite informative. More sophisticated animations, with images of the bones generated from computed tomographic (CT) scans and images of the muscles generated from magnetic resonance imaging (MRI) data, are under development (Chao et al 1997, Delp et al 1988, Lu et al 1998b), and can considerably aid the interpretation of data.

Skin movement

Locating the moving bones from the measured tracks of a set of surface-mounted markers is not a trivial problem. The California studies (Bresler & Frankel 1950) used markers screwed into the subjects' bones (under local anaesthetic), following more accurately the true movements of the bones. Skin-mounted markers move relative to the underlying bones, movements that introduce errors in the calculation of the results. Skin movement is, in part, systematic (Cappozzo et al 1996) and methods of minimising the errors are still being proposed (Lu & O'Connor 1999, Andriacchi & Alexander 2000).

Joint centres

Movements and moments are referred to joint centres. It is reasonably clear that the centre of the femoral head is the centre of the hip joint, about which the bones rotate relative to each other and from which the lengths of the lever-arms of the muscles spanning the joint should be measured. Various methods have been proposed to allow calculation of the position of the centre of the hip from the tracks of the surface markers; recently, a functional method based on circumduction exercises or a sequence of flexion/extension, abduction/adduction exercises has been shown to be most accurate (Leardini et al 1999c). The effects of errors in the location of the hip joint centre have been shown to have profound effects not only on the magnitudes of the moments at the hip, but also on the timing within the gait cycle of changes from flexing to extending moments, abducting to adducting (Stagni et al 2000).

Just what is meant by the centres of the knee and ankle is less clear. Conventionally, in gait analysis, the centre of the knee is taken to be a point fixed halfway between the medial and lateral epicondyles of the femur; the centre of the ankle is taken to be a point fixed midway between the malleoli. However, it has been known since Borelli that the axis of rotation of the knee translates and rotates relative to the bones; similar phenomena have recently been described at the ankle (Leardini et al 1999). Various methods have been proposed for calculating the angles of rotation at the joints that are consistent both with three-dimensional kinematic theory and with the classical descriptions given by anatomists (Grood & Suntay 1983, Cole et al 1993, Woltring 1994). Cheze (2000) showed these methods to be reasonably consistent with each other, apart from calculations of axial rotations. Treating knee and ankle joint centres as fixed makes difficult the study of the effects of ligament injuries in the form of excessive laxity or subluxation. Further developments of the mathematical models of the human musculoskeletal system are needed.

Calculation of muscle forces

Despite their importance as the main moderators of force distributions across the joints and in the bones, the muscle forces are rarely calculated in conventional gait analyses, which limit themselves to the calculation of the resultant moment of the combined muscle, ligament and contact forces at the joints. The main reason for this apparent omission is that the equations of geometry and mechanics are not, in themselves, sufficient to determine the firing sequence and phasing of muscles during activity.

Crowninshield & Brand (1981) stated that 47 muscles contribute to load transmission in each lower limb. Add to these the contact and ligament forces at the joints. While geometric models can determine the directions of the muscles tendons and ligaments spanning the joints and the directions of the contact forces at the knee and ankle (Lu et al 1998a), the total number of unknown forces at the hip, knee and ankle is nearly 60, whereas the total number of equations of mechanics for the foot, the shank and the thigh is only 18, i.e. six each. The locomotor system is therefore mechanically redundant. This implies that there is not a single unique combination of muscle, ligament and interarticular contact forces that can maintain a specified sequence of movements and transmit a specified system of loads. While this may be frustrating to the analyst of gait, it means that individuals can deploy a large number of strategies to accomplish a specified activity, an ability which is useful in the event of injury or disease. However, a study of EMG patterns suggests that normal gait is accomplished with a remarkably consistent pattern of muscle activity across the population.

Pauwels (1935b) used the work of Fick and of Braune & Fisher (1987) to calculate the compressive force acting on the hip during single leg stance. He assumed simultaneous activity of all the hip abductors, using Fick's values for their relative force contributions and also his coordinates of the origins and insertions of the individual muscles, to determine their lines of action relative to the centre of the hip.[1] He used Braune and Fisher's data to determine the position, velocity and acceleration of the centre of gravity of the upper body and suspended leg at a chosen moment during the stance phase of level walking. He then calculated the magnitude of the resultant muscle force and, thence, the contact force on the hip. He found a value of nearly four times body weight as opposed to one-third of body weight during symmetrical double leg support, a spectacular demonstration of the effects of muscle force and the principles enunciated by Leonardo and Borelli.

Paul (1965) used similar methods but performed his own gait analysis with two cinecameras, a force-plate and collection of EMG. He deduced the lines of action of the muscle forces by measuring the coordinates of their origins and insertions on a skeleton. He considered only the action of six muscle groups and, at any instant, calculated the values of only two, guided in his choice by the EMG signals. He found a peak resultant hip contact force of 5.8 times body weight occurring shortly after heelstrike. Morrison (1969) used a similar method of considering only a subset of the muscles to be active at any instant, guided by EMG, in his calculation of the resultant contact force acting at the knee joint during level walking. Procter & Paul (1982) applied similar techniques to the ankle. These are examples of the so-called Reduction method, reducing the number of forces to be calculated to the number of available equations of mechanics.

The alternative is to assume that neuromuscular control is directed towards some optimal choice of phasic muscle activity, particularly during learned motor activities. MacConaill (1967) proposed that 'No more total muscular force is used than is both necessary and sufficient for the task to be performed.' Numerous studies have investigated variants on this theme (Seireg & Arvikar 1973, Crowninshield & Brand 1981, Patriarco et al 1981). An alternative criterion, advanced by the Weber brothers (1836), is that humans walk to minimise energy expenditure (Nubar & Contini 1961).

Recently, we have pursued an approach first taken by Chao et al (1976) by which we calculated all possible sets of 18 unknown forces, rejecting any set in which any of the muscle or ligament forces prove to be compressive or any of the intra-articular contact forces prove to be tensile (Lu et al 1998b). These one-sided constraints greatly reduce the number of mechanically feasible sets of forces. These force sets identify the strategies available to a subject to perform a given movement in the presence of given external loads (Collins & O'Connor 1991). A multiplicity of strategies ensures that activity is possible even after injury to some of the muscles. Using a two-dimensional model of the locomotor system, Collins (1995) showed that this approach gives predictions of muscle phasic activity at least as consistent with EMG data as any of the optimisation procedures so far studied. Using a three-dimensional model, Lu (1997) and Lu et al (1997, 1998b) showed that calculations of the axial force in the proximal femur during a range of activities agree well with measurements telemetered from instrumented massive prostheses. There remains the question how the individual actually selects a particular pattern of muscle activity to accomplish a particular task.

Validation of results

Micro-electronics has made possible the development of instrumented implants, hip and knee prostheses, and internal fixation nails that makes practical the measurement of internal forces *in vivo*. These developments open up the possibility of the validation of the models of force transmission through the human which are a necessary part of gait analysis and could lead to their wider use in a clinical setting.

Clinical gait analysis

Despite the problems yet to be resolved, gait analysis is now used in hundreds of hospitals around the world to help in the assessment of patients and the planning of their treatment. Since Brand's rather depressing review of this work (1992), a number of papers have addressed directly the question whether additional useful information can be obtained. Nene et al (1993) and DeLuca et al (1997) demonstrated that gait analysis can contribute to the planning of the surgical treatment of spastic diplegic children, particularly when simultaneous multiple procedures are being planned, often guiding clinicians away from surgery which would otherwise be contemplated on the basis of a clinical assessment alone. Gait analysis is beginning to meet the Brand test outlined above.

FRIEDRICH PAUWELS

Friedrich Pauwels sought to extend his own understanding of musculoskeletal mechanics and to apply it in his treatment of disease or deformity. His work has largely been ignored in the non-German-speaking world, despite recent excellent translations by Paul Maquet and Roland Furlong (Pauwels 1976, 1980).

In the first of a series of papers, 1935–76, Pauwels (1935b) stated that 'Mechanical forces decisively influence the healing process of fracture of the neck of the femur. From this fact proceeds the possibility to establish concrete directions as to the prognosis and treatment of fractures of the neck of the femur, both recent and old.'

In that 1935 paper, he showed that previous standard treatments of femoral neck pseudarthroses did not work because they did not take mechanics into account. He devised an osteotomy to eliminate tension and shear forces from the pseudarthrosis, using Roux's argument that only compressive force was conducive to fracture repair. He used an analysis of the equilibrium of forces, with mechanical models and vector diagrams, to determine the optimum geometry (site and wedge angle) for the osteotomy. This paper set the pattern for much of his subsequent work: description of the preoperative state, surgical planning based on a mechanical analysis of the individual case together with an hypothesis about the ideal mechanical state to be created, postoperative radiograph and a minimum 2–3-year follow-up to validate the hypothesis. In contrast, in his penultimate paper (Pauwels 1975), he showed how a mild coxa vara resulting from a subtrochanteric fracture at birth and causing eccentric loading of the epiphyseal cartilage resolved without surgery because of increased bone growth on the more heavily loaded concave side until, at 5 years, physiological stressing had been restored, with similar subchondral condensation of bony tissue under both hips.

In the 1935 paper, Pauwels used data from Braune and Fischer's work to deduce that the compressive force acting on the femoral head during the stance phase of gait can reach four times body weight. He attributed this large force mainly to the muscle action needed to balance the horizontal components of the ground reaction force, which lie perpendicular to the limb. There are shades of Leonardo and Borelli.

Pauwels learnt the theory of elasticity and how to analyse stress and strain distributions in eccentrically (non-axially) loaded columns, which he compared with the long bones of the upper and lower limbs; some of his papers even quote the mathematical formulae. Later papers exploited photoelasticity, the technique relating the distribution of optical fringes in loaded birefringent materials to the distribution of stress (Fig. 6.1). A purely axial compressive force produces a uniform distribution of compressive stress in a uniform column; for a given cross-sectional area, the level of compressive stress is as small as possible. When a force of the same magnitude is applied eccentrically, parallel but not coincident with the axis of the column, the column bends as well as compressing and the stress varies from a maximum compressive value on the concave side to its maximum tensile value of the convex side. The maximum stresses with eccentric loading are much larger than with axial loading.

Pauwels used this knowledge in a variety of ways. On the theoretical side, in a series of papers published between 1948 and 1954 (Pauwels 1948, 1949, 1950a, b, 1954a–d), he showed how the shapes of the long bones were ideally adapted to minimise the bending moments and stresses which they transmit. Bending moments can be transmitted along the *limb* by a combination of tension forces in the muscles and axial compression forces in the bones, as demonstrated by Leonardo. However, Pauwels showed that this mechanism greatly reduced the levels of stress, both tensile and compressive, in the bones. Bi-articular muscles were particularly effective in this regard. The combination of muscle tension and bony compression has recently been referred to as the 'Pauwels Couple' (Lu et al 1997).

Where bending moments are unavoidable (as in the femoral neck), Pauwels (1973) showed how the

trabeculae were laid down to transmit either tension or compression. He proposed a very simple bone-remodelling law based on the hypothesis that bone prefers to transmit a certain optimum stress, either in tension or compression. When loaded above this optimum level, new bone forms to increase the load-bearing cross-sectional area appropriately; below this level, bone is resorbed. With this hypothesis, he showed how trabeculae, loaded eccentrically by a change in the loading such as after a fracture, can move and change direction until they are aligned with the new trajectories of the stresses, eliminating uneven stresses due to the presence of bending moments. Comparing the trajectories of the trabeculae in the proximal femur with photoelastic isostatics (or fringes), he concluded 'a cancellous structure constitutes a framework free from bending' with 'the elements of the cancellous bone all stressed axially in compression or tension'. When bending moments in tubular bone are unavoidable, cortical thickness can change, increasing to transmit compression at the optimal level on the concave side and decreasing to transmit optimal tension on the convex side.

On the practical side, one group of examples will suffice to demonstrate his approach: fracture repair of a tubular bone by grafting (Pauwels 1935a). Pauwels considered two cases: when the fragments remain in contact and when they are separated by a gap. Contacting fragments can transmit compressive stress but rotate apart under eccentric loading. A cortical bone graft placed on the concave side is stressed in bending with very high levels of stress, whereas, when placed on the convex side, it prevents rotation while transmitting minimal uniform tensile stress. In the presence of a gap between the fragments, two grafts placed on the convex and concave sides are loaded with minimal uniform tensile and compressive stress, respectively. When the tibia is used to provide the graft, Pauwels showed that secondary fractures must be expected or lengthy splinting of the tibia is necessary when the anterior crest is used as the graft whereas he allowed full weight-bearing after 8 days when he took the graft from the anteromedial cortex. He argued that removing the anterior cortex was akin to removing one of the flanges of an I-beam while removal of the anteromedial cortex merely reduced the thickness of the lightly loaded central web of the beam. He even advised removing the graft by drilling through its corners and using a reciprocating saw, avoiding the hairline fractures inevitable with the use of a chisel! From the theoretical to the practical.

Osteotomy

Correction of deformity by osteotomy has been a traditional practice in orthopaedic surgery (*opθos*, straight;

παιδιον, child). The use of gait analysis to guide the choice of osteotomy to correct developmental deformities in the cerebral palsy patient has been discussed above. This practice aims at creating more normal anatomy, and more normal geometry. McMurray (1935) described an intertrochanteric osteotomy for the treatment of osteoarthritis of the hip; Jackson & Waugh (1961) described a domed high tibial osteotomy for osteoarthritis of the knee. Neither description was based on a study of the mechanics of the joint and its surrounding muscles although Jackson and Waugh speculated that improvements resulting from the operation might be attributed to restoration of more normal mechanics. They noted the changes in trabecular architecture. Coventry (1965) described a wedge osteotomy for unicompartmental arthritis of the knee. His colleagues (Kettelkamp & Chao 1972) provided a general analysis of load sharing between medial and lateral compartments but the analysis of bicompartmental loading did not take account of muscle activity and it appears that the surgeons did not carry out this analysis for each individual patient. More recently, Chao & Sim (1995) provided a computer programme for preoperative planning.

The work of Pauwels and his pupil Maquet was based on detailed study of joint mechanics. For each patient, they chose the appropriate osteotomy based on weight-bearing radiographs. They defined clearly in advance the biomechanical changes to be effected and designed the bone cuts for each operation with meticulous care. Their use of osteotomy to treat osteoarthritic joints was based on the hypothesis that the disease develops when the load-bearing capacity of the cartilage falls below the level of the pressures it is required to transmit. Its progression can be halted and even reversed by reduction of those pressures. Since pressure is calculated by dividing force by area, Pauwels (1976) insisted that an increase in the effective weight-bearing area was as important an objective of surgical treatment as was reduction in load.

Pauwels studied force transmission through the normal hip during single leg stance. Using vector diagrams, he determined the line of action of the hip contact force in the coronal plane on the basis that not only must it pass through the centre of the femoral head, but also it must be concurrent with the lines of action of the hip abductors and the weight force of the proportion of the body supported by the planted limb. The former he obtained from radiographs, the latter from the anthropomorphic data of Braune & Fischer (1985).

Pauwels observed that the sclerotic line (which he termed the *sourcil*, the eyebrow) above the acetabulum in anteroposterior radiographs of normal hips is uniform in width, attributing its uniform thickness to a uniform distribution of compressive stress on the articular surfaces. He deduced that the uniform line implied (1) the line of action of the hip contact force passes through the centre of the weight-bearing area; (2) the presence of cartilage; and (3) a slight incongruence of the articular surfaces in the unloaded state.

On examining the radiographs of osteoarthritic hips, Pauwels observed three main forms of sclerosis associated with three forms of osteoarthritis (OA). Initially the line widens and develops a cup-like shape. Subsequent lateral subluxation with complete loss of joint space is accompanied by a triangular-shaped sclerosis concentrated at the lateral edge of the acetabulum, indicating a reduction in the effective weight-bearing area and an increase in contact pressure. A medial subluxation and loss of joint space has an associated triangular sclerosis and concentration of contact pressure in the depths of the acetabulum. A concentric OA is indicated by a concentric narrowing of the joint space as seen in a lateral view but with a uniform sclerotic line. Surgical alteration of the biomechanics proved successful when the OA was hypertrophic, with evidence of remodelling and osteophyte formation.

For concentric OA, Pauwels deduced that there was no associated reduction in the effective weight-bearing area and that the only option was to reduce the joint contact force by tenotomy, the so-called hanging hip operation. If neutral, abduction and adduction radiographs all demonstrated congruence of the joint surfaces, contact pressure could be reduced by tenotomy of adductor longus, gluteus medius and minimus, and iliopsoas, since the tendons of these muscles are directed more vertically and are mainly responsible for the development of compressive force at the hip. Loss of function may be thought to be one of the hazards of this operation. However, Maquet (1985) showed that with a minimum 3-year follow up, 60% of his patients could walk unlimited distances while another 33% could do so with the help of a stick.

For the laterally or medially subluxed hip, Pauwels proposed varus or valgus intertrochanteric osteotomy. For the former, an abduction radiograph had to confirm that joint congruence could be achieved, while congruence should be seen in an adduction radiograph in the latter. With this vital condition satisfied, Pauwels showed by using vector diagrams that the lever-arm of the abductor muscles could be increased, the magnitudes of the muscle and joint contact forces decreased but, vitally, that the line of action of the joint contact force could be brought back into the centre of the congruent contact area. The angle of the wedge of bone to be removed was determined using vector diagrams traced on the radiograph images from individual patients.

To supplement the increase in lever-arm achieved by a varus osteotomy, Maquet (1985) added a subsequent lateral displacement of the greater trochanter in cases with a short femoral neck and a relatively high greater trochanter.

Joint space, lost during the progression of the disease, was seen to be recovered in many of these patients, presumably by the growth of fibrous tissue layers on the articular surfaces. Maquet's (1985) review of 174 cases at 10-year minimum follow up showed that 73% were pain-free, had a normal range of movement and could walk unlimited distances, while all of the remainder had been improved by the operation, 88% being described as good or excellent.

Maquet (1984) applied similar ideas to the treatment of osteoarthritis of the knee joint. He gave a comprehensive analysis of the biomechanics of the joint in the coronal plane and in the sagittal plane. Whereas the line of action of the contact force at the hip has to pass through the centre of the femoral head, a point fixed in the pelvis as well as the femur, analysis of the knee is more difficult because the joint contact force can pass through any point on the flexion axis. Unlike proponents of the wedge type osteotomy of the proximal tibia, he took full account of the force in the iliotibial tract and demonstrated that, in the normal knee during single leg stance, the line of action of the contact force passes centrally between the medial and lateral condyles and is transmitted over the largest possible contact areas in both compartments, taking account of the load-bearing function of the menisci. He attributed the uniform, thin sclerotic lines found under both compartments in radiographs of the normal knee to a uniform distribution of pressure in the two compartments. Similarly, local concentrations of sclerosis, often with a loss of trabecular structures elsewhere, were attributed to stress concentrations in one compartment or the other, or in the patellofemoral joint, arising from osteoarthritic changes. He described a range of osteotomies aimed at recentralising the joint contact force, diminishing its magnitude by increasing the lengths of muscle lever-arms, and, where possible, maximising the effective areas of contact between the articular surfaces. His anterior displacement of the tibial tubercle was found, alone, to be effective in the treatment of tricompartmental osteoarthritis.

The accumulated experience of Pauwels and Maquet shows that the effects of the disease can be reversed by adjustment of the biomechanics. It may be suggested that the effects achieved were a consequence of more biological factors triggered by the operations: improvement in vascularity, re-initiation of a growth-like process, etc. Maquet (1984) described the treatment of patients with unicompartmental arthritis of the knee, which developed as a consequence of deformities, induced at a distance from the joint, by a malaligned hip arthrodesis or proximal femoral fracture, with demonstrably abnormal knee mechanics. Correction of the deformity at hip level and of knee mechanics resulted in improvement of symptoms and re-establishment of joint space at knee level.

However, osteotomies have not been able to compete with total hip and knee replacements, which can be implanted without any knowledge or understanding of vector diagrams on the part of the surgeon. A recent review (Stukenborg-Colsman et al 2001) compared the outcome of high tibial osteotomy of the Coventry type with unicompartmental arthroplasty in a randomised clinical trial. It was found that the survival rate 7–10 years postoperatively, based on the need for further surgery, was better with the arthroplasty, although the prosthesis used has been found to have significantly lower survival rates than some other designs.

JOINTS

Lubrication

The phenomenally low friction exhibited by healthy joints has attracted the attention of anatomists, engineers and physicists for generations. William Hunter (1743) wrote of the bone ends in articulating joints: 'Both are covered with a smooth crust, to prevent natural abrasion; connected with strong ligaments to prevent dislocation; and enclosed in a bag that contains a proper fluid deposited there, for lubricating the two contiguous surfaces.'[2] Failure of the lubricating mechanism could be a contributing factor in the failure of cartilage and the development of osteoarthritis. Understanding that mechanism could have application to the design of artificial joints.

Reynolds (1866) established the theory of hydrodynamic lubrication. MacConaill (1932) suggested that the joints of the skeleton used a hydrodynamic lubrication mechanism, similar to that achieved in journal bearings, where shear stress gradients through the thickness of the synovial fluid layer separating the articular surfaces were balanced by pressure gradients across the region of contact, thus allowing higher pressures in the gap between the surfaces than in the surroundings and making possible the support of load across the fluid film. Viscosity of the synovial fluid is therefore critical. However, the calculated layer thickness (about 1 μm) was significantly smaller than the asperity height on the surface of hyaline cartilage (2–6 cm), so that complete separation of the surfaces would not be achieved and boundary lubrication would occur. The work of Dowson (1990) and his group in studying the possibility of elastohydrodynamic lubrication (in which deformation of the contacting surfaces plays an important role in the mechanism and increasing load results in increased deformation of the surfaces as well as decreased thickness of the lubricating layer) was eventually rewarded (Dowson & Jin 1986) when they realised that the asperities themselves would flatten under pressure so that a fluid layer, calculated to be only 0.75 μm thick, could nonetheless keep the cartilage surfaces fully apart.

An alternative theory, squeeze-film lubrication, suggested that the lubricating fluid was actually squeezed out of the cartilage layers in contact, cartilage consisting of roughly 80% water held within a collagen network. Mow et al (1987) modelled cartilage as a biphasic layer with fluid transport through a permeable solid matrix. They studied the squeeze-film mechanism (Hou et al 1990) and demonstrated that fluid film thickness was determined by a balance between the rate of fluid imbibed by the cartilage layers in the pressurised region under the load, the rate of its exudation outside the pressurised region and the rate at which the bones approached each other. When load is applied suddenly, several seconds are required to reduce the fluid film thickness to about 1 μm.

Putting these two theories together provides an attractive scenario in which the squeeze-film mechanism deals with the start-up period as load is applied and motion begins and the micro-elastohydrodynamic mechanism operates as the surfaces slide on each other. Dowson (1990) further suggested that artificial joints could be designed to exploit the elastohydrodynamic mechanism by covering their relatively rigid articulating surfaces with compliant layers which enable the elasto-element of the lubrication process to be easily established while providing some squeeze-film action during start-up. A prosthesis embodying this mechanism has not yet appeared.

Kinematics and mechanics

Although all diarthrodial joints utilise the same tissues, more or less as described by Hunter (see above), there are very considerable difference between joints both in the range of movement allowed and in the degrees of freedom and patterns of movement exhibited. Compare the very limited movements possible at the distal interphalangeal joints of the fingers and the wide range of movement allowed at the shoulder. If we were to divide all the soft tissues that hold the tibia to the femur at the knee, we would have given the tibia six degrees of

freedom relative to the femur, unrestricted freedom to rotate about each of three perpendicular axes and unrestricted freedom to translate along each of those axes. The passive structures of joints, the ligaments, the capsule and the articular surfaces suppress most of those degrees of freedom and limit possible movement to a very limited range.

In activity, the joints allow motion under load. In discussing the kinematics and mechanics of joints, it is helpful to distinguish between the way the passive structures interact to allow and control mobility and the way they interact together and with the muscles to resist motion and control stability. It is helpful to distinguish between passive stability, when only the passive structures are involved in resisting motion, as in the drawer test, and active stability when muscle action is used to allow an otherwise unstable skeleton to stand and perform various activities under load. To stand under gravity, muscle action is used to suppress motion at the joints.

Utilising the power of modern computers, several mathematical models of the knee joint have recently been developed that simulate motion under load (Andriacchi et al 1983, Essenger et al 1989, Blankevoort et al 1991), but which may seem difficult to understand and to exploit in clinical practice. In particular, the role of the ligaments in limiting and controlling motion is still not universally acknowledged. Some surgeons take pains to reconstruct the damaged or ruptured ligaments in a young athlete while happily sacrificing the same ligaments when performing a joint replacement in an older patient. Classification of joints according to the shapes of the surfaces alone (Huson 1987) does not bring out the complementary roles of the ligaments.

The ball-and-socket nature of the hip constrains relative motion of the femur and the pelvis to possible rotations about three axes through the centre of the femoral head, the joint centre. The soft tissues serve to hold the bones in contact, suppressing the translatory freedoms of the joint centre, which therefore remains fixed relative to both bones. The hip allows the bones three independent degrees of freedom. Kapandji (1970) demonstrated that the ligaments separately tighten only at the limits of motion and are otherwise slack. The hip, however, seems to be the exception rather than the rule. Most other joints are much more constrained. We will use the knee as the basis of discussion.

The articular surfaces of the knee are of dissimilar non-conforming shapes although it has been realised only recently (Seedhom et al 1974, Walker & Erkman 1975, Shrive et al 1978, Maquet 1984) that the menisci transmit a large proportion of the compressive load across the articulation, a realisation which has prompted the surgical repair of a damaged meniscus as a desirable alternative to meniscectomy. Borelli (1680) described the backwards motion of the menisci on the tibial plateau during flexion and their forwards motion during extension, a description confirmed most spectacularly by Thompson et al (1991) using MRI. The menisci are a pair of mobile and deformable bearings that bring the articular surfaces into effective conformity over the range of motion.

Weber & Weber (1836) described how the femoral condyles roll backwards on the tibia during flexion and forwards again during extension. Meyer (1853) described the so-called screw-home mechanism, the coupling of axial rotation with flexion, the tibia rotating internally on the femur about 30° during 100° of flexion. The question arises how these movements are controlled and guided. Many authors have suggested that these movements are a consequence of the polycentric polyradial shapes of the femoral condyles. In mechanical engineering, low-friction surfaces are guided to move on each other by interdigitating them together with cams or gear teeth or by linking the contacting bodies together to form a single degree of freedom mechanism, such as the crossed four-bar Chebychev mechanism, which produces pure rolling between two low friction surfaces. In many of the joints of the skeleton, the ligaments connecting the bones form such a mechanism.

Brantigan and Voshell (1941) summarised the totally confused state of knowledge about ligament function at that time. The first page of their paper finds ten references in the literature to support each of three propositions about different ligament fascicles in the knee: that the fascicle tightens during flexion; that it slackens during flexion; that it remains isometric during flexion. It is hardly possible to insert an instrument into a ligament that will resolve the matter beyond dispute, but modern methods of instrumentation have been developed that allow the relative movements of the bones to be measured with precision so that, using modern three-dimensional kinematic theory (Cole et al 1993), it is possible to calculate how any point on the surface of origin of a ligament moves relative to any point on its insertion. Using such techniques, Sapega et al (1990) found that the anteromedial fascicle of the Anterior Cruciate Ligament (ACL) remains more or less isometric during passive flexion whereas all other fibres progressively slacken until 90 degrees when they begin to tighten again. The same group found that the more anterior fibres of the Posterior Cruciate Ligament (PCL) are slack in extension but tighten progressively during flexion whereas the more posterior fibres are tight in extension and slacken progressively with flexion. This leaves open the possibility that between these two groups of fibres lies one which remains isometric during passive flexion/extension. These observations and deductions justify the insight of Zuppinger (1904), who proposed that the two bones and two isometric cruciate ligament fibres form a crossed four-bar linkage that controls and guides the movements of the bones on each other. Four-bar linkage theory has been rediscovered by Menschik (1974), Huson (1974) and Goodfellow & O'Connor (1978). It explains why the flexion axis of the joint moves backwards during flexion and forwards during extension. It demonstrates how the shapes of the articular surfaces are compatible with the ligaments in the sense that the ligaments keep the surfaces in contact while the surfaces keep certain fibres within the ligaments isometric over the range of motion. A substantial range of motion is achieved because those fibres can *rotate* about their origins and insertions without stretching or slackening while the articular surfaces roll as well as slide on each other. Unresisted passive motion can be achieved without straining the ligaments or indenting the articular surfaces.

An extension to this theory was described by Zavatsky & O'Connor (1992) and Lu & O'Connor (1996a). Each of the four principal ligaments at the knee joint was represented as an array of fibres joining the bones. As the joint flexes and extends, the attachment areas of the ligaments rotate towards each other and away from each other so that all but the isometric fibres slacken and tighten in a manner quantitatively similar to the descriptions given by Sapega et al (1990). Lu & O'Connor (1996b) showed that the rotations of the model ligament bundles about their insertions on the tibia, and the associated rotations of the origins and insertions of the model muscle tendons are quantitatively similar to the results of measurements made by Hertzog & Read (1993) on cadaver specimens.

Slack ligament fibres are hardly effective load-bearing structures. However, Zavatsky & O'Connor (1992) and Lu & O'Connor (1996a) showed how slack fibres are progressively recruited and the ligaments progressively tighten to transmit increasing load. Huss et al (1999) showed how the passive laxity of the model knee during the drawer test involves a progressive stretch of the ligaments and indentation of the articular surfaces. Thus, mobility is achieved because the ligaments can rotate and the surfaces can roll and slide. Passive stability is achieved because the ligaments can stretch to develop tension forces and the articular surfaces indent to develop compression forces. In activity, both these effects occur simultaneously.

In activity, when muscles apply their forces, Huss et al (2000) showed how increasing load produces forwards or backwards sliding of the tibia on the femur but at a diminishing rate until a configuration is reached where increasing shear forces applied by increasing external loads are balanced by matched components of the muscle forces parallel to the tibial plateau, without further stretch of the ligaments. This explains why the very large loads applied by athletes during extreme activity can be transmitted across the knee without ligament rupture, the ligaments forces remaining relatively small.

While satisfactory experimental confirmation of much of the predictions of the four-bar linkage theory has been found, there is the obvious limitation that the theory is two-dimensional and limited to events in the sagittal plane. Wilson et al (1998) described the three-dimensional analogue of the four-bar linkage model in which isometric fibres in the two cruciates and the medial collateral ligament, together with continuous contact in both medial and lateral compartments, represent five constraints to motion, reducing six possible degrees of freedom to one. Thus, axial rotation is uniquely coupled to flexion, a theory that explains the screw-home mechanism described by Meyer (1853). Modelling the knee as a three-dimensional single-degree of freedom mechanism was justified by the mobility experiments of Wilson et al (2000), which demonstrated the coupling of axial rotation, abduction/adduction and the three components of translation of a chosen point on the femur to flexion angle.

Leardini et al (1999a, 2000) recently showed that the ankle, although a closely conforming joint, behaves in a very similar fashion to the knee and that it can be modelled theoretically in the same way (Leardini et al 1999b). These observations leave open the possibility of using theoretical models as the basis for the design of new prostheses, which will be fully compatible with the geometry of the ligaments.

Mechanical factors in osteoarthrosis

We have discussed the effects of limb malalignment and abnormal biomechanics on the development of osteoarthritis of the hip and knee and the reversal of the effects of the disease using precise osteotomy to re-establish more normal biomechanics. The proponents of osteotomy attribute development of the disease to a failure of cartilage to transmit the loads applied to it, either because of degradation in the mechanical properties of the tissues or overloading and reduction in effective contact area caused by malalignment. While even the most biologically based discussions of the disease recognise a role for mechanical loading in its aetiology (Archer et al 1999), the particular aspects of loading (magnitude, frequency, loading rate) that contribute to cartilage failure remain controversial.

Radin & Paul (1971) suggested that loading *rate* is important. This is an attractive proposition since it would explain why only a proportion of the population is affected by the disease since loading rate is a variable across the population. The entire population transmits large loads through the lower limb joints when running, rising from a chair or climbing and descending stairs so that load magnitude, alone, is less likely to be responsible for cartilage failure. Heelstrike during walking results in repeated rapidly applied loads. Radin & Paul (1971) demonstrated that a group of volunteers with preclinical knee pain had a significantly higher loading rate at heelstrike than a group of age- and sex-matched pain-free volunteers. The localisation of the lesion to the distal femoral condyle and the front half of the tibial plateau in medial osteoarthritis of the knee (White et al 1991), the surfaces which are in contact in extension and therefore at heelstrike, provides some clinical corroboration for the hypothesis. Gill (1996) showed theoretically that minor differences in the timing of the onset of hamstrings and quadriceps action during the swing phase of walking critically affects the vertical downwards velocity of the foot at heelstrike and therefore of the rate of loading. Since walking is a learned activity, it may be possible to identify the young adults with high loading rates and, with biofeedback, to teach them to reduce their loading rates. This hypothesis is not necessarily in conflict with recent evidence (Chapman et al 2000) that there is a genetic link in the incidence of OA. It has been known for some time that there are racial differences in the prevalence of the disease, 7% in Chinese women in the age group 55–64, 15% in Caucasian women in the same age group (Hoaglund et al 1973). Chen et al (2000) recently showed that the loading rate at heelstrike in Chinese women in that age group is significantly lower than that of similarly aged Caucasian women. It could well be that the genetic link lies in associated patterns of walking.

THE FUTURE

Is orthopaedic biomechanics rather old-fashioned and unlikely to contribute further to orthopaedic practice? Is the future with more microbiologically based work? It is my opinion that there are still quite relevant questions for the engineer to answer.

Alfaro-Adrian et al (2001) recently reported the results of migration studies observed by Roentgenstereophotogrammatic Analysis (RSA) at 1–2 years follow up of two different designs of hip replacement implanted by the same surgical teams. They found consistent differences in the patterns of migration with the two designs, particularly in the axes of axial rotation about which the implants rotated relative to the bone. An explanation for these differences is not obvious and requires a more complete understanding of load transmission across the interfaces of the different prostheses. The large body of work carried out so far in this area (Huiskes & Verdonschot 1997) is still too general, using much simplified models of the bones and their loading, to explain the differences (Polgar et al 2001). However, with modern methods of screening (RSA, MRI, fluoroscopy) and with the ability to implant instrumented prostheses, bone nails, spinal discs, etc. and to telemeter the collected data from living patients during various activities, it will become possible to refine our understanding of musculoskeletal mechanics on a patient-by-patient basis. It may then be possible to devise a range of preclinical and early clinical analyses that would allow more precise and reliable evaluation of novel implants to avoid the disasters that continue to occur and which involve thousands of patients (Muirhead-Allwood 1999). With these new tools, orthopaedic biomechanics has entered an exciting new era with direct application to surgical practice.

REFERENCES

Abbott L C, Saunders J Bd C M 1939 The operative lengthening of the tibia and the fibula. A preliminary report on the further development of the principles and technique. Ann Surg 110: 961–991

Alfaro-Adrian J, Gill H S, Murray D W 2001 Should THR femoral components be designed to subside? A RSA study of the Charnely Elite and Exeter stems. J Arthroplasty 16: 598–606

Andriacchi T P, Alexander E J 2000 Studies of human locomotion: past, present and future. J Biomech 33: 1217–1224

Andriacchi T P, Mikosz R P, Hampton S J, Galante J O 1983 Model studies of the stiffness characteristics of the human knee joint. J Biomech 16: 23–29

Archer C W, Caterson B, Benjamin M, Ralphs J R (eds) Biology of the Synovial Joint. Overseas Publishers Association, Amsterdam

Basmajian J V, De Luca C J 1985 Muscles Alive, 5th edn. Williams & Wilkins, Baltimore

Bergmann G, Graichen F, Rohlmann A 1993 Hip joint loading during walking and running, measured in two patients. J Biomech 26: 969–990

Bergmann G, Graichen F, Rohlmann A, Linke H 1997 Hip joint forces during load carrying. Clin Orthop 335: 190–201

Bernstein N 1934 The techniques of the study of movements. In: Couradi G, Forfel V, Slonim A (eds) Textbook of the Physiology of Work. Moscow

Bertram J E A, Swartz S M 1991 The 'Law of Bone Transformation': a case of crying Wolff? Biol Rev 66: 245–273

Blankevoort L, Kuiper J H, Huiskes R, Grootenboer H J 1991 Articular contact in a three-dimensional model of the knee. J Biomech 24: 1019–1031

Boorstin D J 1983 The Discoverers. Random House, New York

Borelli G A 1680 De motu animalium. Rome

Bouisset S 1992 Etienne-Jules Marey, or when motion biomechanics emerged as a science. In: Cappozzo A, Marchetti M, Tosi V (eds) Biolocomotion: A Century of Research using Moving Pictures. Promograph, Rome, pp 71–88

Bourgery J M 1832 Traite complet de l'anatomie de l'homme. I, Osteologie, Paris

Bradley G W, McKenna G B, Dunn H K, Daniels A U, Statton W O 1979 Effects of flexural rigidity of plates on bone healing. J Bone Joint Surg 61A: 866–872

Brand R A 1992 Assessment of musculoskeletal disorders by locomotion analysis: a critical historical and epistemological review. In: Cappozzo A, Marchetti M, Tosi V (eds) Biolocomotion: A Century of Research Using Moving Pictures. Promograph, Rome, pp 227–241

Brantigan O C, Voshell A F 1941 The mechanics of the ligaments and menisci of the knee joint. J Bone Joint Surg 23A: 44–66

Braune W, Fischer O 1985 On the Centre of Gravity of the Human Body. Springer, Berlin

Braune W, Fischer O 1987 The Human Gait. Springer, Berlin

Braune W, Fischer O 1988 Determination of the Moments of Inertia of the Human Body and its Limbs. Springer, Berlin

Bresler B, Frankel J P 1950 The forces and moment in the leg during level walking. Trans Amer Soc Mech Engnrs 72: 27–36

Cappozzo A, Catani F, Leardini A, Benedetti M G, Della Croce U 1996 Position and orientation in space of bones during movement: experimental artefacts. Clin Biomech 11: 90–100

Carter D R, Beaupre G S, Giori N J, Helms J A 1998 Mechanobiology of skeletal regeneration. Clin Orthop 355 (suppl.): S41–55

Chao E Y, Barrance P, Genda E, Iwasaki N, Kato S, Faust A 1997 Virtual reality (VR) techniques in orthopaedic research and practice. Stud Health Technol Inform 39: 107–114

Chao E Y, Hoffman R R 1978 Instrumented measurement of human joint motion. ISA Trans 17: 13–19

Chao EY, Opgrande J D, Axmear F E 1976 Three-dimensional force analysis of finger joints in selected isometric hand functions. J Biomech 9: 387–396

Chao E Y, Sim F H 1995 Computer-aided preoperative planning in knee osteotomy. Iowa Orthop J 15: 4–18

Chapman K, Mustafa Z, Irven C, Carr A J, Clipsham K, Smith A et al 2000 Osteoarthritis susceptibility locus on Chromosome 11q, detected by linkage. Am J Hum Genet 65: 165–174

Chen W L, O'Connor J J, Radin E L 2001 Comparison of the gait of Chinese and Caucasian women with particular reference to their heelstrike transients. Clin Biomech (submitted)

Cheze L 2000 Comparison of different calculations of three-dimensional joint kinematics from video-based system data. J Biomech 33: 1695–1699

Clarys J P, Lewillie L 1992 Clinical and kinesiological electromyography by le Dr. Duchenne (de Boulogne). In: Cappozzo A, Marchetti M, Tosi V (eds) Biolocomotion: A Century of Research Using Moving Pictures. Promograph, Rome, pp 89–114

Codivilla A 1905 Means of lengthening in the lower limbs, the muscles and tissues which are shortened by deformity. Am J Orthop Surg 2: 353–369

Cole G K, Nigg B M, Ronsky J L, Yeadon M R 1993 Application of the joint coordinate system to three-dimensional joint attitude and movement representation: a standardization proposal. J Biomech Eng 115: 344–349

Collins J J 1995 The redundant nature of locomotor optimization laws. J Biomech 28: 251–267

Collins J J, O'Connor J J 1991 Muscle-ligament interactions at the knee during walking. Proc Inst Mech Eng [H] 205: 11–18

Contini R 1972 Body segment parameters, Part II. Artificial Limbs 16: 1–19

Coventry M B 1965 Osteotomy of the upper tibia for degenerative arthritis of the knee. J Bone Joint Surg 47A: 984

Crowninshield R D, Brand R A 1981 A physiologically based criterion of muscle force prediction in locomotion. J Biomech 14: 793–801

Culmann C 1862 Die Graphische Statik. Zurich

Delp S L, Arnold A S, Piazza S J 1998 Graphics-based modeling and analysis of gait abnormalities. Biomed Mater Eng 8: 227–240

DeLuca P A, Davis R B, Ounpuu S, Rose S, Sirkin R 1997 Alterations in surgical decision making in patients with cerebral palsy based on three-dimensional gait analysis. J Pediatr Orthop 17: 608–614

Dempster W T 1955 Space Requirements for the Seated Operator. Report No. WADC-TR-55-159. Wright Patterson Airforce Base

Dowson D 1990 Bio-tribology of synovial joints. In: Mow V C, Ratcliffe A, Woo S L-Y (eds) Biomechanics of Synovial Joints. Springer, New York, pp 305–345

Dowson D, Jin Z 1986 Micro-elastohydrodynamic lubrication of synovial joints. Eng Med 15: 63–65

Drillis R, Contini R 1966 Body Segment Parameters. Report No. 1163-03. Office of Vocational Rehabilitation, Department of Health, Education and Welfare, New York

Egerton J (ed) George Stubbs, Anatomist and Portrait Painter. Tate Gallery, London

Essenger J R, Leyvraz P F, Heegard J H, Robertson D D 1989 A mathematical model for the evaluation of the behaviour during flexion of condylar-type knee prostheses. J Biomech 22: 1229–1241

Fritton S P, McLeod K J, Rubin C T 2000 Quantifying the strain history of bone: spatial uniformity and self-similarity of low-magnitude strains. J Biomech 33: 317–325

Fung Y C 1993 Biomechanics: Mechanical Properties of Living Tissues, 2nd edn. Springer, New York

Furnee E H 1967 Hybrid instrumentation in prosthetics research. In: 7th International Conference on Medical and Biological Engineering, Stockholm

Gill H S 1996 The mechanics of heelstrike during level walking. DPhil, University of Oxford

Goodfellow J, O'Connor J 1978 The mechanics of the knee and prosthesis design. J Bone Joint Surg 60B: 358–369

Goodship A E, Kenwright J 1985 The influence of induced micromovement upon the healing of experimental tibial fractures. J Bone Joint Surg 67B: 650–655

Grood E S, Suntay W J 1983 A joint coordinate system for the clinical description of three-dimensional motions: application to the knee. J Biomech Eng 105: 136–144

Herzog W, Read L J 1993 Lines of action and moment arms of the major force-carrying structures crossing the human knee joint. J Anat 182: 213–230

Hoaglund F T, Yau A C M C, Wong W L 1973 Osteoarthritis of the hip and other joints in Southern Chinese in Hong Kong. J Bone Joint Surg 55A: 545–557

Hou J S, Holmes M H, Lai W M, Mow V C 1990 Squeeze film lubrication for articular cartilage with synovial fluid. In: Mow V C, Ratcliffe A, Woo S L-Y (eds) Biomechanics of Diarthrodial Joints. Springer, New York, pp 347–367

Huiskes R, Verdonschot N 1997 Biomechanics of artificial joints: the hip. In: Mow V C, Hayes W C (eds) Basic Orthopaedic Biomechanics, 2nd edn. Lippincott-Raven, Philadelphia, pp 395–460

Huiskes R, Weinans H, van Rietbergen B 1992 The relationship between stress shielding and bone resorption around total hip stems and the effects of flexible materials. Clin Orthop 274: 124–134

Hunter W 1743 Of the structure and diseases of articulating cartilages. Phil Trans 42: 514

Huson A 1974 Biomechanische probleme des kniegelenks. Orthopade 3

Huson A 1987 Joints and movements of the foot: terminology and concepts. Acta Morphol Neerl Scand 25: 117–130

Huss R A, Holstein H, O'Connor J J 1999 The effect of cartilage deformation on the laxity of the knee joint. Proc Inst Mech Eng [H] 213: 19–32

Huss R A, Holstein H, O'Connor J J 2000 A mathematical model of forces in the knee under isometric quadriceps contractions. Clin Biomech 15: 112–122

Inman V T, Ralston H J, Todd F 1981 Human Walking. Williams & Wilkins, Baltimore

Jackson J P, Waugh W 1961 Tibial osteotomy for osteoarthritis of the knee. J Bone Joint Surg 43B: 746–751

Jarrett M O, Andrews B J, Paul J P 1974 Quantitative analysis of locomotion using television. In: World Congress of IS PO, INTER BOR & APO. Montreaux

Kapandji I A 1970 The Physiology of the Joints, Churchill Livingstone, Edinburgh

Karpovitch P V, Herden E L, Maxim M A 1960 Electrogoniometric study of joints. US Armed Forces Med J 11

Keele K D 1977 Leonardo da Vinci, the anatomist. In: Leonardo da Vinci, Anatomical Drawings from the Royal Collection. Royal Academy of Arts, London, pp 13–21

Kenwright J, White S H 1993 A historical review of limb lengthening and bone transport. Injury (suppl. 2): S9–S19

Kettelkamp D B, Chao E Y 1972 A method for quantitative analysis of medial and lateral compression forces at the knee during standing. Clin Orthop 83: 202–213

Lanyon L E, Rubin C T 1984 Static vs dynamic loads as an influence on bone remodelling. J Biomech 17: 897–905

Leardini A, Cappozzo A, Catani F, Toksvig-Larsen S, Petitto A, Sforza V et al 1999c Validation of a functional method for the estimation of hip joint centre location. J Biomech 32: 99–103

Leardini A, O'Connor J J, Catani F, Giannini S 1999a Kinematics of the human ankle complex in passive flexion; a single degree of freedom system. J Biomech 32: 111–118

Leardini A, O'Connor J J, Catani F, Giannini S 1999b A geometric model of the human ankle joint. J Biomech 32: 585–591

Leardini A, O'Connor J J, Catani F, Giannini S 2000 The role of the passive structures in the mobility and stability of the human ankle joint: a literature review. Foot Ankle Int 21: 602–615

Ling R S M, O'Connor J J, Lu T-W, Lee A J C 1996 Muscular activity and the biomechanics of the hip. Hip International 6: 91–105

Lu T-W 1997 Geometric and mechanical modelling of the human locomotor system. DPhil, University of Oxford

Lu T-W, O'Connor J J 1996a Fibre recruitment and shape changes of knee ligaments during motion: as revealed by a computer graphics-based model. Proc Inst Mech Eng [H] 210: 71–79

Lu T-W, O'Connor J J 1996b Lines of action and moment arms of the major force-bearing structures crossing the human knee joint: comparison between theory and experiment. J Anat 189: 575–585

Lu T-W, O'Connor J J 1999 Bone position estimation from skin marker co-ordinates using global optimisation with joint constraints. J Biomech 32: 129–134

Lu T-W, O'Connor J J, Taylor S J, Walker P S 1998a Validation of a lower limb model with in vivo femoral forces teleme-tered from two subjects. J Biomech 31: 63–69

Lu T-W, Taylor S J, O'Connor J J, Walker P S 1997 Influence of muscle activity on the forces in the femur: an in vivo study. J Biomech 30: 1101–1106

Lu T-W, O'Connor J J, Taylor S J G, Walker P S 1998b Comparison of telemetered femoral forces with model calculations. In: European Society of Biomechanics, J Biomech, Toulouse, p 47

MacConaill M A 1967 Studies in neurological structure VII. Polyneuronal mapping and discrimination. Irish J Med Sci 6: 243–256

MacConaill M A 1932 The function of intra-articular carti-lages, with special reference to the knee and inferior radio-ulnar joints. J Anat 66: 210–227

Maquet P G J 1984 Biomechanics of the Knee. Springer, Berlin

Maquet P G J 1985 Biomechanics of the Hip. Springer, Berlin

Maquet P G J 1992 The 'Human Gait' by Braune and Fischer. In: Cappozzo A, Marchetti M, Tosi V (eds) Biolocomotion: A Century of Research Using Moving Pictures. Promograph, Rome, pp 115–126

Marey E-J 1873 La machine animale. Librairie Germer Bailliere, Paris

Marey E-J 1883 De la mesure dans les differents actes de la locomotion. CR Acad Sci Paris 97: 820–825

Marey E-J 1885 Developpement de la methode graphique par l'emploi de la Photographie. G. Masson, Paris

McMurray T P 1935 Osteoarthritis of the hip joint. Br J Surg 22: 716

Menschik A 1974 Mechanik des Kniegelenkes. Z Orthop 112: 481

Meyer H 1853 Die mechanik des Kniegelenkes. Arch Anat Physiol 497

Morris J R W 1973 Accelerometry – a technique for the meas-urement of human body movements. J Biomech 6: 729–736

Morrison J B 1969 Function of the knee joint in various activ-ities. Biomed Eng 4: 573–580

Mow V C, Hayes W C (eds) 1997 Basic Orthopaedic Biomechanics, 2nd edn. Lippincott-Raven, Philadelphia

Muirhead-Allwood S K 1999 Lessons of a hip failure. Br Med J 316: 644

Muybridge E 1882 The Horse in Motion, As Seen by Instantaneous Photography. London

Nene A V, Evans G A, Patrick J H 1993 Simultaneous multiple operations for spastic diplegia: outcome and functional assessment of walking in 18 patients. J Bone Joint Surg 75B: 488–494

Nigg B M, Herzog W (eds) 1998 Biomechanics of the Musculo-Skeletal System, 2nd edn. Wiley, New York

Nubar Y, Contini R 1961 A minimal principal in biomechanics. Bull Math Biophys 23: 377–391

O'Malley C D, Saunders J Bd C M (eds) 1983 Leonardo on the Human Body. Dover, New York

Patriarco A G, Mann R W, Simon S R, Mansour J M 1981 An evaluation of the approaches of optimization models in the prediction of muscle forces during human gait. J Biomech 14: 513–525

Paul J P 1965 Bio-engineering studies of the forces transmitted by joints, Part (II): Engineering analysis. In: Kenedi R M (ed) Biomechanics and Related Bio-engineering Topics. Pergamon, Oxford, pp 369–380

Pauwels F 1935a Biomechanics of bone grafting. Acta Orthop Belg 37: 701–725

Pauwels F 1935b The fracture of the femoral neck. A mechanical problem. Z Orthop 63(suppl.)

Pauwels F 1948 The principles of construction of the loco-motor system. Their significance for the stressing of the tubular bones. Z Anat Entwickl Gesch 114: 129–166

Pauwels F 1949 The mechanical significance of the gross structure of the cortex in normal and pathologically bent tubular bones. Anat Nachr 1: 53–67

Pauwels F 1950a Principles of construction of the lower extremity. Their significance for the stressing of the skeleton of the leg. Z Anat Entwickl Gesch 114: 525–538

Pauwels F 1950b Significance of the muscular forces for the regulation of the stressing of the tubular bones during movement of the limb. Z Anat Entwickl Gesch 115: 327–351

Pauwels F 1954a Critical examination of the work of Roux: 'Description and explanation of a bony ankylosis of the knee'. Z Anat Entwickl Gesch 117: 528–552

Pauwels F 1954b The static significance of the linea aspera. Z Anat Entwickl Gesch 117: 497–503

Pauwels F 1954c The significance of the mechanical factors acting on the elbow joint for the carrying capacity of the flexed upper limb. Z Anat Entwickl Gesch 118: 35–94

Pauwels F 1954d On the distribution of the density of cancellous bone in the upper end of the femur and its significance for the theory of the functional structure of bone. Morph Jb: 35–54

Pauwels F 1960 Eine neue Theorie uber den Einfluss mecha-nischer Reize auf die Differenzierung der Stutzgewebe. Z Anat Entwickl Gesch 121: 478–515

Pauwels F 1973 Short survey of the mechanical stressing of bone and its significance for functional adaptation. Z Orthop 111: 681–705

Pauwels F 1975 A clinical observation as example and proof of functional adaptation of the bone through longitudinal growth. Z Orthop 113: 1–5

Pauwels F 1976 Biomechanics of the Normal and Diseased Hip. Springer, Berlin

Pauwels F 1980 Biomechanics of the Locomotor Apparatus. Springer, Berlin

Polgar K, Gill H S, Murray D W, O'Connor J J 2001 Physiological strain distributions within the human femur: finite element analysis using the muscle – standardised femur model. J Biomech (submitted)

Procter P, Paul J P 1982 Ankle joint biomechanics. J Biomech 15: 627–634

Radin E L, Paul I L 1971 Response of joints to impact loading. I. In vitro wear. Arthritis Rheum 14: 356–362

Reynolds O 1886 On the theory of lubrication and its appli-cation to Mr Beauchamp Tower's experiments, including an experimental determination of the viscosity of olive oil. Phil Trans 177: 157–234

Roesler H 1987 The history of some fundamental concepts in bone biomechanics. J Biomech 20: 1025–1034

Roux W 1895 Gesammelte Abhandlungen uber Entwicklungsmechanik der Organismen, Wilhem Engelmann, Leipzig

Sapega A A, Moyer M A, Schneck C, Komalahiranya N 1990 Testing for isometry during reconstruction of the anterior cruciate ligament. J Bone Joint Surg 72A: 259–267

Seedhom B B, Dowson D, Wright V 1974 The load-bearing function of the menisci. In: International Congress Series No. 324. Excerpta Medica, Amsterdam

Seireg A, Arvikar R J 1973 A mathematical model for evaluation of forces in lower extremities of the musculo-skeletal system. J Biomech 6: 313–326

Shrive N G, O'Connor J J, Goodfellow J W 1978 Load-bearing in the knee joint. Clin Orthop 131: 279–287

Stagni R, Leardini A, Cappozzo A, Grazia Benedetti M, Cappello A 2000 Effects of hip joint centre mislocation on gait analysis results. J Biomech 33: 1479–1487

Stukenborg-Colsman C, Wirth C J, Lazovic D, Wefer A 2001 High tibial osteotomy versus unicompartmental joint replacement in unicompartmental knee joint osteoarthritis: 7–10 year follow-up prospective randomised study. Knee 8: 187–194

Sutherland D H, Olshen R A, Biden E N, Wyatt M P The Development of Mature Walking. MacKeith, Oxford

Taylor M E, Tanner K E, Freeman M A R, Yettram A L 1996 Stress and strain distribution within the intact femur: compression or bending? Med Engng Physics 18: 122–131

Thompson W O, Thaete F L, Fu F H, Dye S F 1991 Tibial meniscal dynamics using three-dimensional reconstruction of magnetic resonance images. Am J Sports Med 19: 210–215; discussion 215–216

University of California 1953 The Pattern of Muscular Activity in the Lower Extremity During Walking. Report No. Series II, Issue 25

Von Meyer G H 1867 Die architekter die spongiosa. Archs Anat Physiol Wiss Med 34: 615–628

Walker P S, Erkman M J 1975 The role of the menisci in force transmission across the knee. Clin Orthop 109: 184–192

Weber W, Weber E 1836 Mechanik der menschlichen Gehwerkzeuge. Dieterichschen Buchhandlung, Gottingen

White S H, Ludkowski P F, Goodfellow J W 1991 Anteromedial osteoarthritis of the knee. J Bone Joint Surg 73: 582–586

Wilson D R, Feikes J D, O'Connor J J 1998 Ligaments and articular contact guide passive knee flexion. J Biomech 31: 1127–1136

Wilson D R, Feikes J D, Zavatsky A B, O'Connor J J 2000 The components of passive knee movement are coupled to flexion angle. J Biomech 33: 465–473

Winter D A 1995 A. B. C. of Balance During Standing and Walking. Waterloo Biomechanics, Waterloo

Winter D A 1979 Biomechanics of Human Movement. John Wiley, New York

Winter D A, Greenlaw R K, Hobson D A 1972 Television–computer analysis of kinematics of human gait. Computers Biomed Res 5: 498–504

Wolff J 1899 Die Lehre von der Funktionellen Knochengestalt, Viruhav's Archiv 155: 256–315.

Woltring H J 1974 New possibilities for human motion studies by real-time light spot position measurement. Biotelemetry 1: 132–146

Woltring H J 1987 Data acquisition and processing systems in functional movement analysis. Minerva Ortopedica e Traumatologica 38: 703–716

Woltring H J 1994 3-D attitude representation of human joints: a standardization proposal. J Biomech 27: 1399–1414

Zavatsky A B, O'Connor J J 1992 A model of human knee ligaments in the sagittal plane. Part 2: Fibre recruitment under load. Proc Inst Mech Eng [H] 206: 135–145

Zuppinger H 1904 Die aktive Flexion in unbelasteten Kniegelenk. In: Zuricher Habil Schr, Bergmann, Wiesbaden, pp 703–763

Notes

1. I have been unable to find a copy of A Fick's 'Statische Betrachtung der Muskeln der Oberschenkels' and rely instead on the description of it given in Pauwels (1935).

2. Quoted by Dowson (1990), 305–345, who gives a detailed history of the science of animal joint lubrication.

7

Biomaterials

Neil Rushton

The incorporation of biomaterials into the tissues of the body is a fundamental component of surgery. Bell (1804) described galvanic corrosion occurring in body fluids when steel-pointed silver pins were used in wounds. Levert (1829) used dogs to test various metals being considered for use as arterial sutures. The metals tested included silver, gold, lead and platinum and he found that platinum was least irritating.

Repair, or more correctly fixation, of fractures using pins and wires made from iron, gold, platinum or silver was attempted in the eighteenth century. Hansmann (1886) described a method of fracture fixation that was probably the earliest plating system, although other countries have claimed this honour for their own surgeons. He used hardened nickel-plated sheet steel, the plate being constructed so that a right-angle bend allowed it to protrude from the wound for use as a handle for removal, presumably the infective process having loosened the screw fixation. Infection was commonplace and limited the application of these materials. A major contribution was made by Lane (1893) who, having initially used silver wire, described the use of steel screws to produce forcible compression of fractures with delayed union in an attempt to stimulate healing.

In vivo testing was the rule and correlation of results was uncommon, leading to intuitively inspired mistakes. Meyer (1902) described silver mesh reinforcement for closure of large hernial defects. Robb (1907) compared the results of silver wire with catgut used for abdominal fascial closure. Cushing (1911) described the use of silver clips to control the bleeding of otherwise inaccessible vessels.

The introduction of Listerian aseptic techniques allowed further experimentation to be continued. The difficulty of treating fractures of the neck of the femur stimulated much of the development. Hey Groves (1913), as part of a large work, concluded that 'indifferent aseptic

foreign materials' did no harm and that nickel-plated steel produced least tissue reaction but that magnesium plates disintegrated rapidly. His paper contains one of the earliest accounts of the interaction between the insecure prosthesis and the surrounding tissue. 'If a plate is attached to a bone in such a way that slight but constant recurring movement is permitted, it will cause mechanical irritation, fluid collection, sinus formation and finally sepsis.' Lane (1914) introduced a plate that is similar to those used today. It was not strong enough as it was made from high carbon ('stout') steel. Lane's results were good, largely owing to his belief in careful surgery and aseptic technique. Lane's plate was in common use until it was changed by Venable whose design was almost identical with that used today (Venable & Stuck 1947).

Brittle materials and firm fixation led to frequent breakage of the plate. Sherman (1912) realised the inherent weakness of Lane's design, modified its shape and had it manufactured from vanadium steel, a more appropriate alloy. Cotton (1912) addressed the problem of breakage due to fatigue in a different manner believing that it was the rigidity of Lane's plate that resulted in failure of screw fixation. He advocated the use of slightly flexible plates made from aluminium, phosphor bronze, silver or wrought iron. He would be gratified to know of the very recent developments in flexible plates (Bradley et al 1980, Claes et al 1980, Tayton et al 1982), although contemporary reasoning is related to the physiology of fracture healing rather than to the avoidance of failure of materials. The Lambotte brothers experimented with the principles of fracture fixation including careful aseptic surgery, adequate fixation and early movement without weight bearing (Lambotte 1913).

Metal interaction became apparent when magnesium plates disintegrated when fixed to bone using steel screws. Non-reactive materials were considered and stainless steel (18% chromium, 8% nickel) was intro-duced into surgery in the mid-1920s but it was found to corrode when in contact with electrolytic body fluids (Speed 1935, Harris 1938, Raagaard 1939). A more recent alloy incorporating 24% molybdenum is now used extensively as its corrosion resistance is superior. The advantage of this material had been demonstrated by Large (1926) but it was not adopted until after the Second World War when the most popular implant alloy was probably chrome-cobalt steel. A similar material, Stellite, was investigated by Zierold (1924). Venable and Stuck (1947) experimented with chrome-cobalt steel in 1936, although by then it had been in use by dentists for several years.

Hey Groves (1926) pointed out the inadequacy of screw grip in the cancellous bone of the femoral head and advocated the use of pegs made from bone or ivory. Smith-Petersen et al (1931) produced a trifin nail to replace the bone or ivory peg and with the addition of a plate (Thornton 1937) the now familiar internal fixation device was created. This evolving design has been modified by many surgeons and engineers to produce a multitude of similar devices. There remained a worrying group of patients with non-union of the fracture and an avascular femoral head. The range of treatments for this condition available at that time was summarised by Wiles (1958): 'Methods available for treatment of painful hip are those applying to most orthopaedic problems – move it, keep it still, cut it out.' Interposition arthroplasty became popular, using many different materials. Jones (1908) used gold foil which he later supplemented with soft tissue. Baer (1926) recom-mended chromalised pig bladder and claimed 82% good results in one hundred hips. Other materials were used: Carnochan (1860) inserted a wooden block as a spacer following resection of the neck of a mandible. Ollier (1885) is given credit for creating new interest in the method. Tensor fascia lata was used by Murphy (1905, 1913a, b), Lexer (1908) and Payr (1910), skin was used by Loewe (1913) and Kallio (1957), Page (1939) and McKeever (1943) used cellophane, whilst Kuhns and Potter (1950) and Kuhns (1953, 1964) used nylon, but without much success. The vogue for inter-position arthroplasty exceeded all expectations and most tissues and materials were used. Putti (1921) operated on a vast number of patients with surprising materials for his interposition experiments. Wiles (1958) repeated his attempts to produce a sprayed molten metal surface coating applied directly to the femoral head. He was unsuccessful because of the unsuitability of the metals that could be melted using an oxyacetylene flame. The most successful development was that of Smith-Petersen (1939, 1948) who used a

glass mould in a patient's hip in order to reshape and reinforce the joint. This prosthesis was too fragile, but Pyrex and plastics were a little better. Only when a Vitalium mould was used did the success of the method become apparent.

Theophilus Gluck (1891) used ivory femoral head replacements to treat soldiers injured in Bulgaria; he used intramedullary stems for added strength and cemented the prosthesis in the femur using californium, pumice and plaster of Paris. A preserved specimen shows changes that resemble osteomyelitis of the eroded bone stock. A precise history of the progress of this specific patient is, unfortunately, not available but such information as does exist suggests that the patient may have died from septi-caemia owing to a late infection of the hip.

The Judet brothers (1950, 1952) introduced a methyl methacrylate prosthesis that had an initial appeal but poor long-term results. Subsequently a stem was added in an attempt to overcome the failure of the prosthesis owing to breakage and bone resorption; it was not widely used as an all-metal prosthesis had been devised by this time. Devas (1954) reported on 110 cup and replacement arthroplasties and was generally discouraged by the results, no more than half of the Judet prostheses being satisfactory compared with success in five of every six of the cups. He commented: 'the easier an operation is to do the easier it is to do badly'! The Judet brothers produced a more detailed review of their results in 1952 including accounts of failures and a description of a modification incorpo-rating a metal rod within the acrylic stem. Scales and Zarek (1954), in a combined laboratory and clinical examination of the biomechanical problems associated with the Judet prosthesis, studied mechanical failure, material failure and manufacturing variations. They concluded that these factors together with imperfect operative technique were likely to lead to failure. Some of these prostheses, however, functioned well. Rushton et al (1979) reported three patients with mobile hips who had had Judet prostheses for more than twenty years before revision was required.

During the 1940s and 1950s experimentation was directed towards hemi-arthroplasty. Peterson (1951) reported results using his short-stemmed steel pros-thesis which was fixed to the femoral shaft with screws. McBride (1951) produced his screw-fit 'doorknob' prosthesis. Thompson produced and reported on his intramedullary prosthesis (1952, 1954, 1966). Austin Moore produced his similar design (Moore & Bohlman 1943, Moore 1952) and reported later on its progress (Moore 1957). This prosthesis had a fenestrated stem; designed initially for lightness, it was later found useful for its locking action as tissue grew into the interstices.

When used for the treatment of osteoarthritis, hemi-arthroplasties were no better than pseudarthroses (Heywood-Waddington 1966). Thomson et al (1953) described the development of the 'light bulb' type of replacement for the femoral head which was fixed by being screwed into the prepared femoral neck. The prosthesis was abandoned because of the difficulty of obtaining sufficient bony support and its consequent loosening. Haboush (1953) reported the use of dental cold-curing acrylic cement to fix a femoral prosthesis but was not impressed by the results; he is believed to have made no further similar attempts.

Wiles (1958) carried out the first total hip replacement in 1938 at the Middlesex Hospital. His prosthesis (Fig. 7.1) was made from stainless steel; the acetabular component was fixed with screws whilst the femoral component was a 'lollipop' shape. The stem penetrated the lateral femoral cortex where it was attached to a plate and thence to the femur with screws. He performed six operations on young patients with Still's disease with reasonable results, although he was not particularly encouraged. New bone formation resulted in loss of movement in two patients. Other prostheses became loose but at least one patient had active use of the hip for ten years postoperatively.

McKee (1951, 1970, McKee & Watson-Farrar 1966) and Charnley (1960, 1964, 1974) developed their prostheses concurrently. McKee used Vitallium for both components, which was a fortunate choice as it is the only biocompatible alloy that when forming both components of a joint produces a satisfactory mechanical joint which functions within the environment of the body. Charnley initially used Teflon spacers unsuccessfully, and when used as an acetabular component the results were disastrous causing a massive tissue response resulting in loss of bone followed by loosening of the prosthesis. Two major advances are attributable to Charnley: the use of high-density polyethylene for the acetabular cup and 'bone cement' (polymethylmethacrylate or cold-curing dental acrylic) to act as a space filler, or grout, to stabilise the prosthesis in the femur. The combination of a metal intramedullary femoral component with a high-density polyethylene acetabular cup, both of which were cemented in position using bone cement, is now accepted as the classic design for modern total hip arthroplasty. Modifications of this basic design are legion and far too numerous to list here. The justification for so many designs is elusive, perhaps representing commercial or egotistical interests rather than a desire for improvement in patient care.

In recent years relatively small changes to the design of successful hips have resulted in dramatic differences in prosthetic survivorship. Rough-finish Exeter hips

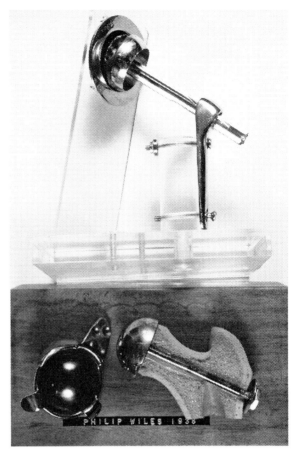

Fig. 7.1 Philip Wiles' prosthesis, 1938. By kind permission of the British Orthopaedic Association, London

were much less satisfactory than the polished version. A Charnley copy, the Capital hip, has been shown to be much less durable than the original. The precise reasons for these differences in performance are a matter of conjecture rather than of fact.

Bone cement has played a major part in the success of joint replacement; this is slightly surprising as the material is relatively brittle and the monomer toxic. Kaier described fixing plastic cups to the femoral head using acrylic cement in 1951. Charnley and D. C. Smith, a lecturer in material sciences at the Turner Dental Hospital in Manchester, experimented with self-curing acrylic cement (Nu-Life). This dental repair material was a mixture of polymethylmethacrylate powder and methylmethacrylate. Charnley used the bone cement to anchor a Moore prosthesis in a femur in 1958. He commented that the addition of 25% barium sulphate was needed to make the cement visible on radiographs. The cement was marketed as CMW⁸ Bone

Cement from 1966. Other cements were available at the time were Palacos[g] and Surgical Simplex[g], which was used by neurosurgeons to fill defects in the skull and by McKee in Norwich for hip replacements.

Polymethylmethacrylate (PMMA) bone cements are polymers of methyl methacrylate with a molecular weight of about 200,000. They are supplied as a liquid monomer that combines with pre-polymerised particles. Spontaneous polymerisation is controlled by the addition of hydroquinone and N,N-dimethyl-p-toluidine is added to promote curing. Setting time is influenced by many factors including temperature, humidity, liquid-to-powder ratio and the amount of material. The reaction is exothermic; volumetric changes also occur during curing. In the first third of the curing process the monomer molecules form chains causing polymerisation shrinkage of 7% without a change in temperature. In the middle third the temperature rises quickly causing thermal expansion. During the final period the cement cools producing volumetric shrinkage of about 5% owing to thermal contraction. The radial shrinkage is less than 0.5%, which is important for the interface (Jasty 1995). During polymerisation the local temperature may exceed 67°C at which point the proteins will coagulate.

Commercially available bone cements vary in composition. Some have methylmethacrylate copolymer; others are powdered PMMA polymers, mixtures of PMMA and methylmethacrylate-styrene or copolymers of PMMA and polybutyl methacrylate. In order to make them visible on radiographs barium sulphate or zirconium dioxide are added. Variation in the powder particle size changes the viscosity and working time. Antibiotics have been added to cements in an attempt to reduce infection. The fatigue life and tensile strength is not affected by inclusion of up to 4% by volume (Maloney 1998). Palacos[g], which contains gentamicin, has the lowest risk for revision of all the cements studied in the Swedish Hip Registry (Malchau & Herberts 1998).

PMMA is a brittle polymer with an elastic modulus of 2.3 Gpa compared with cancellous bone (1 Gpa) and cortical bone (16 Gpa). The fatigue life of PMMA varies between cements. One study demonstrated that Simplex[g] P had a significantly better fatigue life than Zimmer[g] LVC cement but had a similar tensile strength (Davies et al 1989). PMMA is also known to creep. Brittle fracture can cause failure of fixation (Jasty 1995). Pores within the cement can act as stress raisers (Maloney 1998). These can be reduced by using vacuum mixing and centrifugation leading to improved laboratory measurements. Paradoxically the clinical results from the Swedish Hip Registry indicate a worse result with vacuum mixing (Malchau & Herberts 1998).

Charnley (1960) noted that the cement acts as a grout rather than glue. It does not bond chemically with the bone or with the surface of conventional components. Fixation, therefore, depends on the penetration of PMMA into the interstices of the bone and with the textured surface of the prostheses. The viscosity and pressure of the cement at insertion determines the depth of penetration. Medium viscosity cements penetrate about 5 mm into the bone when delivered using a standard gun (Jasty 1995). It is important that the cement continues to be pressurised for as much of the process as is possible otherwise the hydrostatic pressure produced by the blood will push the cement out of the bone. The use of bone cement effectively seals the interface at operation. This situation is in contrast to the implantation of an uncemented prosthesis where no satisfactory particle-resistant seal is available. This is particularly important as an increased incidence of particle generation is seen immediately after implantation of the prosthesis owing to the polishing process as the articulation is 'run in'. The interface may be sealed using other methods, for example tissue glue or occlusive films made from synthetic material or the patient's own tissue.

As mentioned above, the first prostheses used either metal on metal articulations or metal on plastic. Charnley first used polytetrafluorethylene (PTFE), which produced disastrous results and led to a large number of revisions. He went on to use HDPE, a material that has been used in the majority of prosthetic hips for many years. It is expected that at the soft counterface it will wear to produce multitudes of particles per step! The cellular reaction to this deluge of particles can result in osteolysis, prosthetic instability and revision surgery. All particles contribute to this process: cement, metal, plastics, soft tissue and bone. Initially Willert et al (1974) and Willert and Semlitsch (1975) felt that PMMA was the major contributor to aseptic loosening and it was largely their influence that resulted in the ban on bone cement in the USA. It is now generally agreed that HDPE particles are the principal cause of aseptic loosening in the majority of instances. They went on to explore the role of metal particles at the interface (Willert & Semlitsch 1976).

The development of osteolysis is influenced by a number of factors, each of which can operate alone or together with one or more of the other factors. The cellular response to wear particles is well known to be a potent cause of osteolysis and has been investigated frequently, but there are other potent reasons for bone loss. Osteolysis takes different forms. It may be a very localised event, for example the lacunae that contain wear particles and phagocytic cells found close to the surface of the implant. The mechanical effect of the prosthesis can have a marked effect on the bone cell response, producing profound bone loss within a few weeks of implantation. Contamination with endotoxin and overt infection are very potent causes of peri-prosthetic osteolysis.

An immediate cause of bone loss, often ignored in clinical studies, is the effect of the surgeon as he prepares the bone at the time of initial implantation. Stability of the prostheses also has a very strong influence on the development of osteolysis, either as a mechanical-wearing processor, the so-called type II wear (where parts of the prosthesis not designed to articulate move against the tissue). This can result in two effects: the accumulation of wear products at the interface and changed strain rates imposed on the adjacent cells. These local effects need to be considered in the context of the dynamics of systemic bone; that is the rate of loss of bone in the whole skeleton, which is particularly relevant in elderly women and patients who have disuse atrophy owing to enforced rest. A more widespread reduction in bone mass is frequently seen after implantation of an otherwise successful prosthesis and is presumed to be due to the differences in material properties of the bone and prosthesis, particularly the difference between the bulk modulus of elasticity of the implant and that of the bone.

The general level of osteoporosis may have a profound influence on this phenomenon in particular Kroger et al (1996, 1997). It is characteristic of the osteoporotic process that there is endosteal bone removal and periosteal bone deposition. This has the effect of making the bony tube wider and thinner walled. Unless there is some effective bone remodelling at the bone/prosthesis interface it is inevitable that the prosthesis will become loose, leading to early failure of the joint. The degree of osteoporosis of the bone at the time of implantation is very important for survival of the prosthesis but possibly even more important is the continued development of osteoporosis throughout the working lifetime of the artificial joint.

For important relevant findings to be derived from this work in the context of osteolysis, see Aspenberg & Herbertsson (1996). They demonstrated that movement of a metal prosthesis against bone caused osteolysis. In the presence of particles when the movement was stopped the osteolytic lesion did not heal, but if there were no particles in the osteolytic lesion then the bone defect healed. This clearly indicates the 'symbiosis' between different mechanisms causing bone loss. Kobayashi et al (1997) studied specimens retrieved from revision arthroplasties and demonstrated that a specific concentration of particles is required to produce, or maintain, an osteolytic lesion close to a prosthesis. The mechanical effect of an unstable prosthesis can range from mild to disastrous as far as bone loss at the bone prosthesis interface is concerned. When there is a type II wear process particles can be generated from bone, soft tissue or the prosthesis.

It has been clear for some years that implantation of a prosthesis has a considerable effect on bone activity (Cohen & Rushton 1994, 1995a). Radioisotope methods give a good indication of bone activity, but care has to be taken to differentiate between the metabolic changes caused by mechanical effects and those caused by infection. The use of dual energy X-ray absorptiometry, related to Gruen zones (Gruen et al 1979), has produced a remarkable insight into the effect of successful implantation in the proximal femur. It was further shown that the continuing loss of bone postoperatively was not uniformly distributed and that by twelve months the overall pattern of change in bone mineral density was resorption which increased from the distal to the proximal part of the femur with an increase in bone density below the tip of the prosthesis (Cohen & Rushton 1995b). The distribution of change of bone mineral density in the proximal femur may have a number of explanations. It may follow the postoperative change in strain or it may represent the effect of the destruction of the complex trabecular pattern within the proximal femur (Field et al 1990).

All articulations will wear but improvements may be able to be made thereby reducing the amount of wear debris (Fig 7.2). Recently HDPE manufacture and processing has been modified in the hope of improving the wear characteristics. It is known that the routine methods of sterilisation lead to subsurface oxidation of the HDPE, which in turn reduces the resistance to wear. If the HDPE is irradiated in an inert atmosphere and subsequently heated to a temperature close to its

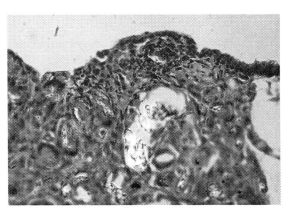

Fig. 7.2 The Synovial response is wear particles

melting point several changes occur. First the long molecules are broken to some extent, weakening the material. Hydrogen bonds are formed between the molecules that stabilises the molecular structure. It is particularly important that free radicals formed in the irradiation process are allowed to escape in the annealing phase thereby reducing the damaging oxidation that occurs during storage. It is not clear whether this changed material will lead to an improvement in the wear properties of the components in clinical use in the long-term but almost all manufacturers have adopted some variation of the process.

Most orthopaedic biomaterials are in contact with bone which provides structural support for the implant. The whole construct is surrounded by soft tissue that is probably much more influenced by the implant than is the bone. Bone can be considered as an organ involved in calcium metabolism or as a repository for bone marrow. However, its unique characteristic is the structural function provided by its mechanical properties. Currey (1975) made an extensive study of bone and concluded that bone appeared at least two hundred million years ago. There is little variation between species. The mechanical properties vary depending on the composition of the bone, e.g. the amount of mineralisation and also the porosity and Haversian remodelling. The modulus of elasticity of cortical bone is about 15 Gpa and for cancellous bone 1 Gpa, the exact figure depending on site. In contrast, a metal alloy femoral component would be expected to have a modulus in the order of 25 Gpa.

The strength of the whole bone depends on many factors in addition to the properties of the individual components. Cross-sectional size, shape, the relative proportion of trabecular to cortical bone and the internal architecture all have an influence. Bones also adapt to the forces that act on them, a process often referred to as Wolf's Law. This remodelling can be measured using dual-energy X-ray absorptiometry (Cohen et al 1995).

The ability of the bone to respond to outside forces is both its major advantage and its downfall. Fracture repair and structural reorganisation after injury are clear advantages. The loss of bone density after implantation of a prosthesis is not advantageous to the longevity of the artificial joint. This bone loss is thought to be due to a mismatch of the material properties between bone and the prosthesis and presumably is a cellular response to reduced strain. It is the change in bulk modulus of the whole construct that seems to be important. The loss of bone from the proximal femur after hip replacement can be dramatic and is often characteristic of specific prostheses. Unfortunately the

more osteoporotic the bone, the more the patients are affected by the loss of bone density (Kroger et al 1996). Studies of serial DEXA scans can predict early failure of new prostheses within a few months of implantation and may allow early withdrawal of poor prostheses as well as early rollout of the more successful. The advantage of the method is that it indicates bone structure rather than measuring movement of the prosthesis within the bone.

Many new materials are being introduced and existing materials are being used in new ways. Composites can be tailored to have specific properties thought to be relevant to the desired application. Most manufacturers are testing new structural materials for bone plates and joint replacements. Compliant bearings may revolutionise the practice of joint replacement by reducing wear. The most dramatic change is likely to be in the use of *resorbable* biomaterials to produce sophisticated scaffolds for tissue engineering purposes. These devices may be so effective that a supply of exogenous cells may not need to be artificially introduced into the construct thereby limiting the concerns about infection as well as reducing expense. Some of these constructs may consist of bone mineral and be suitable for bone substitute materials: a holy grail for orthopaedic surgeons with the potential to produce a major change in surgical techniques which are currently limited by lack of suitable donor bone.

'Natural' incorporation of prostheses has been influenced by the use of coatings, the most commonly used being hydroxyapatite but others, for example diamond-like carbon, are currently being tested. The use of surface texturing may have the potential to direct growth of tissues in this and many other applications, both in orthopaedics and in other surgical specialities. These new techniques are part of the development of tissue engineering that has dominated the last decade of the twentieth century. Further refinements already include the production of complex substrate scaffolds using sophisticated technology such as multiple-pass ink-jet printing to produce liver architecture and three-dimensional fabric manufacturing methods to produce bioresorbable formers for cartilage culture. The original concept of external tissue/organ culture followed by surgical implantation is already being modified in favour of a method whereby biomaterials with the correct geometry are implanted in the recipient site to be colonised by the local cells. This route for tissue regeneration circumvents many of the problems of the external culture method and may lead to a completely new form of restorative orthopaedic surgery this century where plastics and alloys of metals will have little place.

REFERENCES

Aspenberg P, Herbertsson P J 1996 Peri-prosthetic bone resorption. Particles versus movement. J Bone Joint Surg 78B: 641–646

Baer W S 1926 Arthroplasty of the hip. Bone Joint Surg 8: 769–802

Bell B A 1804 A System of Surgery, Ed Perriman, Troy, New York

Bradley J S, Hastings G W, Johnson-Nurse, C 1980 Carbon fibre reinforced epoxy as a high strength low modulus material for internal fixation plates. Biomaterials 1: 38–40

Carnochan J M 1860 Archives of Medicine, p 284; cited in Thompson F R 1966 An essay on the development of arthroplasty of the hip. Clin Orthop 44: 79–82

Charnley J 1960 Anchorage of the femoral head prosthesis to the shaft of the femur. J Bone Joint Surg 42B: 28–30

Charnley J 1964 The bonding of prosthesis to bone by cement. J Bone Joint Surg 46B: 518–521

Charnley J 1974 Total hip replacement. J Am Med Assoc 230: 1025–1028

Claes L, Curri C, Kinzl L, Fitzer E, Hutter W 1980 Less rigid fixation with carbon fibre reinforced materials: mechanical characteristics and behaviour *in vivo*. In: Uhthoff J D (ed) Current Concepts of Internal Fixation of Fractures. Springer, Berlin, pp 215–263

Cohen B, Millett P J, Mist B, Laskey M A, Rushton N 1995 Effect of exercise training programme on bone mineral density in novice college rowers. Br J Sports Med 29: 85–88

Cohen B, Rushton N 1994 A comparative study of peri-prosthetic bone mineral measurement using two different dual-energy X-ray absorptiometry systems. Br J Radiol 67: 852–855

Cohen B, Rushton N 1995a Accuracy of DEXA measurement of bone mineral density after total hip arthroplasty. J Bone Joint Surg 77B: 479–448

Cohen B, Rushton N 1995b Bone remodeling in the proximal femur after Charnley total hip arthroplasty. J Bone Joint Surg 77B: 815–819

Cotton F J 1912 Discussion. J Am Med Assoc 49: 354

Currey J D 1975 The effects of strain rate, reconstruction and mineral content on some mechanical properties of bovine bone. J Biomech 8: 81–86

Cushing H 1911 The control of bleeding in operations for brain tumours with the description of silver 'clips' for the occlusion of vessels inaccessible to ligature. Ann Surg 54: 1–19

Davies J P, Jasty M, O'Connor D O, Burke D W, Harrigan T P, Harris W H 1989 The effect of centrifuging bone cement. J Bone Joint Surg 71B: 39–42

Devas M B 1954 A review of 110 cup and replacement arthroplasties. J Bone Joint Surg 36B: 561–566

Field R E, Dixon A K, Lawrence J P, Rushton N 1990 Bone density distribution within the femoral head and neck. An examination by high resolution computed tomography. Skeletal Radiol 19: 319–325

Gluck T 1891 Referat uber die Ch VIII Archiv fur klinische chirurgie. Von August Hirschwald, Berlin, pp 41, 186

Gruen T A, McNice G M, Amstutts H C 1979 Modes of failure of cemented stem type femoral components: a radiographic analysis of loosening. Clin Orthop 141: 17–27

Haboush E J 1953 New operation for arthroplasty of the hip, based on biomechanics, photoelasticity, fast setting dental acrylic and other considerations. Bull Hosp Joint Dis 14: 242–277

Hansmann H 1886 A new method of fixation of fragments in complicated fractures. Verein Deutsches Gesellschafftur Chirugie 15: 347

Harris R I 1938 Experiences with internal fixation in fresh fractures of the neck of the femur. J Bone Joint Surg 20: 114–123

Hey Groves E W 1913 An experimental study of the operative treatment of fracture. Br J Surg 1: 438–501

Hey Groves E W 1926 Some contributions to the reconstructive surgery of the hip. Br J Surg 14: 486–517

Heywood-Waddington M B 1966 Use of the Austin Moore prosthesis for advanced osteoarthritis of the hip. J Bone Joint Surg 48B: 236–244

Jasty M 1995 Polymethylmethacrylate. In: Callagan J, Dennis D, Paprosky W, Rosenberg A (eds) Orthopaedic Knowledge Update Hip and Knee Reconstruction. American Academy of Orthopaedic Surgeons, Rosemont, pp 43–47

Jones, R 1908 On the production of pseudoarthrosis of the hip without disarticulation of the head. Br Med J 1: 494–495

Judet J, Judet R 1950 The use of an artificial femoral head for arthroplasty of the hip joint. J Bone Joint Surg 32B: 166–173

Judet J, Judet R 1952 Technique and result with the acrylic head prosthesis. J Bone Joint Surg 34B: 173–180

Kaier S 1951 Experimental investigation of the tissue reaction to acrylic plastics. In: Proceedings of the Vth Congres International de Chirurgie Orthopédique, Stockholm

Kallio K E 1957 Arthroplastia artanea. Proceedings of the Nordisk Ortopedisk Forenings Twenty-eighth Assembly in Helsinki, June 1956. Acta Orth Scand 26: 327

Kobayashi A, Freeman M, Bonfield W, Kodoya Y, Yamac T, Al-Saffar N, Scott G, Ravell P 1997 Number of polyethylene particles and osteolysis in total joint replacements. J Bone Joint Surg 78B: 844–848

Kroger H, Miettinen H, Arnala I, Koski E, Rushton N, Suomalainen O 1996 Evaluation of periprosthetic bone using dual x-ray absorptiometry – precision of the method and effect of operation on bone mineral density. J Bone Mineral Res 11: 1526–1530

Kroger H, Vanninen E, Overmyer M, Miettinen H, Rushton N, Suomalainen O 1997 Periprosthetic bone loss and regional bone turnover in uncemented total hip arthroplasty: a prospective study using high resolution single photon emission tomography and dual energy x-ray absorptiometry. J Bone Mineral Res 12: 487–492

Kuhns J G 1953 Nylon membrane arthroplasty of the knee in chronic arthritis. J Bone Joint Surg 35A: 929–936

Kuhns J G 1964 Nylon membrane arthroplasty of the knee in chronic arthritis. J Bone Joint Surg 46A: 448–449

Kuhns J G, Potter I A 1950 Nylon arthroplasty of the knee joint in chronic arthritis. Surg Gynec Obstet 91: 351–362

Lambotte A 1913 Chirurgie Operatoire des Fractures. Masson & Cie, Paris

Lane W A 1893 On the advantage of the steel screw in the treatment of ununited fractures. Lancet 140: 1500–1501

Lane W A B 1914 The Operative Treatment of Fractures, 2nd edn. Medical Publishing Co., London

Large M 1926 Krupp steel wire as a bone suture material. Z Orthop Chir 47: 520

Levert H S 1829 Experiments on the use of metallic ligatures as applied to arteries. Am J Med Sci 4: 17

Lexer, E 1908 Uber Gelenkransplantation. Med Klin Berlin 4: 817–820

Loewe O 1913 Uber hautimplantation an stelle der frein Faszienplastik. Munch Med Wochenschr 60: 1320

Malchau H, Herberts P 1998 Prognosis of total hip replacement. American Association of Orthopaedic Surgeons, March

Maloney W 1998 Polymethylmethacrylate. In: Sedal I, Cabanela M (eds) Hip Surgery: Materials and Developments. Martin Dunitz, London, pp 57–65

McBride E D 1951 A metallic femoral head prosthesis for the hip joint. J Intl Coll Surg 15: 498

McKee G K 1951 Artificial hip joint. J Bone Joint Surg 33B: 465

McKee G K 1970 Development of total prosthetic replacement of the hip. Clin Orthop 72: 85–103

McKee G K, Watson-Farrar J 1966 Replacement of arthritic hips by the McKee-Farrar prosthesis. J Bone Joint Surg 48B: 245–259

McKeever D C 1943 The use of cellophane as an interposition membrane in synovectomy. J Bone Joint Surg 25: 576–580

Meyer W 1902 The implantation of silver filigree for the closure of large hernial apertures. Ann Surg 36: 767–778

Moore A T 1952 Metal hip joint – new self locking Vitallium prosthesis. South Med J 45: 1015–1019

Moore A T 1957 The self-locking metal hip prosthesis. J Bone Joint Surg 39A: 811–827

Moore A T, Bohlman H R 1943 Metal hip joint – a case report. J Bone Joint Surg 25: 688–692

Murphy J B 1905 Ankylosis; arthroplasty, clinical and experimental. J Am Med Ass xiiv 1573; 1671; 1749

Murphy J B 1913a Arthroplasty. Ann Surg vii: 593–647

Murphy J B 1913b Old ununited fracture of anatomic neck of femur. South Med J vi: 387–400

Ollier L X E L 1885 Traite des resection et operations conservatrice qu'on peut practiquer sur le system osseus. Masson & Cie, Paris

Page I H 1939 Production of persistent arterial hypertension by cellophane perinephritis. J Am Med Assoc 113: 2046–2048

Payr E 1910 Blutige Mobilisierung rersteifler Gelenke. Zentrabl Clin 37: 1227

Peterson L I 1951 The use of a metallic femoral head. J Bone Joint Surg 33A: 65–75

Putti V 1921 Arthroplasty. J Orthop Surg 3: 421–430

Raagaard O 1939 Some comments on complications occasioned by a rustless surgical nail. Acta Chir Scand 82: 475–479

Robb H 1907 The comparative advantage of catgut and silver wire sutures for closing the fascia after abdominal incisions. Surg Gynec Obstet: V: 193–195

Rushton N, Hart G M, Arden G P 1979 The Judet prosthesis: a long term follow-up of three cases and a review of the literature. Injury 11: 49–51

Scales J T, Zarek J M 1954 Biomechanical problems with the original Judet prosthesis. Br Med J 1: 1007–1013

Sherman W O 1912 Vanadium steel plates and screws. Surg Gynec Obstet 14: 629

Smith-Petersen M N 1939 Arthroplasty of the hip: a new method. J Bone Joint Surg 21: 269–288

Smith-Petersen M N 1948 Evolution of the mould arthroplasty. J Bone Joint Surg 30B: 59–83

Smith-Petersen M N, Cave E, Vangorder G W 1931 Intracapsular fractures of the neck of the femur: treatment by internal fixation. Arch Surg 23: 715

Speed K 1935 The unsolved fracture. Surg Gynaec Obstet 60: 341–343

Tayton K, Johnson-Nurse C, McKibbin B, Bradley J, Hastings G 1982 The use of semi-rigid plates for fixation of human fractures. J Bone Joint Surg 64B: 105–111

Thompson F R 1952 Vitallium intramedullary hip prosthesis – preliminary report. NY State J Med 52: 3011–3020

Thompson F R 1954 Two and a half years experience with a Vitallium intramedullary hip prosthesis. J Bone Joint Surg 36A: 489–502

Thompson F R 1966 An essay on the development of arthroplasty of the hip. Clin Orthop 44: 73–86

Thomson J E M, Ferciot C F, Bartels W W, Webster F S 1953 The 'light-bulb' type of prosthesis for the femoral head. Surg Gynaec Obstet 96: 301–304

Thornton L 1937 The treatment of trochanteric fractures: two new methods. Piedmont Hospital Bull 10: 21

Venable C S, Stuck W G 1947 The Internal Fixation of Fractures. C C Thomas, Springfield

Wiles P 1958 The surgery of the hip joint. Br J Surg 45: 488–497

Willert H G, Ludwig J, Semlitsch M 1974 Reaction of bone to methacrylate after hip arthroplasty a long term gross, light microscopic and scanning electron microscopic study. J Bone Joint Surg 56A: 1386–1382

Willert H G, Semlitsch M 1975 Reaction of articular capsule to plastic and metallic wear products from joint endoprostheses. Sulzer Technical Review 2

Willert H G, Semlitsch M 1976 Tissue reactions to plastic and metallic wear products of joint endoprostheses. In: Total Hip Prosthesis. Gschwend N, Debrunner HU (eds), Bern, Huber H pp 205–239

Zierold A A 1924 Reaction of bone to various metals. Arch Surg 9: 364

8

History of orthopaedic radiology

Peter Renton

The discovery of the 'X'- or Röntgen ray is a good example of the aphorism that 'chance favours the prepared mind'. The man credited with the discovery, Wilhelm Conrad Röntgen (Fig. 8.1), was born on 27 March 1845 in Lennep, a town in the Rhineland. His mother, who was a first cousin to his father, was Dutch. At the age of three his family moved to Appledorn where he received his basic education, but he was expelled from school because he refused to tell tales on a fellow pupil who had drawn a caricature of a teacher. He thus did not matriculate, but spent some time at the Technical School in Utrecht. At twenty years of age he went to Zurich where in 1869 he gained a doctorate and became associated with Kundt, whom he followed to Würzburg and subsequently Strasbourg. In 1879 Röntgen was appointed Professor of Physics at Giessen and, in 1888, he returned to Würzburg.

Röntgen's research on the use of Crooke's tubes commenced in 1895, but he was also working with Lenard tubes – i.e. Crooke's tubes with a small aluminium foil window inserted – designed by a younger assistant, Philipp Lenard. The window allowed the cathode rays produced in the tube to escape and to be detected on a fluorescent screen a short distances from the tube.

On the evening of 8 November 1895 in his darkened laboratory Röntgen put black cardboard around the tube to prevent light emanation and supplied power to the tube. A cardboard plate coated with barium platinocyanide lay a short distance away. In the dark Röntgen saw the plate glowing (as he was colour blind he could not see that the glow was green). Kevles (1998) writes that the glow was in the shape of a letter 'A', which a student had written after dipping his finger in the platinocyanide solution (a phosphor that emits light when impinged upon by X-rays), but Röntgen himself 'noticed a peculiar black line across the [coated] paper. The line was the effect of one which only could be produced … by the passage of light. No light

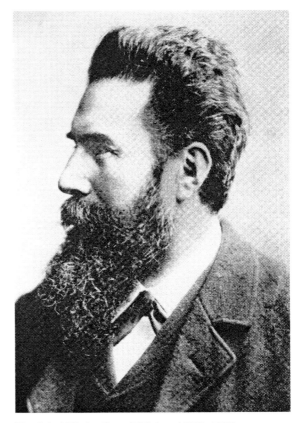

Fig. 8.1 Wilhelm Conrad Röntgen (1845–1923)

could come from the tube, because the shield which covered it was impervious to any light known' (quoted in Burrows 1986).

When the current was disconnected, the glow disappeared, only to reappear again when the current was switched on, in short, related to something – not a cathode ray because of the greater distance – emanating from the tube.

The rays were thus noted to pass through opaque matter – the cardboard box – and subsequently to leave shadows on the screen, for instance of coins inside a wooden box. Röntgen noted that the phosphorescent screen was equally bright when a book was placed between it and the Crooke's tube or when no book was present, and it did not matter if the book was thick or thin. When he placed his hand between the tube and the screen he saw the shadow of his bones. Röntgen soon divided substances into those opaque to the X-ray and those not, and showed that magnets could not divert the beam.

Röntgen let his wife into the secret on 22 December 1895, exposing her hand for 15 minutes on a photographic plate – the first orthopaedic use of X-rays. Mrs Röntgen herself – *die Frau Professorin* – was not too happy with this, having intimations of her own mortality.

On 28 December he presented a 'preliminary communication' to the President of the Medical Physics Society of Würzburg. The paper, entitled 'On a new type of rays', was not read then but was immediately printed and the reprints sent out on New Year's Day 1896 with specimens of X-ray photographs. One copy was sent to Franz Exner, Professor of Physics in Vienna, and another to Arthur Schuster, a Manchester-based, but German-born, physicist.

Exner showed the pictures at a dinner party during the first week of January 1896. A physicist from Prague was present whose father was the Editor of *Die Presse* – Vienna's leading newspaper. On 5 January the discovery made front-page news (Fig. 8.2).

In England news of the discovery was published in the *Daily Chronicle* of 6 January 1896 and in the *Standard* the next day. That evening, having read the report in the *Standard*, an electrical engineer, A. A. Campbell Swinton, produced X-ray pictures of his hands which he showed later that evening to his friends at the Camera Club. *The Times* reported this the following day. On 7 January the Manchester Literary and Philosophical Society was shown the film of Frau Röntgen's hand as well as images of a compass, a coil and shadows of different metals.

On 8 February 1896 the *British Medical Journal* announced that it had commissioned Sydney Rowland to enquire about the practicality of Röntgen's discovery. An illustration in the *British Medical Journal* of 29 February shows a patient being 'skiagraphed' by Rowland (Fig. 8.3) (Saxton 1973). Five days earlier he had demonstrated X-rays to the Medical Society of London. Using a vacuum tube and coil, he produced an image of a hand on film in 20 seconds. Between February and June Rowland contributed thirteen weekly reports on the developing science while he was still an undergraduate at St Bartholomew's Hospital (Fig. 8.4).

According to Saxton (1973), the first clinical use of X-ray in England was the demonstration of a needle in a woman's hand by two Birmingham General Practitioners, J. R. Ratcliffe and J. Hall-Edwards. Burrows (1986) notes that the March issue of the *Photographic Review* was filled with photographic prints made by Hall-Edwards.

The other recipient of Röntgen's original paper had been Sir Arthur Schuster, whose daughter Nora described the 'early days of Röntgen's photography in

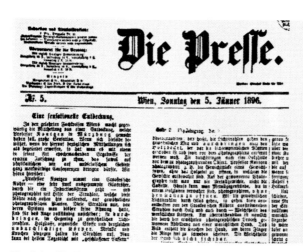

Fig. 8.2 *Die Presse* (Vienna) for Sunday, 5 January 1986, together with the first English report which appeared in the *Daily Chronicle* on 6 January 1896 (right)

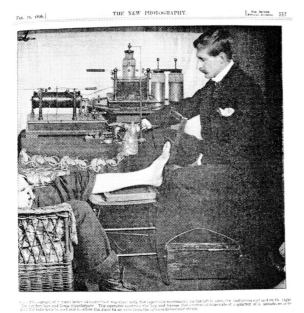

THE NEW PHOTOGRAPHY. 557

Fig. 8.3 Sidney Domville Rowland (1872–1917). After qualifying, Rowland gave up radiology and, according to Burrows (1986), went on to a career in laboratory medicine. He died of cerebrospinal fever in 1917 when in France during the First World War. Reproduced from the *British Medical Journal* (1896)

Britain' (Schuster 1962). Schuster had been born in Frankfurt but he emigrated to Manchester in 1870 when nineteen years of age, becoming first a student and eventually Professor of Physics there (Burrows 1986). He later became President of the Royal Society. His first radiographic patient had been a dancing girl from a local pantomime with a needle in her foot, the photograph of which he kept on this desk for thirty-eight years until he died in 1934. On 7 March 1896 the *British Medical Journal* reported from Manchester:

Professor Schuster gave in Owens College on March 2nd a lecture on Professor Röntgen's discovery. A skiagraph of an opaque object was taken, and after it was developed it was exhibited to the audience on the screen. Professor Schuster expressed the opinion that the new rays are possibly, but not certainly, like the rays of light. If they are, they are of very much shorter length than any of those which we at present have any knowledge. The opacity of different bodies to these rays was not, he said, a difference in kind but only in degree. Some photographs taken in Owens College were shown, including a hand, part of which had been photographed through a sovereign. The bone was distinctly visible through the gold. A very interesting slide was that showing the bones in the hand of a child of 6 years of age. The epiphyses could be seen quite distinctly, as cartilage is very transparent. Another showed the presence of a needle in a girl's foot. The usefulness

of the discovery will largely depend on the possibility of increasing the intensity of the rays. The present method of using a photographic plate was, he said, very clumsy, for by far the greatest amount of the rays passed through the plate.

Meanwhile, in London, by March 1896, Campbell Swinton at 66 Victoria Street had opened a laboratory offering a diagnostic and later therapeutic service. Burrows (1986) maintains that Swinton was the first man in the world after Röntgen to image a part of the human body. He was not a medical man but an electrical contractor and keen photographer and as a radiological pioneer he greatly improved X-ray apparatus. He was later appointed a Fellow of the Royal Society even though he had left school at seventeen and had never taken an examination.

Posner (1970) relates that a copy of *Die Frankfurter Zeitung* reached a Mrs Wimpfheimer who assisted Robert Jones in a Free Clinic in Rodney Street, Liverpool. She showed it to Jones and to Charles Thurston Holland (1863–1941) who at that time was a general practitioner and who also assisted Jones at his Sunday clinic (see Chapter 1).

Dr Thurston Holland had received his medical training at University College Hospital, London, entering general practice in Liverpool in 1889, even though he was a West Country man (Fig. 8.5). Jones suggested that Thurston Holland should obtain an X-ray apparatus and take up radiography.

On 29 May 1896 Thurston Holland took his first radiograph – that of his own hand – with an exposure time of 2 minutes. (Later in September he obtained a radiograph of Lord Lister's hand.) He saw his first pathology on 5 June 1896 – a subungual exostosis. On 16 June he took radiographs of a boy's forearm with exposures of 4–5 minutes. Necrosis with loss of bone was seen but, although the X-ray pathology was gross, no one knew what it implied.

By October 1896 Thurston Holland was in post as radiologist at the Royal Southern Hospital, Liverpool. His department there between the Wars was said to be one of the most advanced in the country, but when I saw it, just prior to closure, it was derelict, probably unaltered for fifty years. Within the year, Thurston Holland had taken 261 plates and had seen:

A number of plates for testing purposes.
Several cases of exostoses.
Congenital deformities of various kinds – club hand, talipes equino-varus, cases of deformities of the bones and hands.
Fractures, old and recent, to show cause of non-union, follow-up cases.
Pieces of needles, mostly hands and feet.
Rheumatoid arthritis.

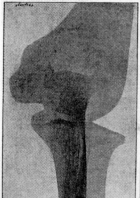

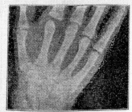

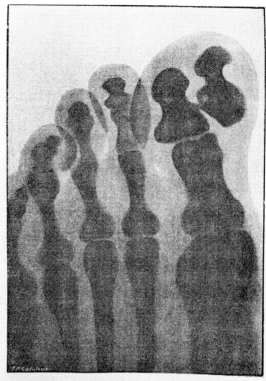

(a)

(c)

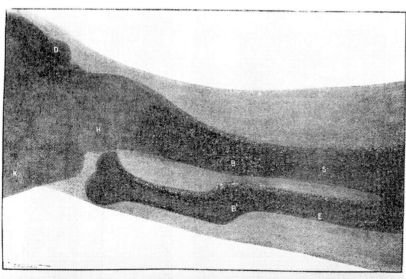

(b)

Fig. 8.4 (a) A dislocated elbow and a hand with a gap between the base of the proximal phalanx and the second metacarpal head. (b) A fracture with malunion. (c) Supernumeracy phalanx of the great toe. Reproduced from the *British Medical Journal* (1896)

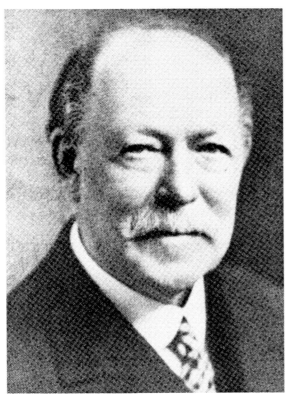

Fig. 8.5 Charles Thurston Holland (1863–1941)

Osteitis.

Hypertrophic pulmonary osteo-arthropathy.

Strumous dactylitis.

Tuberculous disease of various joints.

Various dislocations, traumatic.

Congenital displacement of the patella.

Congenital dislocation of the hip.

Enchondromata.

Osteoma.

Foetuses.

Coins in the oesophagus.

Foreign bodies such as bullets, swallowed coins, swallowed tooth plate, foreign body in the eye (an attempt to show), a swallowed trouser button (seen in the rectum and afterwards passed).

A series of children's hands to show bone growth.

Rickets.

Metatarsalgia.

A piece of an iron fork in a bone and resulting bone changes.

Attempts to examine chests and even the abdomen.

To show the density of various stones.

To show the density of diamonds and paste.

To demonstrate a 'mummy bird'.

X-ray of a fish to show the bones.

Sprengel's deformity.

Osteomalacia, etc. (Burrows 1986)

Most of the cases were orthopaedic and involved the appendicular skeleton, which was inevitable given the limitations of early radiology.

According to Burrows (1986), Thurston Holland was a leader of British and world radiology. In 1925 he was elected President of the First International Radiological Congress. His collaboration with Jones gave a status to radiology it might not otherwise have achieved.

The first radiological journal to appear in Britain was *Archives of Clinical Skiagraphy* in April 1896, edited by Sydney Rowland who provided all the copy (Fig. 8.6). The journal is the direct forerunner of *British Journal of Radiology*, which is still in print. The major paper by Rowland in the first issue was a review of the brief history of radiology and a description of the materials in use at that time. The first issue otherwise consisted of case reports, but of course everything was a 'first': Plate 3, a needle in an index finger from the Royal Free Hospital (2-minute exposure) (Fig. 8.7); Plate 4, multiple exostoses at the knee (9-minute exposure) from the Children's Hospital, Shadwell; Plate 5, syphilis in a fifteen-year-old boy showing a radial pseudarthrosis and ulnar periostitis with osteolysis; Plate 7, a case of hypertrophic osteosclerosis of the fibula – possibly a stress fracture – in a seventeen-year-old boy from St Thomas's Hospital; Plate 8, a bullet in the palm of a hand; Plate 9, a fracture of the femur extending to the knee.

The next issue, in June 1896, already had a section entitled 'Answers to Correspondents'. Plates included: Plate 8, a fracture of the olecranon treated by wiring, taken by A. E. Morison, FRCS, of Hartlepool; Plate 14, left hip joint disease, possibly following an old fracture, taken by H. McLean of Glasgow, in a seven-year-old (not a very good film); Plate 18, skiagraphy of the soft and hard tissues, including the first 'photograph' of the heart; Plate 21, congenital dislocation of the left hip with a 10-minute exposure (Fig. 8.8); and, on page 37, a paper on cineradiography of moving frog's legs by John Macintyre, another great British pioneer of diagnostic radiology. He was the 'Medical Electrician' to the Glasgow Royal Infirmary, later also becoming an ENT surgeon there. He was a pioneer of fluoroscopy, using a screen of potassium platinocyanide and subsequently calcium tungstate. Röntgen himself corresponded with Macintyre and gave him one of his original X-ray tubes.

By 1897 and 1898 cases had been shown of gout, acromegaly and of a five-year-old child with a cat scratch who had developed pyaemia and septic dislocation of the right hip. In February 1898 Thurston Holland showed a shot in the right orbit, in May 1898 an 'ossifying sarcoma' and in November 1898, from the London

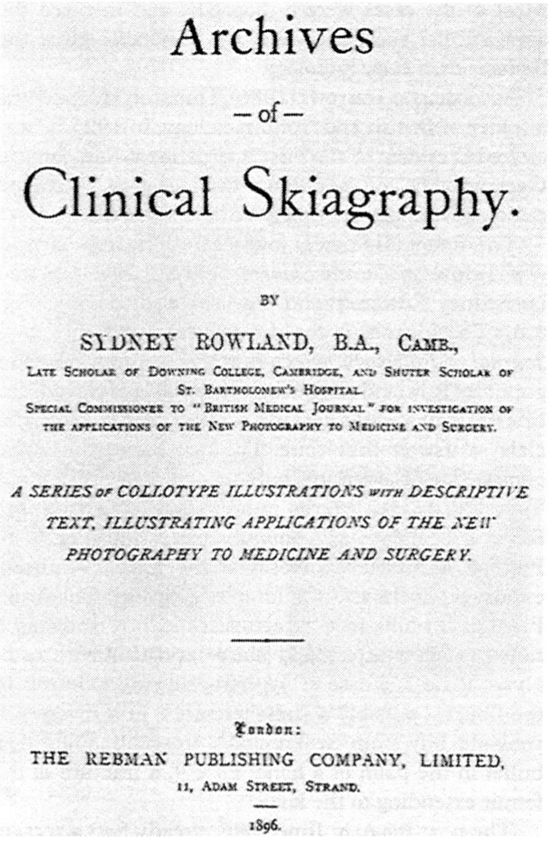

Archives

— of —

Clinical Skiagraphy.

BY

SYDNEY ROWLAND, B.A., CAMB.,

LATE SCHOLAR OF DOWNING COLLEGE, CAMBRIDGE, AND SHUTER SCHOLAR OF
ST. BARTHOLOMEW'S HOSPITAL.
SPECIAL COMMISSIONER TO "BRITISH MEDICAL JOURNAL" FOR INVESTIGATION OF
THE APPLICATIONS OF THE NEW PHOTOGRAPHY TO MEDICINE AND SURGERY.

A SERIES of COLLOTYPE ILLUSTRATIONS with DESCRIPTIVE

TEXT, ILLUSTRATING APPLICATIONS OF THE NEW

PHOTOGRAPHY TO MEDICINE AND SURGERY.

London:

THE REBMAN PUBLISHING COMPANY, LIMITED,

11, ADAM STREET, STRAND.

1896.

Fig. 8.6 Title page of the first radiological journal to appear in England – *Archives of Clinical Skiagraphyii* (1896). Courtesy of the British Institute of Radiology, London

Hospital, absence of the clavicles (presumably a case of cleidocranial dysostosis) in which the shoulders could be brought together in front of the body.

What is evident from the early issues of the first British radiological journal is the rapid acceptance of the new technique. Everything came together at one time. Electricity, photography and physics were no longer quite in their infancy and the necessary ingredients were all readily – and cheaply – available. X-ray departments rapidly sprang up all over the UK. (This is similar to the situation with computed tomography in the 1970s when computers made axial imaging possible. The expense involved in an underfunded health service, however, inhibited the spread of this modern technology, many of the machines in early use being funded from non-governmental sources.) It is also evident that most of the images obtained were musculoskeletal and related to the limbs. This was partly because of the great inherent contrast between a bone (or opaque foreign body) and the surrounding soft tissues. The limbs were more suited to early radiography than deeper parts, that is, the pelvis and spine; initial exposure times were long and the images of poor quality, but the Victorian spirit of inventiveness ensured the rapid advance of technology and the diagnostic quality of images soon improved.

The early pioneers could – and did – easily make a name for themselves. Every week must have brought about a new discovery. Thus, before the use of the X-ray many fractures were believed to be dislocations, while so-called 'reduction' often showed no change from the initial films.

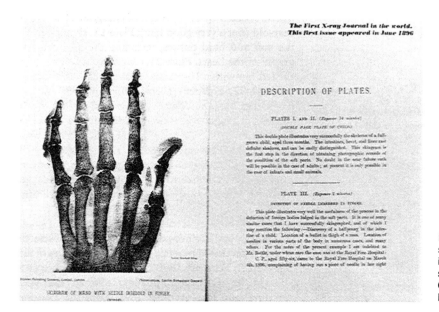

Fig. 8.7 The needle is difficult to see on the early skiagraph, but it is adjacent to the letter 'X' in the soft tissues of the index finger. Courtesy of the British Institute of Radiology, London

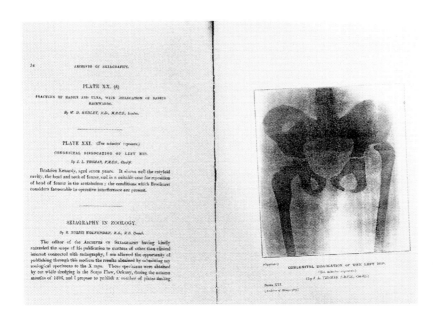

Fig. 8.8 Congenital dislocation of the left hip from an early issue of *Archives*, pl. XXI. Courtesy of the British Institute of Radiology, London

Wilbert (1904) wrote:

It not infrequently happens that even an extensive injury to the osseous framework may be, and sometimes is, mistaken for a more simple lesion. That many cases of actual fracture, particularly at or near the articulating portion of the long bones, have gone unrecognized and untreated, is evidenced by the well-known popular saying that 'A sprain is ofttimes worse than a fracture.' This saying is well founded on the fact that, when a fracture has been diagnosed as a sprain, and treated as such, it usually results in an exuberance of callus that, almost invariably, causes subsequent impairment of function.

With the advent of the new discovery, both normal and abnormal growth and the size and morphology of bone could be assessed, and change in newly discovered diseases recognised.

Amongst the earliest surgeons to make use of X-rays was Sir John Poland, surgeon to the City Orthopaedic Hospital, Hatton Garden, the forerunner of the Royal National Orthopaedic Hospital. This pioneering spirit published his *Skiagraphic Atlas Showing the Development of the Bones of the Wrist and Hand* in 1898. In order to publish at that time he must have started collecting much earlier – possibly at the start of radiology – at his other hospital, the Miller in Greenwich, which had installed an X-ray department in 1896. Poland's book shows radiographs of the hands of children of both sexes from twelve months to sixteen years of age, with a description of each age (Fig. 8.9) (as Greulich and Pyle did later in 1959). In Germany, similar books appeared *c.*1905 (Hueck 1995).

GROWTH AND DEVELOPMENT OF BONES AND CARTILAGE

Alban Köhler, a radiologist in Germany, was aware that females matured earlier and that the order in which the osseous centres in the bones of the wrist could vary (Köhler 1928). He was of the opinion, as was Poland, that

the children of the well-to-do are wont to exhibit even in their earliest childhood an acceleration in growth in regard both to increase of length and more particularly the early appearance of the osseous nuclei. It would appear as if an early stimulation of the spirit and the intellect had elicited an early maturing of the organism, in which doubtless the same kind of influence had acted for many generations. The country child is slowest in development.

The idea is not too far-fetched – presumably poor nutrition played a part in delayed skeletal maturity.

Poland had also published in 1898 *Traumatic Separation of the Epiphyses*, which had a thousand pages and 292 illustrations (of which more later). He wrote:

The most valuable aid in the treatment as well as in the diagnosis of epiphysial separations at the elbow-joint has been recently developed under the Röntgen rays and in the additional use of the fluoroscope. ... Not only is the diagnosis greatly facilitated, but, what is of more value, the position of the fragments can be inspected from day to day with the fluoroscope after the application of non-metallic splints. Subsequent taking down of the dressings, with its accompanying pain and disturbance, can thus be often avoided. So, too, the approximation of the fragments may be accurately accomplished under the guidance of the eye.

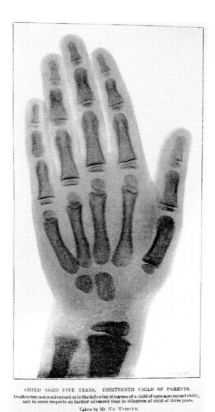

CHILD AGED FIVE YEARS. THIRTEENTH CHILD OF PARENTS.
Ossification not so advanced as in the following skiagram of a child of same age (second child), and in some respects no further advanced than in skiagram of child of three years.

Taken by Mr Wm. Webster.

Fig. 8.9 The bone age of a five-year-old child (Poland 1898a)

Poland showed that fractures through the growth plate could be classified (as did Salter and Harris much later in North America) and pointed out that the mechanism of these lesions was well established by experiments on the dead. Poland's foresight is also evident in his Hunterian Lecture for 1901:

In all *deformities* involving the bones the method plays an important *rôle* in determining the character of the lesion, whether congenital absence of radius or tibia, polydactylism or syndactylism, hallux valgus, congenital club foot, and deformities due to defective growth of the shafts of the bone after injury or disease of the epiphyses.

The use of the X-rays is still in its infancy, but skiagraphy will, I am sure, develop into a science worthy of surgery, provided its study be prosecuted by medical men, or by men having a thorough anatomical training, who would study it in a scientific spirit, with time and opportunity to make it a speciality. I can only hope that it may fall to the lot of some member of this Society to take up this fascinating study in a true Hunterian spirit. It should not, as I have already said, be allocated to the mechanician or photographer, for thereby its development and assistance to the surgeon will be manifestly checked. (Poland 1901)

Premature fusion was known to result in deformity (Fig. 8.10). Nonetheless, in the early days of radiology some epiphyses were believed to represent fractures, for example at the olecranon, while similar confusion existed with accessory bones, for instance in the foot – the epiphysis at the base of the fifth metatarsal and the local os Vesalianum in particular causing some confusion. Thomas Dwight, in his atlas *Variations of the Bones of the Hands and Feet* of 1907 (Fig. 8.11), called the apophysis at the base of the fifth metatarsal the os Vesalianum which, if it occurs at all as described by Vesalius, is possibly the whole tuberosity of the metatarsal developing separately, perhaps after a fracture (Thurston Holland 1928).

OSGOOD–SCHLATTER'S DISEASE

One of the first abnormalities of ossification in disease to be described was osteochondritis of the tibial tuberosity in adolescence, which was separately described by both Osgood and Schlatter in 1903.

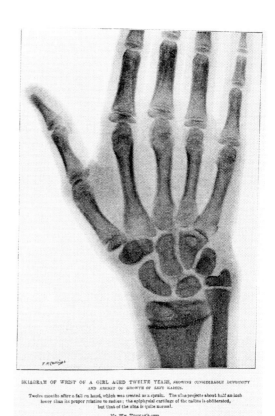

SKIAGRAM OF WRIST OF A GIRL AGED TWELVE YEARS, SHOWING CONSIDERABLE DEFORMITY AND ARREST OF GROWTH OF LEFT RADIUS.

Twelve months after a fall on hand, which was treated as a sprain. The ulna projects about half an inch lower than its proper relation to radius; the epiphysial cartilage of the radius is obliterated, but that of the ulna is quite normal.

Mr. Wm. Thomas's case.

Fig. 8.10 Premature fusion of the distal radial epiphysis following trauma (from Poland 1898a)

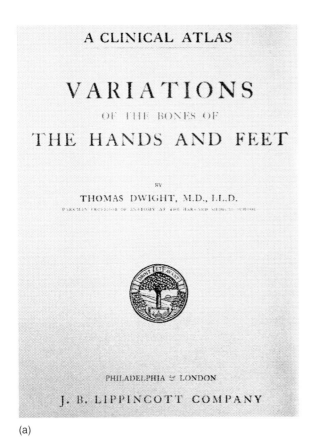

A CLINICAL ATLAS

VARIATIONS

OF THE BONES OF

THE HANDS AND FEET

BY

THOMAS DWIGHT, M.D., LL.D.

PARKMAN PROFESSOR OF ANATOMY AT THE HARVARD MEDICAL SCHOOL

PHILADELPHIA & LONDON

J. B. LIPPINCOTT COMPANY

(a)

Schlatter believed the condition was due to incomplete separation of the epiphyseal process (Köhler 1928). According to Kienböck (1910) the disease was an osteochondritis increased by crushing or tearing, probably of tuberculous nature and accompanied by a primary pretibial bursitis. Some German authors believed that 'late rickets' was the main cause or important predisposition. Köhler (1928) thought it was due to an inflammatory process, but pointed out that occasionally real fractures occurred locally and should not be confused with Osgood–Schlatter's disease. None of the early authors are quoted as commenting on the overlying soft tissue thickening – perhaps it could not be appreciated on early radiographs.

Alban Köhler (1874–1947) of Wiesbaden began his radiological career in 1899 showing the usual fractures and foreign bodies (Fig. 8.12). His major work, *Lexicon der Grenzen des Normalen im Röntgenbilde* was first published in Hamburg in 1910, then subsequently as *Grenzen des Normalen und Anfänge des Pathologischen im Röntgenbilde des Skelettes*. It was translated into English and published in 1928 as *Röntgenology. The Borderlands of the Normal and Early Pathological in the Skiagram*. (The eighth edition, published in 1948, had 809 pages.)

Köhler's first eponymous disease, avascular necrosis of the tarsal navicular, was described in 1908 ('concerning a frequent, up to now unknown disease of particular children's bones') (Köhler 1908, Cockayne 1919). By 1928 he still was uncertain as to the aetiology of the disease but noted that it cleared up within one or two

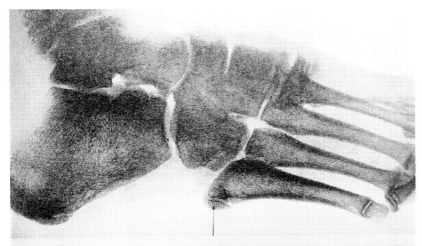

FIG. 75. *Vesalianum.* An X-ray of the foot of a girl (?) aged 13, showing a separate element very clearly. There is no suspicion of injury, for the skiagraph was taken on account of a bullet wound in another part of the foot. I have placed a question mark after the word "girl" because my record of the sex is lost, but there is very little doubt on the point.

(b)

Fig. 8.11   (a) Title page of Thomas Dwight's *Variations of the Bones of the Hands and Feet* (1907). (b) The wrongly described os Vesalianum. Dwight obviously did not recognise that there was a local apophysis

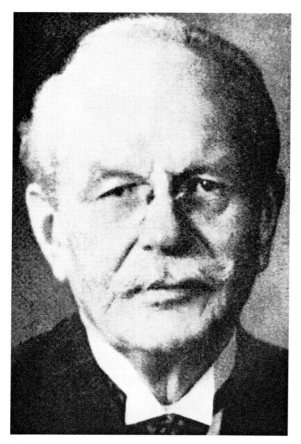

Fig. 8.12 Alban Köhler (1874–1947)

years with rest, and had nothing to do with tuberculosis. He also realised that it did not necessarily follow a fracture but was initially of the opinion that it occurred in poorly developed children, especially those who had been debilitated in early life, or who even had osteomalacia, but he subsequently retracted this belief. Some patients, however, were said to have rachitis (rickets) and, occasionally, gonorrhoea, tuberculosis or syphilis.

Köhler initially believed the disease to be an interruption or delay in development since other bones could be similarly affected, for example, 'osteochondritis coxae' in the hip. He noted 'remarkable results' following treatment with thyroid preparations! Perhaps some of his patients did indeed have congenital hypothyroidism, which causes delay and abnormality of skeletal maturation, or perhaps the hormone accelerated the healing process.

His second eponymous disease, Freiberg-Köhler disease of the second metatarsal head, was described in 1920. Köhler noted that this occurred more commonly than his eponymous navicular disease, usually in the

second, occasionally in the third, or in both, metatarsal heads, generally in the right foot and more commonly in females (rather than in males, as did Köhler's disease of the tarsal navicular). Some patients (about one-fifth) had flat feet and this was thought to be a predisposing factor, as 'coxa vara' was, he thought, to Perthes' disease. In summary, he wrote:

it can be said: there are certainly anatomical-physiological conditions for the localisation of the disease at the second (or third) metatarsophalangeal joint. The body weight is on the second metatarsus, and it is exposed to all manner of strains and stresses, as is shown by the swelling of soldiers' feet affecting the second in the highest percentage of all the metatarsals. This factor of exposed position, however, is never alone sufficient. There must be in addition a factor of a general pathological nature which in particular produces a certain debility of the bony system, perhaps not so much infectious as of a toxic or toxic-infectious, dyscrasic, diathetic, hormonic, or similar nature, by which a diminished resistance of the organs is produced, especially those exposed under physiological conditions of the greatest work and strain, as also here in the head of the second metacarpal bone. Or there arises a particular predisposition somewhat in the sense of a constitutional anomaly, possibly also analogous to the so-called weight-deformities (nor can phylogenetic factors be entirely excluded; they, too, play a rôle). Then with slight repeated strains or greater overstrain a form of osteochondritis malacia is produced (Köhler 1928).

Freiberg, an American, published 'Infraction of the metatarsal head' in *Surgery, Gynaecology and Obstetrics* in August 1914 at around the same time as Köhler wrote his earlier communication (Freiberg 1914).

LEGG–CALVÉ–PERTHES' DISEASE (OSTEOCHONDRITIS DEFORMANS COXAE, PSEUDOCOXALGIA, COXA VARA CAPITALIS)

Köhler stated that the first Röntgen pictures of this disorder, together with a description of the clinical findings, were given by him in March 1905 in his *Atlas of the Hip Joint and Thigh*. He noted a discrepancy between the advanced destructive process in the femoral head and the clinical findings, which were relatively minor and improved after a short rest. Le Vay (1990), however, states that the first radiographs of Perthes' disease were made in 1898 but not published until 1914 by Perthes' assistant, Schwarz, though Köhler's case was presumably the first to be published.

Jacques Calvé lived long into the modern era (1875–1954). Le Vay (1990) writes that Calvé and the X-ray machine arrived simultaneously in the town of Berck. Köhler (1928) noted that Calvé realised that some children with coxa plana recovered with full movement except adduction, with no adenopathy or abscess formation, and no relapsing disease, and so could not have had tuberculosis (Calvé 1910).

Legg noted an 'obscure affection of the hip joint which … radiologically and clinically simulated TB, but did not pursue the usual destructive course'. He described this condition and presented five cases at the Hartford, Connecticut, meeting of the American Orthopaedic Association in June 1909, and published them the following year (Legg 1910). Perthes did not describe the disease until later (Perthes 1913).

The Swedish orthopaedic surgeon Waldenström wrote on tuberculosis of the upper part of the neck of the femur, but some of his cases were due to Perthes' disease (Waldenström 1909, also Delitala 1914–15, Taylor & Frieder 1915, Allison & Moody 1915. Incidentally, Allison and Moody's Cases 10 and 11, showing 'similar pathologic condition', are of premature growth plate fusion following trauma, already shown by Poland in 1898).

Köhler noted that Perthes' disease could be distinguished from 'arthritis deformans of youth' by the preservation of the joint cartilage (presumably he refers to juvenile chronic arthritis).

OSTEOCHONDRITIS OF THE SPINE

According to Köhler (1928), H. W. Scheuermann of Copenhagen described a disease 'appearing from the fifteenth to the seventeenth year with a dorsal kyphosis … which clears up entirely, or almost entirely' (Scheuermann 1921). He noted 'irregularity and deformity of the discs (that is, the end-plates), irregularity especially at the anterior edge of the vertebral body, with atrophy and wedging, in extreme cases arousing a suspicion of tuberculosis. As the lower dorsal region is exposed to the greatest compression, it was there that the greatest changes occurred' (Fig. 8.13). Agricultural workers were the most frequently affected – 'peasant back'. Scheuermann classified the disease with *osteochondritis juvenilis coxae*, i.e. Perthes' disease, whilst others considered it analogous to *coxa vara adolescentium*, i.e. slipped epiphysis.

Interestingly, spondylitic exostoses at the edges of one or more vertebral bodies (the reproduced diagrams of which resemble syndesmophytes) were said by Köhler (1928) to be related to tumours of the spinal cord, more often extramedullary than intramedullary: 'the vertebral column should be opened … at the level of the exostosis formation. If a tumour is not found at this spot, the laminectomy should be extended downwards'.

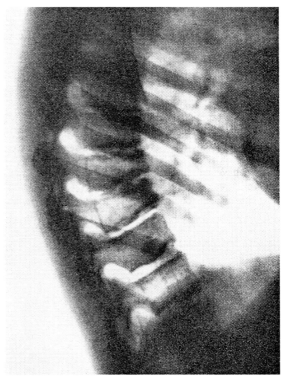

Fig. 8.13   Osteochondritis of the spine (Scheuermann's disease) (Köhler 1928, p 209)

GENETIC DISEASES OF BONE

The term 'chondrodystrophy' appears in both Köhler (1928) and Goldthwait et al (1910). The latter authors illustrate a case with diaphyseal flaring, femoral bowing and coxa vara. Clinically, these children – if they survived – were 'weaklings for varying periods, but if they survive seem to develop a normal resistance'. Some of these cases resemble achondroplastic dwarfs with retracted noses and short, thick limbs, but the disease is further divided into three different types according to the epiphyseal shape:

- Chondrodystrophia foetalis hypoplastica.
- Chondrodystrophia foetalis hyperplastica – with large epiphyses.
- Chondrodystrophia foetalis malica, where the epiphyses are soft and gelatinous (perhaps rickets?).

Heinrich Albers-Schönberg (1865–1921) was a founder member of the German Röntgen Association in 1900 (Fig. 8.14). Originally a gynaecologist, he became the first full-time radiologist in Germany, opening a private radiological clinic in Hamburg in February 1897. He published his first book on techniques in rontgenology in 1903 and made many technical innovations in radiography, as well as describing the disease that bears his name. He developed a radiation sarcoma of his right middle finger and died thirteen years later, having had many amputations for malignant metastatic disease. He is inscribed as a Röntgen martyr on the obelisk in the garden of the St George Hospital, Hamburg, where he was the radiologist. By 1903 he had also demonstrated experimental evidence of the harmful effects of X-rays on rabbit testes.

Albers-Schönberg disease (osteopetrosis, marble bones) was first described at a medical meeting in Munich in 1903, but the text was not illustrated with an example of the disorder (Fig. 8.15) (Albers-Schönberg 1903–04). In 1915 Albers-Schönberg also described osteopoikylosis (Albers-Schönberg 1915). Köhler (1928) thought the distribution of the latter 'similar to that seen in haematogenous tuberculosis, the distribution of the spots in the bones coinciding with the embolism points on end-arteries'.

Some cases of osteopoikylosis, however, seem to have been complicated in Köhler's description by spontaneous fractures, hepatosplenomegaly and anaemia, together with dense bands at the diaphyses and necrosis of the jaws, in one instance of the disease affecting three sisters. There seems to have been some confusion therefore between the two separate sclerosing dysplasias of bone – one, osteopoikylosis, entirely innocent, the other osteopetrosis, often not.

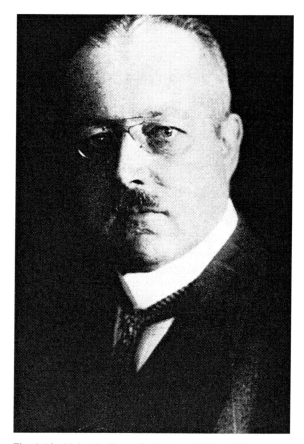

Fig. 8.14 Heinrich Albers-Schönberg (1865–1921)

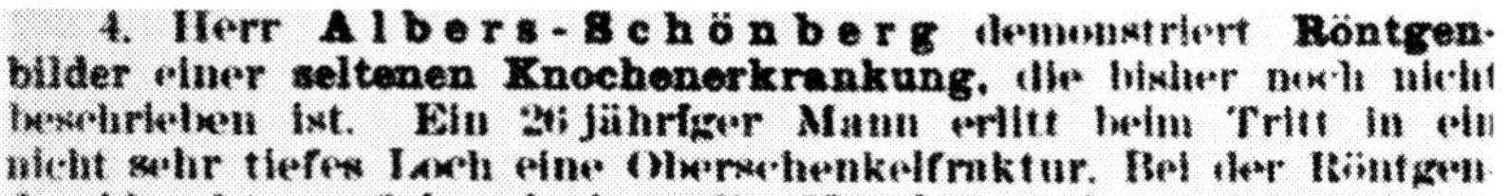

4. Herr **Albers-Schönberg** demonstriert **Röntgenbilder einer seltenen Knochenerkrankung**, die bisher noch nicht beschrieben ist. Ein 26 jähriger Mann erlitt beim Tritt in ein nicht sehr tiefes Loch eine Oberschenkelfraktur. Bei der Röntgendurchleuchtung fiel auf, dass die Knochenstruktur nicht erkennbar war. Die Knochen geben tiefschwarze Schatten, die Markhöhle fehlte, die Kortikalis war verbreitert. Eine Durchleuchtung des ganzen Skeletts ergab eine Fraktur des anderen Oberschenkels und des einen Olekranon, von deren Entstehung und Vorhandensein Pat. nichts wusste, sowie den gleichen Knochenbefund an sämtlichen Skelettabschnitten. Neben der tiefschwarzen Farbe der Knochenbilder sind besonders an den kürzeren Extremitätenknochen, sowie an den Rippen eigentümliche, quer verlaufende Ringe erkennbar. Der ganze Befund entspricht einer ausserordentlich starken Verkalkung des ganzen Skeletts. — Vortr. demonstriert dann **Röntgenbilder einer 3000 Jahre alten ägyptischen Mumie,** einer Neuerwerbung des Hamburger kulturhistorischen Museums.

Fig. 8.15 The case report from the medical meeting in Munich. The text reads: 'Mr Albers-Schönberg demonstrated Röntgen pictures of a rare bone disease that has not previously been described. A twenty-six-year-old man tripped over a not very deep hole and sustained a fracture of the femur. The X-ray examination showed that the bone structure was not recognisable. The bones gave deep black shadows, the marrow cavity did not exist and the cortex was thickened. Examination of the entire skeleton showed a fracture of the other femur and of one olecranon, about which the patient knew nothing, nor of the identical bone change in other parts of the skeleton. Besides the deep black colour of the X-ray pictures there are also strange, transverse rings to be seen especially on the small bones of the extremity as well as on the ribs. The whole find speaks of a most unusually strong calcification of the whole skeleton.'

Köhler described a case of osteopetrosis in an eighteen-day-old child but reports another causing a fracture of the calcaneus in a thirty-four-year-old doctor, otherwise well, inadvertently therefore describing both recessive and dominant forms of the disease (Schell-Lund 1922). Incidentally, he reports a similar looking case 'developing on the basis of rachitic osteomalacia' – presumably renal osteodystrophy with a rugger-jersey spine.

Robert Osgood does not mention his eponymous disease in his co-authored book *Diseases of the Bones and Joints* (Goldthwait et al 1910). Over one-third of the book is on tuberculosis. He does however discuss osteogenesis imperfecta, first named thus by Vrolik (1849), but which had already been described in 1763 by Bordenave. Lovett had also described a case in 1906 in the *British Medical Journal*. The bones, as seen on these images from 1910, are

bent and twisted from the fractures which have occurred *in utero* [Fig. 8.16]. The cranial sutures were noted to be often widely open. Non-union of the intrauterine or extrauterine fractures is rare and callus formation ... gives a bone a nodular feel. The spine is often curved.

Many of the cases reported as idiopathic fragilitas ossium should be considered instances of osteogenesis imperfecta.

A small residue of reported cases in which the fragility occurred later in life and was not associated with congenital disease ... it seems improbable that the process in osteogenesis imperfecta is identical with acquired fragilitas ossium. (Goldthwait et al 1910)

The link between tarda and congenita forms seems not, therefore, to have been recognised, but it was understood that *if early years were survived*, the bones became less brittle and fractures less frequent.

METABOLIC DISEASE
Rickets and osteomalacia

Thurston Holland seems to have had images of rickets and osteomalacia in 1896. E. Muirhead Little, surgeon to the Royal National Orthopaedic Hospital, drew attention to 'cupping of the ends of the diaphyses', especially at the ends of the radius and ulna (Muirhead Little, quoted in Tubby 1912, p 405). (See also the hand of a three-year-old after Köhler (1928, p 406).)

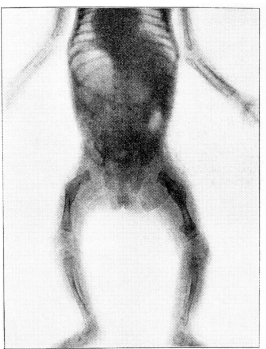

Fig. 226. Observe the numerous fractures, which were spontaneous, also the bowing of the long bones, the flaring diaphyses, and the rarefication of the medullary tissue in certain places.

(a)

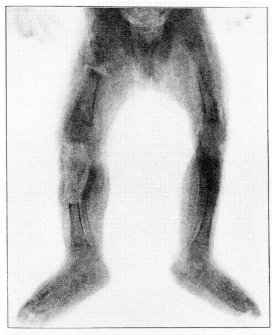

Fig. 227. As in Figure 226 there have been numerous spontaneous fractures with much overriding of fragments in places. There is also a marked rarefication of the upper portion of the right tibia and bowing of the other long bones.

(b)

Fig. 8.16a, b Osteogenesis imperfecta was clearly well recognised in Goldthwait et al (1910)

Henry O. Feiss, a surgeon of Cleveland, Ohio, described a three-and-a-half-year-old child seen in November 1904 with typical severe clinical rickets and who had transverse fractures across the ulna and humerus (Feiss 1905–06). The joints showed typical rachitic features. The lesion in the ulna certainly looks like a Looser zone which has extended transversely across the whole width of the bone, as is known to occur.

Emil Looser wrote his classic paper on rickets and osteomalacia in 1920. The blockade of the Central European powers by the Western Allies during and after the First World War caused mass starvation and his paper must have reflected the dietary deficiencies of the patients. His clinical photographs show gross bony deformity due to bone softening of a type totally unknown today. Figure 8.17a shows the child unable to hold his head erect, presumably because of the myopathy. Figure 8.17b shows what are now termed *Looser's zones*, with healing on treatment, while Fig. 8.17c shows bone softening, bowing and a tibial pseudarthrosis reminiscent of neurofibromatosis. One wonders if any of his patients had osteogenesis imperfecta, but I assume that the differentiation could have been made even in those days.

Certainly before the Second World War, people in poor districts in Britain, such as Glasgow, commonly had rickets, and the ricketty rosary was well known.

Scurvy (Barlow's disease, Barlow-Möller's disease)

According to Köhler (1928), Möller regarded this as acute rickets. Köhler recognised subperiosteal haemorrhages with periostitis and metaphyseal fragmented Trummerfeld zones – 'Trummerfeld' meaning 'wasteland' – while the epiphysis has a 'sharply contained fragmented nucleus' (Wimberger 1925). Instead of 'fragmented zone', the term 'scorbutic line' was proposed by Pelkan (1925). These terms are still in current use.

RADIOLOGY IN MEDICO-LEGAL PRACTICE

John Poland gave the Hunterian oration of the Hunterian Society (of London) in 1901. His lecture was entitled 'A Retrospect of Surgery During the Past Century' (Poland 1901). The committee of the American Surgical Association had drawn up a largely negative review of the routine use of radiology in cases of fracture (report of the Committee of the American Surgical Association 1900). Poland roundly decried such a view: 'Indeed, it may be questioned whether treatises on fractures written before the Röntgen era

may now be regarded as authentic. *A distinct skiagraphic plate will always tell the truth.*' Space does not allow the complete reproduction of his prophetic words, but he notes that before the introduction of the Röntgen ray, many fractures, especially of the carpus, tarsus and metatarsus, were actually unknown.

In the early days of the Röntgen rays, he notes (in 1901) the normal sesamoid bones were a frequent source of error, for example the os trigonum tarsi, which had been mistaken for a fragment severed from the astralagus (talus). Skiagraphs in a recent case brought before the courts in Germany proved that this process of bone existed normally on both feet, and that no fracture had taken place. Shepherd, who mistook this bone for a fracture fragment, 'tried to produce this fracture on the dead body, but in every case ... failed, even where the greatest force was used, to break off the little process of bone'.

The case, mentioned by Carl Beck in *Fractures* (1900), was of a German labourer injured by an iron bar on 20 January 1897 and who complained of continual pain below the lateral malleolus. He was thought to be a malingerer but a skiagraph showed him to have a 'fracture' of the talus. The labourer received an annuity of 30%. He was later seen to be walking normally, however, and the clinician insisted that both feet be examined radiologically. The os trigonum was seen on both sides and the labourer was forced to repay his annuity.

The first occasion in which an X-ray image was used in the USA was in Denver, Colorado, in 1896, alleging failure to diagnose a femoral fracture (Stafford Withers 1931). Kevles (1998) describes the case fully. James Smith, a law student, had fallen off a ladder while painting a wall. Three weeks later, still in pain, he went to a surgeon, W. Grant, who had earlier performed the first appendicectomy in the country. He diagnosed a contusion and prescribed exercise. Pain continued, and the limb became shorter.

Smith found a photographer with an interest in X-rays six months after their discovery. After *80 minutes* of exposure an impacted fracture was shown. Several judges had refused to accept X-ray plates as evidence because there was no proof that such a thing was possible: 'It is like offering the photograph of a ghost, where there is no proof that there is any such thing as a ghost' (Stafford Withers 1931).

RADIOLOGY IN WAR

The Royal Army Medical Corps had a primitive X-ray machine in the Sudan in 1896 (Battersby 1989–99). Power was obtained by means of a tandem cycle, operated by two men, in a temperature of 110°F. Major Battersby

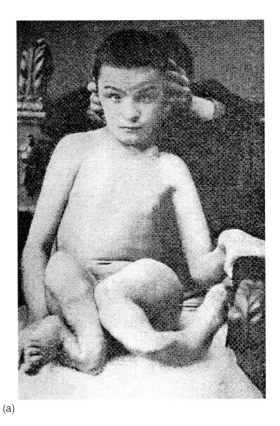

(a)

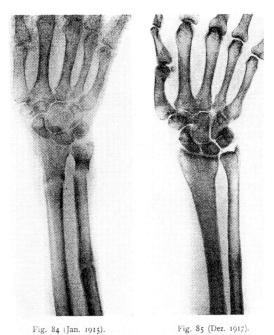

Fig. 84 (Jan. 1915).   Fig. 85 (Dez. 1917).

(b)

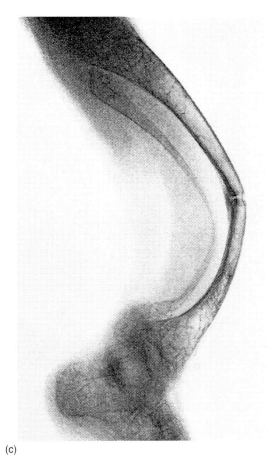

(c)

Fig. 8.17 Gross skeletal deformity (Looser 1920).
(a) The patient presumably has a myopathy as he is no
doubt unable to hold his head erect. (b) Healing Looser's
zones are noted between January 1915 and December
1917. (c) Gross osteopenia together with bowing and a
pseudofracture of the tibial shafts, so reminiscent of
osteogenesis imperfecta

concluded that the X-ray was useful for locating foreign
bodies and diagnosing fractures (Fig. 8.18).

In 1898 the US military had equipped hospital
ships with X-ray machines for use off Cuba in the
Spanish-American war. Radiographs obtained showed
bullet wounds and fractures (Borden 1900).

Meanwhile the Boer War also proved the merits of the
Röntgen ray. *A Civilian War Hospital – Experience of Wounds
and Sickness in South Africa* by Bowley (1901) shows
numerous examples of bullet wounds and fractures (Fig.
8.19), as does *Surgical Experiences in South Africa
(1899–1900)* (1901) by George Henry Makins, surgeon to
St Thomas's Hospital. Makins's case No. 47 clearly shows
a Mauser bullet in the 'nasal fossa'. The soldier had been

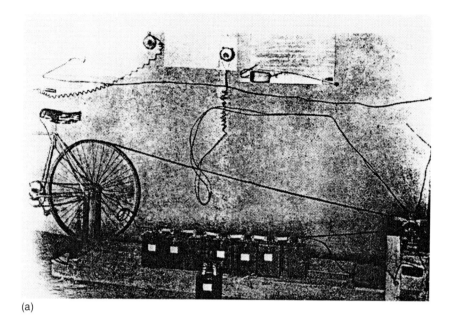

(a)

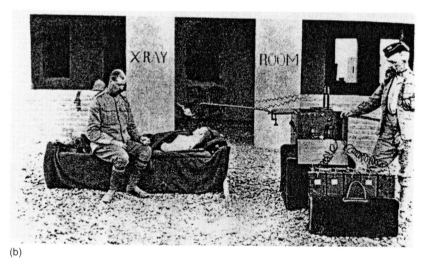

(b)

Fig. 8.18a, b Major Battersby in the Sudan (Battersby 1898–99). Courtesy of the British Institute of Radiology, London

wounded at 'Poplar Grove' (the name given to a local area in South Africa by the troops stationed there; presumably they had either come from Poplar or perhaps Shepherd's Bush), the wound being ¾ inch above the right eyebrow and a similar distance from the midline (Fig. 8.20). He subsequently developed pyrexia and was operated on by Mr Watson Cheyne, of King's College Hospital, the bullet having been localised with the aid of Röntgen rays.

Later, in Vietnam, the American Forces in the field were to use portable fluoroscopes powered by isotopes!

NEOPLASMS

Mention has already been made that Plate 4 of the first volume of *Archives of the Rontgen Ray* (21 April 1898) was of multiple exostoses at the knee, while in February 1898 an ossifying sarcoma of the humerus was illustrated. This was literally 'stamp collecting' with, of course, no possibility of a systematic approach to radiology.

A. H. Tubby was a consultant surgeon at the Royal National Orthopaedic Hospital, London. His textbook *Deformities, Including Diseases of the Bones and Joints* was

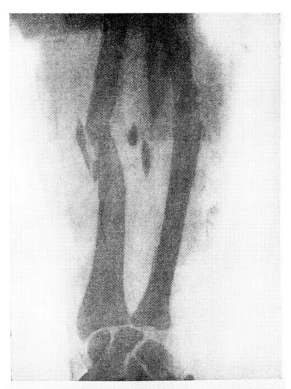

EXPANDING BULLET WOUND OF BONES OF FOREARM, showing the separation of the Bones by the explosive effect of the projectile.

Fig. 8.19 Comminuted fractures following a bullet wound in the Boer War (Bowley 1901)

first published in 1896, prior to the advent of the Röntgen ray. The second, much larger, edition of 1912 was profusely illustrated with numerous X-ray images. Much of the second volume is taken up with tuberculosis and rickets (Fig. 8.21), while there are only seventeen pages on neoplasms of bone. Of course, Tubby was aware of the division into primary and secondary tumours, and benign and malignant lesions. He illustrated a 'pedunculated exostosis' of the distal femur in a case of multiple exostoses, and two cases belonging to Thurston Holland – a chondrosarcoma clearly breaking through the femoral cortex (Fig. 8.22) and a parosteal sarcoma under the care of Robert Jones (Fig. 8.23). He notes that the periosteum at the periphery of the tumour is lifted away from the bone and gradually lost in the substance of the growth. The *Codman triangle* should perhaps better be called the *Tubby triangle*. He also advocated biopsy prior to amputation: 'It is not always easy to differentiate chronic periostitis, osteitis, myelitis or inflammation of bone from new growth; and we have known surgeons to be in error, who have relied upon the clinical signs alone.'

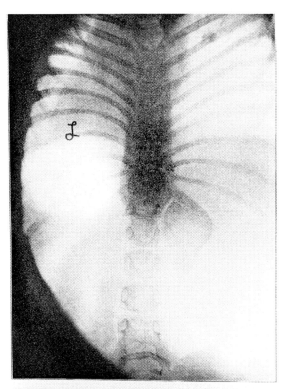

Skiagram, taken by Mr. Mackenzie Davidson, of a case of Dorso-Lumbar Caries, under the care of Dr. Ford Anderson and the author, showing the outline and connection with the spine of a psoas abscess on the right side. L, is a wire placed on the left side.

Fig. 8.21 Spinal tuberculosis. Note the mineralised psoas abscess on the right (Tubby 1912)

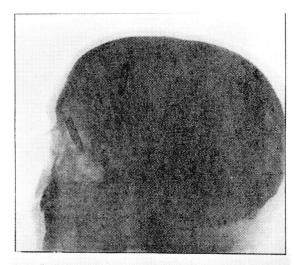

FIG. 60.—Mauser Bullet in Nasal Fossa. (Skiagram by H. Catling.) Case No. 47

Fig. 8.20 A bullet near the eye (Makins 1901)

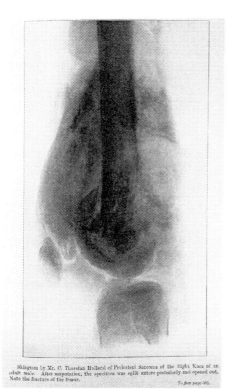

Skingram by Mr. C. Thurstan Holland of Periosteal Sarcoma of the Right Knee of an adult male. After amputation, the specimen was split antero-posteriorly and opened out. Note the fracture of the femur.

To face page 583.

Fig. 8.22 Osteosarcoma (Tubby 1912)

A further image is of a secondary deposit in the humerus and there is a description of an aneurysmal bone cyst.

In 1910 Goldthwait et al showed an image of bone proliferation thought to be a sarcoma but proved to be osteomyelitis (Fig. 8.24), and described Röntgen changes in myeloma. They referred to Coley's paper of 1907 on sarcoma of long bones. Plate 185 is of a Paget's sarcoma Goldthwait et al (1910) (Fig. 8.25).

Fränkel used a more systematic approach in the study of tumours of the spinal column in 150 patients. He also described both lytic and sclerotic metastases (Fränkel 1910), as did Pfahler (1917). Spontaneous fracture in secondary carcinoma of the bones (Fig. 8.26) was also discussed by G. W. Hawley (1913–14); this paper gives a lengthy biography of metastatic disease in bone.

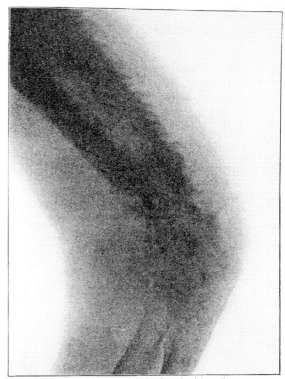

FIG. 180. This shows the close resemblance of certain of the malignant sarcomata to chronic diffuse osteomyelitis. This was thought to be a sarcoma but proved to be osteomyelitis.

Fig. 8.24 Osteomyelitis with close resemblance to osteosarcoma (Goldthwait et al 1910)

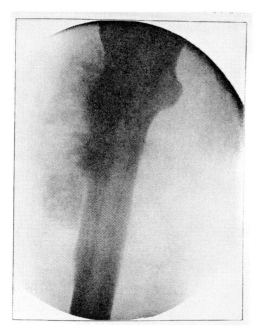

Fig. 8.23 Parosteal sarcoma (Tubby 1912)

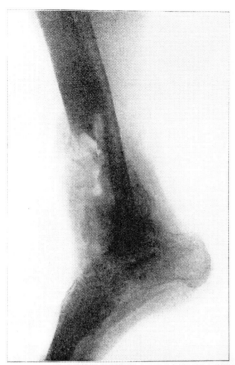

Fig. 165. This specimen was X-rayed after amputation. The new growth in the popliteal space is very marked. Case XIV.

Fig. 8.25 Paget's sarcoma (Goldthwait et al 1910)

INFECTIONS OF BONE

Infections were similarly imaged from the beginnings of radiology, tuberculosis in particular. 'Spina ventosa' or tuberculous disease of the smaller long bones was one of the first radiographs in a child. Alban Köhler also reported spina ventosa. Until the early 1920s images of the spine were more difficult to obtain. Calvé and Lelievre (1913–14) first recommended the use of lateral radiographs of the spine in Pott's disease. Excellent radiographs were obtained showing the progress of Pott's disease (Fig. 8.27). (Incidentally some of the radiographs are printed upside down!) Presumably until then only anteroposterior views had been obtained.

Cotton gave a good radiological overview of bone disease, demonstrating tuberculous septic arthritis (Fig. 8.28), simple osteomyelitis, syphilitic bone disease, parosteal sarcoma (Fig. 8.29), giant-cell tumour (then called giant-cell sarcoma) (Fig. 8.30) and simple bone cyst (Cotton 1915). He pointed out that these were different diseases in which the rontgenograms were similar, and that the diagnosis must be made with the aid of clinical data.

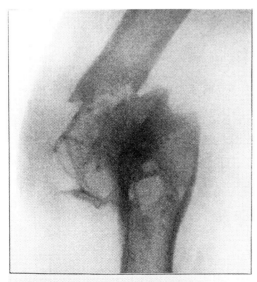

Fig. 4.—Radiograph loaned by Dr. L. G. Cole, of New York. Case of metastases from mammary carcinoma with spontaneous fracture of femur. Fracture had occurred at same site two years previously. Union resulted after each inquiry.

Fig. 8.26 Metastases with pathological fracture (Hawley 1913–14)

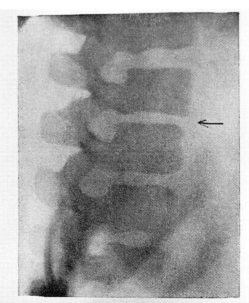

Fig. 1.—Radiograph of beginning Pott's disease. Thinning of an intervertebral disc.

(a)
Fig. 8.27a Progression of Pott's disease: (a) is printed upside down (Calvé & Lelievre 1913–14)

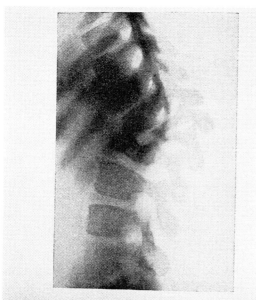

Fig. 6.—Pott's disease insufficiently treated. Shows that the superior fragment has decapitated the first vertebra of the inferior fragment and penetrated into the anterior part of the underlying vertebra.

(b)

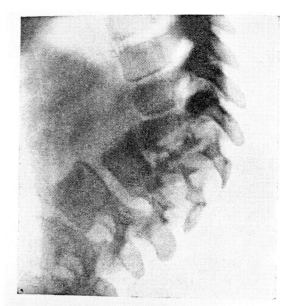

Fig. 7.—Untreated Pott's disease. Kyphos considerable through slipping of the inferior fragment in front of the superior fragment. Three vertebræ are destroyed.

(c)

Fig. 8.27b-c

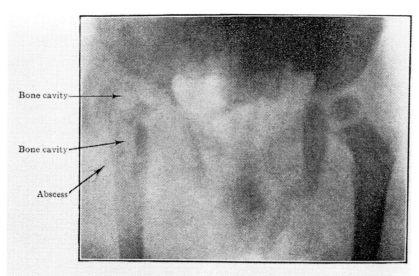

Fig. 1.—Tuberculosis of hip-joint. Active tuberculosis with erosion and abscess formation; extension to shaft of femur. Bone cavities indistinctly outlined; very little periosteal bone formation.

Characteristic "fuzzy" appearance. Rarefaction of bone and bone destruction confused in röntgenogram.

Fig. 8.28 Tuberculous septic arthritis (Cotton 1915)

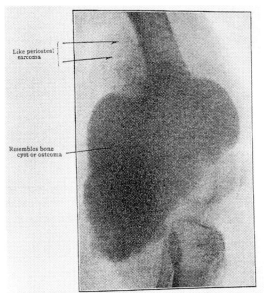

Like periosteal sarcoma
Resembles bone cyst or osteoma
FIG. 14.—Osteo-chondro-sarcoma lower end femur beginning as small osteoma; gradual growth during ten years, finally becoming sarcomatous. Amputation middle thigh; recurrence in grain and death three years later. Note resemblance to bone cyst; also at upper portion to periosteal sarcoma. Diagnosis by history, clinical data, X-ray, and exploratory incision. Amputation above exploratory incision.

Fig. 8.29 Parosteal sarcoma (Cotton 1915)

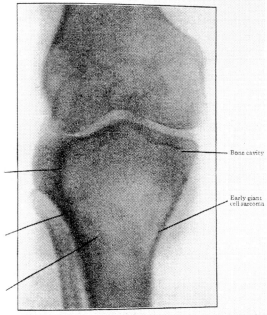

Bone cavity
Early giant cell sarcoma
FIG. 20.—Giant cell sarcoma (early) before operation showing area of rarefaction but no new periosteal bone or trabeculæ. Impossible at this stage to differentiate from bone cyst or abscess of bone by röntgenogram alone.

Fig. 8.30 Giant-cell tumour (Cotton 1915)

CONTRAST MEDIA

The discovery of the X-ray enabled an image to be made that utilised the differing densities and absorptive patterns of four substances: bone, soft tissue, fat and air. Generally, however, all types of soft tissue – muscle, blood, pus and urine – cannot be distinguished on plain radiography.

The first contrast medium to be used in radiology was air. In 1905 Werndorff and Robinsohn examined the knee after insufflation of air into the joint, and Hoffa (1906) used pure oxygen. In later years carbon dioxide was used. The gas separated the internal structures of the knee from the articular surfaces so that menisci and cruciate ligaments could be visualised. I was still performing pneumo-arthrography until fairly recently in patients with a history of allergy to contrast media (Renton 1991). Arthrography did not however take off until the advent of contrast media in the 1930s.

Air in the brain, and especially in the ventricles, following communicating external trauma had already been reported by Luckett and Stewart in Harlem in 1912 (Bruwer 1964), and by Gilbert Scott in London (Bull & Fischgold 1989). Walter Dandy, a surgeon at the Johns Hopkins Hospital, injected air directly into the ventricles in 1918, a process more difficult in adults than in children with hydrocephalus, whose fontanelles were not yet united.

Dandy (1925) subsequently imaged the spine and brain by injecting air at lumbar puncture, taking care to remove an equal amount of cerebrospinal fluid (CSF).

Kevles (1998) describes the first use of a positive contrast medium. *Lipiodol* had previously been used as a painkiller in muscles, but was inadvertently injected into the CSF by a student of Sicard who rushed to tell his chief of the mishap. Sicard, in turn, put the patient on to a screening table and saw the spinal nerve roots outlined (Sicard & Forestier 1921, 1922).

That there were drawbacks to the use of Lipiodol was evident early on, especially the fact that only incomplete filling of the canal could be obtained, while in those early days 'meningitis' apparently resulted if the oil was old. Arachnoiditis would follow later. Oil was however used for shoulder arthrography in 1938 by Lindblom (1939).

Apparently even the radioactive contrast medium *Thorotrast* was used intrathecally, but it could not easily be removed and caused major reactions, ultimately including sarcomas.

Water-soluble ionic contrast media, *Conray* and *Hypaque*, could be used for arthrography, but were not very useful in the CSF because of toxicity. Similarly, *Dimer-X* could only be used to show the lumbosacral roots because of brain and cord toxicity.

Amipaque, the first low osmolar water-soluble non-ionic contrast medium, could be used to examine the entire spinal canal with a high iodine dose. Because it was unstable and could not be sterilised in solution, it had to be made up before each examination. It became the standard intrathecal and intra-articular contrast medium in the 1980s, but was then replaced by second-generation low osmolality contrast media *Omnipaque* and *Niopam*, which are easy to synthesise and relatively cheap.

With the introduction of new dimeric non-ionic contrast media, perfection has apparently been obtained. They are isotonic with blood and CSF, with a very low rate of central nervous system side-effects. While of equal use in arthrography, contrast studies of joints have largely been superseded by magnetic resonance imaging (see below).

DEVELOPMENT OF OTHER IMAGING MODALITIES

Tomography – 'slice writing'

A single layer of varying thickness of the patient can be imaged by moving the film and tube around the patient, the layer imaged lying at the centre of the axis of rotation of tube and film. This level can be altered in a vertical direction. The thickness of the 'slice' obtained is altered by changing the angle of the arc during which the continuous exposure is obtained, a longer arc giving a thinner slice.

Two Frenchmen first described the principle in 1921. In 1930 Vellebona in Italy built a 'stratigraph' that imaged a phantom heart in a phantom body. In 1931 Ziedses des Plantes designed a 'planigraph' that showed a body section inside a patient (Grigg 1965).

In 1928 Jean Kieffer, a French immigrant into America, suffered a relapse of tuberculosis whilst working in the X-ray department of a tuberculosis santorium (Grigg 1965, Kelves 1998). His lesions could not be clearly imaged because they were mediastinal. While lying in his bed, he worked out the principles described above but, having patented his invention, could not persuade anyone to develop a model.

The first machine was built in America by Andrews and Stava in Cleveland, Ohio, but apparently the images were not good. Kieffer's version was finally built by the Mallinckrodt Institute of Radiology in St Louis, Missouri, in 1937.

Tomography was commonly in use in orthopaedic work until computed tomography (CT) became available. Indeed, it still has a role in those patients who have much metal in them as the technique is not hindered by metal artefact.

Ultrasound

Ultrasound shows up alterations in soft tissue texture and organ size. We are all familiar with Second World War movies showing 'sonar'. When I started in radiology, all foetal dating was by radiological examination of the maternal abdomen and, indeed, had been so since the beginning of radiology.

Kevles (1998) notes that in 1877 the Curie brothers, Pierre and Jacques, discovered the piezoelectric effect of crystals, by which they convert electrical to mechanical energy, and vice versa.

It seems the stimulus to ultrasound was the sinking of the *Titanic* in 1912 and the need to detect icebergs under water. Pierre Langevin, a student of the Curies, showed that the crystal, a transducer, resonates when placed in a field of alternating current and that the ultrasound waves produced are transmitted in water. Their reflection back up to the transducer was used in the Second World War to detect submarines by SONAR (SOund Navigation And Ranging).

Pioneering medical work in Austria was interrupted by the War but taken up in America. Initial ultrasound probes were used to show gallstones.

Early attempts at ultrasound imaging had the patient sitting in a waterbath with a water/soft tissue interface. The patient had to be held down in the water by lead weights because of the buoyancy of the body – so seriously ill patients could not be imaged. Laundry tubs, cattle troughs and aircraft parts were all used as water containers, the water being used as a 'coupling agent' with transducers in the container wall.

Kevles (1998) notes that John Wild, an English graduate working in America, realised that ultrasound signals change where two different tissues meet, and so malignant tissue could be distinguished from normal tissue. Wild also incorporated 'a water column sealed with rubber into the transducer, dispensing with the need for water baths'. He further developed miniature transducers for intravaginal and intrarectal scanning, and for breast ultrasound.

'Real time' ultrasound, the great advance in scanning in the 1970s, gives the operator two-dimensional images at a rate of over fourteen images per second, so that the consequential images seem to blend and not flicker. Dynamic and functional images could thereby be obtained.

Ultrasound is now widely used in orthopaedic radiology. The equipment is much cheaper than magnetic resonance imaging (MRI) and computed tomography (CT) scanning, does not involve ionising radiation, but is operator-dependent. The images obtained are not perhaps as easily interpreted by the surgeon as are MRI and CT scans.

Nuclear medicine

We are once again indebted to Kevles (1998) for a succinct, yet dramatic, overview of the history of nuclear medicine. It seems that George Hevesy, a young Hungarian physicist, came to Manchester in 1911 to work with Ernest Rutherford and found that isotopes could be used as tracers.

His landlady, he believed, was in the habit of recycling meat, so one evening he added radioactive lead to the fresh meat pie. Three days later, he used a Geiger counter to show radioactivity in the soufflé! In 1943 Hevesy was awarded the Nobel Prize for Chemistry for showing that radioisotopes are involved in the same normal biological processes at cellular levels as do conventional chemicals.

In 1934, Irene and Frederic Juliot-Curie had produced artificial (as opposed to naturally occurring) isotopes by bombarding natural elements with high-energy particles. Isotopes thus made could be sent via the blood stream to many organs in the body, including the skeleton, where the radiopharmaceutical would incorporate into the target organ and give off a tracer which could be detected from a hand-held Geiger counter, and subsequently a rectilinear scanner with a motorised arm, passing in a transverse mode over the body from top to bottom picking up the gamma-rays emitted from the target organ and imaging the varying intensity of the counts on X-ray film or paper (Fig. 8.31).

The gamma camera, with an array of photomultiplier cells linked to a computer, gives a cheap and rapid overview of the skeleton, showing blood flow to and incorporation of a radiopharmaceutical in bone. Pathology is shown as a deviation in uptake from normal adjacent bone. The technique is highly sensitive.

Computed tomography (CT)

Just as radiography came about with the coming together of electricity, physics and photography, so did computed tomography (CT) with the development of the silicon chip and the computer industry.

Conventional X-ray images are two-dimensional, so that a lateral view, or view in another plane, is needed to give a three-dimensional aspect. Axial imaging was first developed by Watson, of the radiographic equipment firm W. Watson & Co. (Watson 1939, Friedland & Thurber 1966).

Friedland and Thurber (1966) summarised the technical developments that lay behind Sir Geoffrey Hounsfield's working model of the CT scanner, first used at the Atkinson Morley Neurological Hospital in conjunction with J. Ambrose, a neuroradiologist.

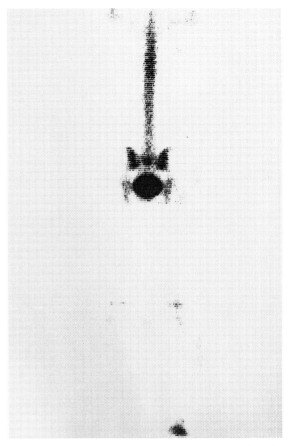

Fig. 8.31 Rectilinear scan with transversely orientated bands of varying density relating to the level of radioactive emission. The abnormality of the left ankle was an osteoid osteoma

The CT scanner provides axial images of variable thickness over a chosen length (Fig. 8.32). As opposed to conventional linear tomography, the X-ray tube moves *around* the patient rather than length-wise. The attenuated beam is received by an array of detectors (instead of film) opposite the rotating tube. The received data are converted by computer to images which may be seen on a visual display unit (VDU) or printed as hard copy on to film. The computer-generated image gives a much broader grey-scale than conventional film, so that soft tissues of different densities do not appear of the same density as they would on a radiograph. Pus or tumour have a different attenuation than that of muscle, especially after enhancement by an iodine-based water-soluble contrast medium. Moreover, electronic manipulation of the data is possible where the images are available so that inherent differences in visual contrast can be heightened. Further advances in computer technology

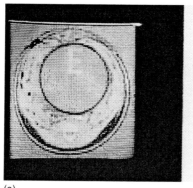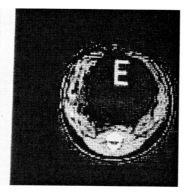

(a)

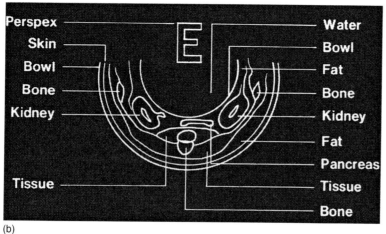

(b)

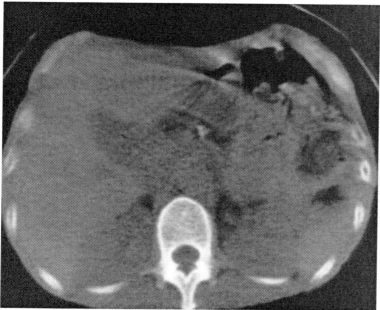

(c)

Fig. 8.32 CT scanning.
(a) Primitive images (from 1970) showing a section of a pig imaged with a water-filled bag.
(b) Representation of a pig slice phantom with a water bag.
(c) CT scan (dated 1975) of one of the first patients imaged at Northwick Park Hospital. The high-density focus within the vertebral body represented a metastatic deposit from a testicular seminoma. Courtesy of Dr David Katz, Northwick Park Hospital

enable reconstructions to be made in any plane chosen by the operator. Three-dimensional or holographic images can also be obtained from the computer-based data (Fig. 8.33).

Images obtained and held on computer can be used to guide the orthopaedic or neurosurgeon to a lesion with millimetre accuracy.

Early use of CT in orthopaedics was in the field of disc disease, with or without added contrast in the disc and theca, and in bone tumour management, where extension of a tumour through the cortex and into soft tissues could be assessed. However, with the advent of MRI, the CT scanner is currently used less for the investigation of disc disease or malignant disease of bone and soft tissue, that is, soft tissue change, but still may be the primary investigation for hard tissue disease. Certainly, bone – and especially the cortex – is better imaged by CT than with MRI. Patients, of course, may end up being investigated by both modalities.

Current advances in X-ray tube technology and computers, together with 'slip ring' distribution of current to the scanner, enable continuous rather than single-slice axial images to be obtained. The actual scanning time is often less than that needed to get the patient on and off the table!

Magnetic resonance imaging (MRI)

To the radiologist who started practice, as I did, in the 1960s, CT, ultrasound and isotope scanning are significant advances, but not beyond the scope of the imagination. Magnetic resonance imaging (MRI), however, is something so wondrous that amazement is the only possible reaction to the theory and practice of this new imaging modality. CT utilised X-rays, and we are accustomed to the use of radiation in everyday life ever since the A-bomb and, indeed, since Madame Curie and radium. MRI, however, is totally different in the kind of images it produces, while the physics remains difficult to comprehend (at least to me!).

The whole dramatic story of the development of clinical MRI has been fully described by Kevles (1998) and is too long to be discussed here. Many workers in both the UK and USA were aiming for the same thing, that is, sectional images of the human body, as in CT, using the long-known principle that nuclei with odd

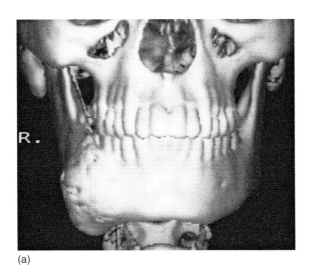

(a)

(b)

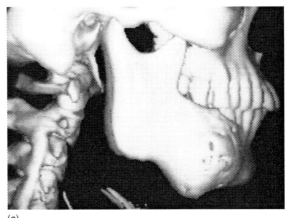

(c)

Fig. 8.33a-c Three-dimensional reconstructions following axial CT imaging. The lesion in the right body of the mandible is especially apparent. Courtesy of the Department of Medical Physics, University College London

numbers of protons and neutrons align themselves when exposed to a strong magnetic field.

The nucleus usually imaged is that of hydrogen, which is in water, the commonest compound in the body. When the magnet is turned off, the protons in the nuclei relax to their original state, giving off T_1 and T_2 relaxation time radiofrequency signals. Differences in the water concentration of various tissues can thus be appreciated.

The cortex of bone is low in water and is imaged as a 'black' or low-signal structure. Fat is high in water content and so gives out a high-signal 'white' image. Tissues can be differentiated not only in dimension and situation (as in CT), but also by their pathophysiology so that alterations in texture are reflected by alterations in signal.

CONCLUSION

Progress in science can never be said to have ended. Just as the physician could not have imagined MRI before its advent into clinical practice, so most of us have no conception of what lies ahead, but something new and more wondrous will turn up – it always does!

REFERENCES

Albers-Schönberg H E 1903–04 Projektions-Röntgenbilder einer seltenen Knockenerkrankung. Fortschr Röntgenstr 7: 158–159

Albers-Schönberg H E 1915 Eine seltene, bisher nicht bekannte Structur-Anomalie des Skelettes. Fortschr Röntgenstr 23: 174–175

Allison N, Moody E F 1915 Osteochondritis deformans juvenalis (Perthes' disease). Am J Orthop Surg 13: 197–216

American Surgical Association 1900. Report of the Committee of the American Surgical Association on the medico-legal relation of the X-rays. Trans Am Surg Assoc 18: 429–461

Battersby J C 1898–99 The present position of the Rontgen rays in military surgery. Arch Rontgen Ray 3: 74–78, 89–91

Beck C 1900 Fractures, with an Appendix on the Practical Use of the Röntgen Rays. W B Saunders, Philadelphia

Borden W C 1900 The Use of the Rontgen Ray by the Medical Department of the United States Army in the War with Spain (1898). Government Printing Office, Washington, DC

Bowley A 1901 A Civilian War Hospital – Experience of Wounds and Sickness in South Africa. John Murray, London

Bull J W, Fischgold H 1989 A short history of neuroradiology. In: Cabanis E (ed) Contribution à L'Histoire de la Neuroradiologie Européenne. Pradel, Paris

Burrows E H 1986 Pioneers and Early Years: A History of British Radiology. Colophon, Alderney

Calvé J 1910 Sue une forme particulière de pseudo-coxalgie greffée sur des déformations caracteristiques de l'extremité supériere du fémur. Rev Chir 42: 54–84

Calvé J, Lelievre H 1913–14 Radiography of the vertebral column in profile in Pott's disease. Am J Orth Surg 11: 193–206

Cockayne E A 1919 Isolated disease of the scaphoid. Lancet ii: 1086

Coley W B 1907 Sarcoma of the long bones. Ann Surgery Phil: 321–368

Cotton A 1915 The limitation of the X-ray in the diagnosis of certain bone and joint diseases. Am J Orth Surg 13: 216–240

Dandy W E 1918 Ventriculography following the injection of air into the cerebral ventricles. Ann Surg 68: 5–11

Dandy W E 1925 Diagnosis and localisation of spinal cord tumours. Ann Surg 81: 223–254

Delitala F 1914–15 Contribution for the study of a typical disease of the upper end of the femur (Perthes' disease). Am J Orthop Surg 12: 555–588

Dwight, T 1907 Variations of the Bones of the Hands and Feet. Lippincott, Philadelphia

Feiss H 1905–06 Spontaneous fractures with rickets. Report of a case. Am J Orth Surg 3: 271–278

Fränkel, E 1910 über Wirbelgeschwulste im Röntgenbilde. Forsch Röntgenstr 16: 245–257

Freiberg A H 1905–06 Coxa vara adolescentium and osteochondritis deformans coxae. Am J Orthop Surg 3: 6–14

Freiberg A H 1914 Infraction of the second metatarsal head. Surg Gynae Obstet 19: 191

Friedland G W, Thurber B D 1966 The birth of CT. Am J Rontgenol 167: 1365–1370

Goldthwait J E, Painter C F, Osgood R B 1910 Diseases of the Bones and Joints. Leonard, Boston

Greulich W W, Pyle S I 1959 Radiographic Atlas of Skeletal Development of the Hand and Wrist. California University Press, Stanford

Grigg E R W 1965 The Trail of the Invisible Light. C C Thomas, Springfield

Hawley G W 1913–14 Spontaneous fracture in carcinoma of the bones. Am J Orth Surg 11: 139–150

Hoffa A 1906 Über Röntgenbilder nach Sauesstoffeinblasung in das Kniegelenk. Berlin Klin Waschr 43: 941–945

Hueck F H W 1995 Entwicklung der Skelettradiologie von 1895 bis 1995. Radiologe 35: 337–353

Kevles B H 1998 Naked to the Bone: Medical Imaging in the Twentieth Century. Addison-Wesley, Reading

Kienböck R 1910 Abbruch der Tuberositas tibiae samt Teil des Condylus. Fortschr Röntgenstr: 15

Köhler A 1905 Atlas of the Hip Joint and Thigh. Graefe & Sillem, Hamburg

Köhler A 1908 Über eine häufige, bisher anscheinend unbekannte Erkrankung einzelner kindlicher Knochen. Münch Med Wochenschr 55: 1923

Köhler A 1920 Eine typische Erkrankung des zweiten Metatarso-Phalangealgelenkes. Münch Med Wochenschr 67: 1289–1290

Köhler A 1928 Röntgenology. The Borderlands of the Normal and Early Pathological in the Skiagram. Baillière, Tindall & Cox, London

Le Vay D 1990 The History of Orthopaedics. Parthenon, Carnforth

Legg A T 1910 An obscure affection of the hip joint. Boston Med Surg J 162: 202

Lindblom K 1939 Arthrography and röntgenography in ruptures of tendons of the shoulder joint. Acta Radiol 20: 548–562

Looser F 1920 Über Spätrachitis und Osteomalacie. Klinische, röntgenologische und pathologisch-anatomische Untersuchungen. Dtsch Z Chir 152: 210

Lovett R G, Nichols E H 1906 Osteogenesis imperfecta. Br Med J: 915–920

Luckett W H 1964 Air in the ventricles of the brain following a fracture of the skull. In: Bruwer A J (ed) 1964 Classic Descriptions in Diagnostic Rontgenology. C C Thomas, Springfield

Makins G H 1901 Surgical Experiences in South Africa (1899–1900). Smith Elder & Co, London

Muirhead Little E Clin Soc Trans 40: 1 quoted in Tubby

Osgood R B 1903 Lesions of the tibial tubercle occurring during adolescence. Boston Med Surg J 148: 114–117

Pelkan K F 1925 Rontgenogram in early scurvy. Am J Dis Child 30: 174

Perthes, G C 1913 Über osteochondritis deformans juvenilis. Archiv Klin Chir 101: 779

Pfahler G E 1917 The rontgen diagnosis of metastatic disease of bone, with special reference to the spinal column. Am J Rontgenol 4: 114–122

Poland J 1898a Skiagraphic Atlas Showing the Development of the Bones of the Wrist and Hand. Smith, Elder & Co., London

Poland, J 1898b Traumatic Separation of the Epiphyses. Smith, Elder & Co., London

Poland, J 1901 A Retrospect of Surgery During the Past Century. Smith, Elder & Co., London

Posner E 1970 Reception of Röntgen's discovery in Britain and U.S.A. Br Med J iv: 357–360

Renton P 1991 Arthrography. In: Watson M S (ed) Surgical Disorders of the Shoulder. Churchill Livingstone, Edinburgh, pp 97–117

Saxton H M 1973 Seventy six years of British radiology. Br J Radiol 46: 872–884

Schell-Lund A 1922 A case of a rare skeleton anomaly. Acta Radiologica 1

Scheuermann H W 1921 Kyphosis dorsalis juvenilis. Zeitsch Orth Chir 41: 305

Schlatter C 1903 Verletzungen des schnabelförmigen Fortsatzes der oberen Tibia-epiphyse. Bruns Beitr Klin Chir 38: 874–887

Schuster N H 1962 Early days of Rontgen photography in Britain. Br Med J ii: 1164–1166

Sicard J A, Forestier J 1921 Méthode radiographique d'exploration de la cavité épidurale par le lipiodol. Rev Neurol 28: 1264

Sicard J A, Forestier J 1922 Méthode générale d'exploration radiologique par huille iodée (Lipodol). Bull Mem Soc Méd Hop Paris 46: 463–469

Taylor H L, Frieder W 1915 Quiet hip disease. Am J Orthop Surg 13: 192–196

Thurston Holland, C 1928 The accessory bones of the foot. In: Fairbank H A T (ed) The Robert Jones Birthday Volume. Oxford University Press, Oxford

Tubby A H 1912 Deformities, Including Diseases of the Bones and Joints. Macmillan, London

Vrolik W 1849 Tabulae ad Illustrandam Embryo-Genesin Hominus et Mammalium, tam Naturatem quam Abnormen. Tab 91. Amstelodami

Waldenström H 1909 Tuberculous foci of upper part of neck of femur. Zeitsch Orth Chir 24: 3–4

Watson W 1939 Improvements in or relating to X-ray apparatus. British Patent 50838, UK Patent Office, London

Werndorff R, Robinsohn I 1905 Kongress verhandl Deutsch Gesellsch Orthop Chir: 9–11

Wilbert M I 1904 A comparative study of fractures of the extremities. Trans Am Rontgen Ray Soc: 195–204

Wimberger H 1925 Klinisch-radiologische Diagnostik von Rachitis, Skorbut und Lues congenita im Kindesalter. Ergebn im Med u Kinderh 28: 264

Withers S, 1931 The story of the first Rontgen evidence. Radiology 17: 99–100

SECTION 3:

Fragmentation of
Orthopaedic Surgery

9

The development of hand surgery

Nicholas Barton

WHAT IS SO SPECIAL ABOUT HAND SURGERY?

Surgery of the hand differs in several ways from general orthopaedic surgery.

The clinical approach is different

The diagnosis may be obvious at a glance, but only by taking a history can one learn how the pathology is affecting the function of the hand and the life of the patient, and thus whether an operation might help. Similarly, the examination may be not so much to discover the diagnosis as to decide exactly what operation is needed.

In addition, the hand is one of the emotionally charged areas of the body and patients may develop emotional and psychiatric disturbances when it is disabled. Orthopaedic surgeons are apt to overlook the cosmetic aspect of the hand. In ordinary life, the only visible parts of the body are the face, hands, and sometimes, in women, the lower part of the leg. The hand is thrust forwards and draws attention when giving and receiving objects, and in greeting. Rheumatoid patients, although they may not say so, are often very concerned about this.

The structures are small and need different surgical techniques

Internal fixation in the hand is very different from plating a tibia. The small radius of the bone means that it has a sharply curved surface on which a drill or wire can easily slip, yet a slip of only 1 or 2 mm may fracture one cortex and make internal fixation impossible.

Hand surgery is surgery in miniature. The flexor tendons are less than 1 cm in diameter, and a digital nerve is only about 1.5 mm across. Thus, very fine carefully placed sutures are necessary to appose the epineurium

without penetrating the nerve itself. Magnification should be used for such work. Magnifying spectacles ('loupes') giving about two and a half times magnification make a surprising difference. An operating microscope is even better and is, of course, essential for microvascular surgery. However, very fine micro-instruments and sutures are also needed. One must also become familiar with the operating microscope and its controls, and undergo supervised practice on synthetic materials or animal tissue to learn how to make the fine movements.

Some of the techniques needed for the hand derive from plastic surgery. Ideally a hand surgeon should be trained in both orthopaedic and plastic surgery; if not, surgeons from each side should work together in combined clinics. In the British Society for Surgery of the Hand, plastic and orthopaedic surgeons co-operate harmoniously and happily.

A lot of time and patience is needed

Impatient surgeons should not operate on the hand. The delicate dissection and suture of fine tissues with the necessary accuracy can only be done slowly and carefully.

Complex microvascular operations (in which a tourniquet is not used or is used only at the beginning) may go on for 14 hours or more, so endurance is also needed. It is best to have two teams of trained surgeons who can relieve each other before fatigue begins to impair performance.

Higher standards are required

This applies not only to the surgeon, but also to the mobility and function of the hand that are achieved. The normal hand is an exceptionally mobile structure, and to restore full function all this mobility must be restored. After a quadricepsplasty the aim is to achieve perhaps

120° flexion, but 90° is satisfactory. Following a flexor tendon repair or graft, the aim is a total of 180° flexion at the interphalangeal joints and 90° is not really useful.

In reduction of fractures of the shafts of long bones imperfect apposition may be acceptable, but fractures of the shaft of the proximal phalanx of a finger must be exactly reduced; the phalanx forms the floor of the fibrous flexor tendon sheath, and a step of even 1 mm will impair the gliding of the tendon.

Failure is more acceptable

This appears paradoxical in view of what has been said above, but the hand, like a spacecraft, has built-in reserve capacity so that if one system fails another can take its place. The index finger is used a great deal, especially in precision handling, but if it is amputated, the middle finger can take over its functions. A leg would not be amputated just because it is stiff, but it may be wise to amputate a stiff finger if it interferes with the function of the rest of the hand. A harder decision, but one which may save a patient much unnecessary surgery and time off work, is to amputate a finger because it is *going* to be stiff following a severe injury.

The organisation of a hand surgeon's work is different

He can see more new patients in an outpatient clinic than a general orthopaedic surgeon. Although some will be complex (to assess a pair of rheumatoid hands properly takes at least 30 minutes) many will be simple matters which can be dealt with quickly (e.g. a trigger finger). Moreover, patients do not need to undress and can thus pass through the clinic more quickly.

A hand surgeon will obtain a larger yield of patients from the clinic who need operations – perhaps 50%, compared with 10 or 20% in a general orthopaedic clinic. He will therefore need more operating time but, as most of his patients go home within 48 hours of operation, he needs fewer beds. Many patients can be operated on as day cases and need not occupy a bed at all.

At the end of an operation the hand surgeon should apply the dressings himself to be sure of getting the hand in the correct position. The so-called non-adherent dressings, such as Melolin, become hard, blood-soaked and adherent after release of the tourniquet, and tullegras or one of its variants should be used instead. I prefer Sofra-tulle because it is less greasy.

ORIGINS OF HAND SURGERY

The *anatomy* of the hand was studied in some detail by Leonardo da Vinci (1452–1519) who dissected

cadaveric arms and hands. His drawings show the flexor tendons in their pulleys (Fig. 9.1), the intrinsic muscles, the arteries, the cutaneous nerves and the bones of the carpus and hand. Leonardo's accompanying notes say 'Remember that to be certain of the point of origin of any muscle, you must pull the sinew from which the muscle springs in such a way as to see that muscle move, and where it is attached to the ligaments of the bones.' Further on, he asks himself, 'Which nerves or sinews of the hand are those which close and point the fingers and toes laterally?'

'However, the first serious study of the hand as a functional entity was motivated by religious impulse when Sir Charles Bell (1784–1842), while Professor at the Royal College of Surgeons of England, was charged under the will of the Earl of Bridgewater to write a treatise on '*The Hand: Its Mechanism and Vital Endowments as Evincing Design*' and this was published in 1833. This was indeed a tour de force and was a milestone in the growing concept of the hand as a uniquely human organ' (Fisk 1990). This book was republished in 1979 by Graham Stack. The skin-retaining ligaments of the hand, so beloved of hand surgeons, were described much later: by Cleland in 1867 and Grayson in 1941.

As regards *disorders* of the hand, Hippocrates of Kos (*c.*460-*c.*377 BC) described pain, redness, numbness,

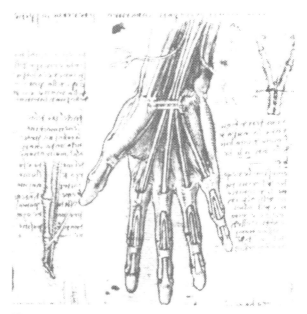

Fig. 9.1 Leonardo da Vinci's drawing (*c.*1500) of the flexor tendons and their pulleys. Courtesy of The Royal Library, Windsor Castle and reproduced by gracious permission of Her Majesty the Queen

hotness, twitching and shaking of the hands as features of systemic disease, usually indicating a bad prognosis and how to treat fractures and dislocations in the hand (Verdan, 2000). Infections of the hand must have been treated from the earliest times. Prehistoric cave paintings, done by putting a hand against the wall and blowing paint around it, show amputated and partly amputated fingers, but we do not know whether these resulted from accidents or fights or were carried out for religious or magical reasons (as still happens in certain African tribes).

Compensation for hand injuries was laid down in seventh-century Ireland on a scale depending upon which digit and how much of it was affected (Mooney & Prendiville 1991). Three centuries later, King Canute issued a similar schedule corresponding quite closely with that used in our own time by the Ministry of Pensions! (Capener 1959). It is therefore not surprising that medico-legal reports appeared early. For example, in 1569 four surgeons in Edinburgh (it was an agreed report!) concluded: 'After long consultation we find John Farrer neither to be mutilated nor impotent of his arm or hand but that it would be daily better if he would make labour upon it' (Lamb 1994). *Plus ça change ...*

In modern times, the first important text on hand disorders was *Infections of the Hand* by Allen Kanavel of Chicago in 1916. His successor, in 1932, was Sumner Koch who 'increasingly turned his attention to injuries of the flexor tendons and nerves, burns and other hand conditions such as Dupuytren's disease. He developed an interest in plastic surgery and skin cover which arose as a result of the problems created by the many cases of skin cancer of the hand resulting from the injudicious use (particularly by dentists) of the crude x-ray equipment in use at that time' (Bolton 1991). He also recognised that, if allowed to, the hand will become stiff with the MP joints straight and the IP joints flexed: the position of failure. It was, however, many years before the corollary of this was applied, by Professor J. I. P. James of Edinburgh (who had visited Koch): he taught us that the hand should be immobilised with the MP joints flexed and the IP joints straight. Koch's colleagues, Mason and Allen, also made important contributions to flexor tendon surgery but the later Chicago school published most of their papers in local journals and never produced a book, so their contribution became overshadowed by that of Sterling Bunnell of San Francisco (Fig. 9.2) who was undoubtedly the father of hand surgery.

Sterling Bunnell (1882–1957) had that quality which, in most walks of life, distinguishes the great from

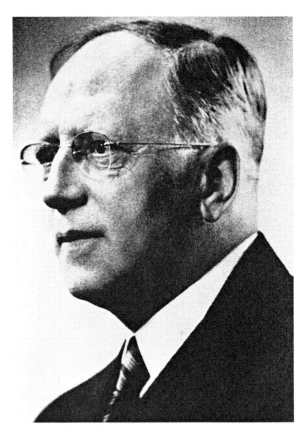

Fig. 9.2 Sterling Bunnell, the father of hand surgery. Courtesy of Andrew Palmer as President of ASSH

the ordinary: not so much exceptional intelligence as exceptional drive and energy. Paul Brown, who described him as tireless, recalled that he and his wife went to dinner with Dr Bunnell. 'Our host greeted us at the gate and cautioned my wife "Please don't step on the alligators." We glanced at one another wondering if our host might be a bit tipsy, but my wife then clutched my arm in fright and nodded at her foot where reposed a four-foot alligator. Bunnell thought this hilarious' (Brown 1989). He had always been interested in natural history and at the time was studying the foreleg of the larger reptiles. Brown also mentions Bunnell's 'ferocious concentration' and 'his willingness to take suggestions from anybody – even a student nurse. I have heard him observe that some of the best suggestions come from the least sophisticated sources and he said this was so because they were the least prejudiced and had the most open minds' (Brown 1989).

We shall return to Bunnell, but it seems best to describe the development of hand surgery by selecting a few topics and considering them in detail.

TENDON INJURIES

Galen (129–201 AD), a Greek physician from Pergamon in Asia Minor (in what is now western Turkey) who later practised in Rome, considered that the white cord at the end of a muscle, which is in fact the tendon, was the termination of a bundle of nerves 'and stated that a prick of a nerve or tendon will induce convulsions' (Adamson & Wilson 1961). In addition, it has been suggested that Galen may have had the unhappy experience of suturing the median nerve to a flexor tendon (Chamay 1997), perhaps in one of the gladiators of Pergamon to whom he was medical officer. He therefore advised that cut tendons should not be repaired. His authority prevailed for eight centuries (and even longer in some places; the first lectures in Anatomy at Oxford in 1624 were based on his readings) until challenged by Avicenna (980–1037), who is usually described as an Arab. He did write in Arabic and was known as Ibn Sina before his name was Latinised, but he was born near Bokhara in Central Asia then capital of the Persian-based empire of the Sassanids, and never went outside that empire though he had access to the superb royal library in Bokhara. 'In a wandering life driven by burning intellectual curiosity, Ibn Sina held positions as a jurist, a teacher of philosophy, an administrator, and as physician to various courts. His autobiography boasts that his writing was done on horseback during military campaigns, in hiding, in prison and even after drinking bouts. The outcome was 270 titles' (Porter 1997), which became as influential as had been the works of Galen. Remarkably, Avicenna's *Canons of Medicine* became a required textbook even in the hospitals of Christian Europe for five hundred years. He advocated that every time a tendon was cut through or ruptured, it must be sewn together.

This practice, however, remained uncommon. For example, Pietro de Marchetti (1589–1675), professor at Padua, wrote: 'Nerves and tendons must never be sutured, for this practice is often followed by fatal tetanus.' He was consulted by

'a distinguished Marshal of France, of the family of Montmorency. He received a sword cut on the right wrist, dividing the extensor tendons of the thumb. When the wound healed the thumb was drawn across the palm of the hand, so that he could not hold sword, dagger or lance, and was entirely incapacitated for the profession of arms, apart from which he declared life was not worth living. So he consulted me about amputating his hand to which I could in no wise consent, but devised an iron case to hold the thumb out, fixed by two cords to bracelets round the wrist, and so he was able to hold and use all kinds of weapons' (Bishop 1960)

A century later, Jean Louis Petit (1674–1750), working in Paris, described a method of repair that included the skin in the tendon suture to avoid direct contact with the tendon (Adamson & Wilson 1961); he deplored the practice of holding the tendon ends with toothed forceps. He was also the first surgeon to divide the tissues at different levels when amputating a limb, as opposed to the previous guillotine amputations.

At the same period in Germany, Lorenz Heister (1683–1758) was suturing tendons by several different techniques (Nigst 1997) and using instruments illustrated in his famous textbook on *Chirugie*, first published in 1718. As a young man Heister had enlarged his knowledge by visiting hospitals in The Netherlands, France and England. 'So keen was he on seeing operations that he frequented the great fairs to which itinerant operators resorted in large numbers. Some of these wandering surgeons undertook operations which the more regular practitioners of the time did not dare to perform' (Bishop 1960), including those for hernia, cataract, the stone and hare lip! 'Heister was not too proud to learn from them' (Bishop 1960). Later he became Professor of Surgery and Anatomy at Altdorf where in 1711 he dissected the body of a malefactor in the public anatomical theatre and found a gangrenous appendix: the first time that the diagnosis of appendicitis was established.

'The Galenian concept of the complications that are associated with tendon damage was finally refuted by the classic work of Albrecht von Haller who, in 1752, published his work on the sensibility and irritability of the various tissues of the body and demonstrated the insensibility of tendons' (Adamson & Wilson 1961). Following this, repair of tendons became acceptable. Syme, for example, who was Professor of Surgery in Edinburgh from 1833 to 1870, did a number of successful repairs of tendons, mainly the Achilles tendon.

There are several papers on the history of surgery to the flexor tendons in the hand, but they glide imperceptibly from the repair of tendons in general into the repair of flexor tendons in the fingers, without making it clear who first undertook the latter (Kleinert et al, 1995). One would think that this could only be after the introduction of anaesthetics. According to Verdan (1980), it was Konrad Biesalski of Berlin in 1910 and Erich Lexer of Jena (130 miles south-west of Berlin) in 1912 who not only first repaired flexor tendons, but also carried out the first flexor tendon grafts, the latter in late cases and ruptures. (Biesalski also researched into the nutrition of tendons and Lexer into bone grafts and transplants of joints, in whole or in part.)

However, Biesalski was an orthopaedic surgeon and in Germany these did not (and do not) treat acute trauma, and his papers concern tendon transfer rather than grafts. It probably was Lexer who first did tendon grafts, but I have been unable to discover who first repaired cut flexor tendons in the fingers.

The cut flexor tendon is the classic problem of hand surgery, which illustrates well some of the ways in which hand surgery differs from the rest of orthopaedics. In essence, there are two difficulties in treating this injury. The first we may call *secure fixation*: the flexor muscles, contracting strongly, exert a powerful force tending to pull apart the repair. No other common suture-line in the body is exposed to such a strong distracting force. We therefore need a strong suture material and a strong form of stitch. Early suture materials made of organic fibres such as silk and cotton were fairly strong but produced a tissue reaction. Stainless steel wire, favoured forty years ago, is difficult to use: it kinks easily and then loses much of its strength. Most surgeons today favour a braided polyester or something similar. There is a current vogue for absorbable materials but we know that it takes weeks before the tendon heals to its greatest strength, so it seems foolish to risk using a material which may weaken before then. A simple through-and-through suture will pass between the longitudinally running strands of the tendon and will cut out quickly. Bunnell devised his zigzag suture to overcome this, but it has a tendency to strangulate the tendon. Kirchmayr from Vienna described in 1917 a method of suture that was modified by Kessler, and further modified by Tajima almost back to Kirchmayr's original technique. Variations on these are the usual core sutures today, to which is added a fine surface suture that not only apposes the edges, but also increases the strength.

Secure fixation is, however, a less formidable difficulty than *sliding function*. Tendons that pass across joints where they might bowstring are restrained by semi-rigid fibrous sheaths (Fig. 9.1) within which the tendon and its thin synovial visceral sheath glide up and down. The cut goes through skin, fat, tendon sheath and tendon and the resultant scar runs through all these tissues, so that the tendon becomes stuck down and its excursion is diminished.

Bunnell vividly described the effect of this in a classic paper finally published in 1918. ('Mrs. Bunnell said that he submitted it many, many times for publication and each time it was rejected he doggedly rewrote it and resubmitted it. After more than a dozen and a half rejections *Surgery, Gynecology and Obstetrics* finally accepted it. "But by then", she said, "I was so sick of seeing that thick brown envelope returned again and again in the mail, that I wanted to hear no more of it". This paper was, of course, just the beginning'; Brown 1989.) In it Bunnell wrote:

'My first attempts at repair of tendons in the fingers resulted in immediate successes, but as the succeeding days went by the motion became less and less until at the end of a few weeks it became nil. The tendons had become firmly imbedded in scar tissue and had united to the finger in a solid mass. Such failures as these prompted me to work out a method of treatment which would yield better functional results in these cases.' (Bunnell 1918)

This method was the tendon graft, introduced recently in Germany for 'hopeless cases' (Adamson & Wilson 1961) but applied more widely by Bunnell. Its purpose was to avoid having a suture-line within the fibrous flexor sheath. The distal suture is close to or at the insertion of the tendon where there is little or no excursion, and the proximal one is in the palm where it is surrounded by softer and more yielding tissues (not in so-called 'no man's land', originally referring to the dangerous area between the front-line trenches in the First World War. Bunnell may have used this term, but it does not appear in his writings). Bunnell stressed the importance of atraumatic technique to avoid adhesions; Galen had been right about the danger of handling the tendon, but for the wrong reason! This tendon graft was not done immediately, but about three months later, when the original injury had healed fully and a soft, supple finger had been regained by passive exercises. The doctor who first treated the patient was advised simply to sew up the skin and not interfere with the tendon at all: physiotherapy was then started and the patient referred to the specialist hand surgeon which, as it happened, was Bunnell.

This doubtless helped Bunnell's practice but was also good for the patient: once scar tissue has developed in the finger, it can never be removed and if a surgeon is not trained in this type of work (which nobody was in 1918) it is better he does nothing: this at least avoids making matters worse.

In his 1918 article Bunnell actually said that 'suturing of freshly severed tendons will give a far better result than repairing such cases when old', though he suggested a routine tenolysis six weeks later. He himself continued to carry out primary repair of flexor tendons when he got the chance, but the accepted treatment elsewhere became a delayed flexor tendon graft. This was carried to a high pitch of excellence by Guy Pulvertaft in England (Fig. 9.3), who was then a Consultant Orthopaedic Surgeon in Grimsby, a fishing port where the fishwives who gutted the fish frequently cut their flexor tendons. The young Pulvertaft had been advised that the best thing to do was to amputate the finger, but he felt it must be possible to do better and proved that it was. Later, on the advice of Sir Reginald Watson-Jones, Pulvertaft moved to the larger town of Derby where Bunnell himself came to visit him and was so impressed by the results that he concluded that British patients must be more limber (i.e. supple) than American ones!

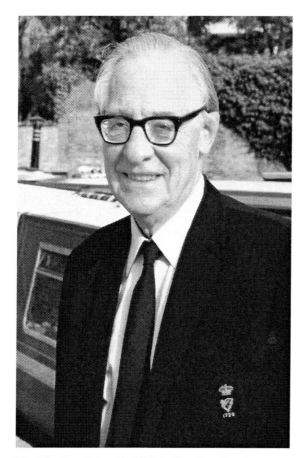

Fig. 9.3 Guy Pulvertaft, CBE, the founder of hand surgery in the UK

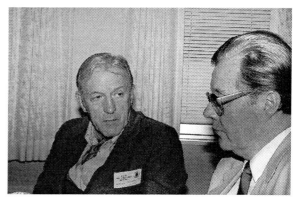

Fig. 9.4 Harold Kleinert (left), a pioneer of hand surgery in our own time, with Dieter Buck-Gramcko (right).

Since then things have changed. A few surgeons, such as Verdan in Switzerland, Brunelli in Italy and Bolton in England, had long practised and recommended primary repair but the widespread return to this method is attributable to the work of Harold Kleinert (Fig. 9.4) in Louisville, Kentucky, and particularly his postoperative management.

In his 1918 paper, Bunnell had also said, 'Movement should be instituted with care and judgement'. This should not be in the first week but not too late; the paper did not specify a period, but Bunnell seems to have settled on three weeks because this became accepted as the period for which tendons should be immobilised. However, he anticipated further developments by saying, 'It would seem that a moderate amount of intermittent motion, with as long an excursion as practical, interspersed by rest, will yield the best results'. Progress in the last forty years has been in this direction.

In 1960 Young and Harmon in Columbus, Ohio (where so many terrible things happened to James Thurber!), advocated fastening the fingernail to a rubber band which was then secured to the wrist, holding the finger in a partly flexed position. The patient used his other hand to carry out passive extension against the elastic band. From this, developments occurred in two directions: Duran and Houser (1975) pursued passive movements without the elastic band, whereas Kleinert and colleagues, starting in the late 1950s, retained the elastic band but required the patient to extend the finger *actively* against the pull of the elastic band which should abolish tone in the flexors (Lister et al 1977). When Kleinert's results were first presented to the American Society for Surgery of the Hand, it was questioned whether such results could possibly be accurate. A committee of three led by Bill Littler was sent to Louisville to review the cases. In his report to the Society, Littler said that not only was the presentation accurate, but also, if he should injure a flexor tendon, he would get on a plane to Louisville to have it repaired! (This echoes the advice of Ronald Furlong in England that patients should buy a railway ticket to Derby.)

Harold Kleinert (Fig. 9.4), a great man, gathered gifted colleagues from all over the world and made Louisville into the foremost centre of hand surgery in the 1970s and 1980s.

Later, in the Plastic Surgery Department in Belfast (Small et al 1989), the elastic band was discarded and patients carried out both passive and active movements within the confines of a dorsal splint; this programme has been widely adopted in Britain. All these methods of mobilisation can produce good results if carried out enthusiastically but carefully, though in a few cases the repair comes apart and has to be done again. This has sent us back to the problem of secure fixation and led to a search for stronger methods of suture.

Savage devised an ingenious six-strand suture; other surgeons find this difficult but the principle is now accepted that the more strands of suture-material that join the tendon ends, the stronger will be the repair.

'In the light of this rekindling of enthusiasm for active mobilisation after tendon repair, it is pertinent to ask why previous experience was so much less satisfactory and led for a time to its abandonment. There is no reason to suppose that the contrasting results could be accounted for by different levels of surgical skill: perhaps instead we should be looking at those changes in technique which have crept in and may be exerting a favourable influence on tendon healing. Notable amongst these is the trend to the repair of both superficialis and profundus tendons when both have been divided, the more conservative approach towards the tendon sheath and more effective methods of suture to maintain opposition of the cut ends of the tendon. In this latter context, the use of a circumferential suture to supplement the main core stitch has become almost universal and offers distinct advantages. As well as adding to the strength of the repair and discouraging gapping, the approximation of the visceral synovial layers "tucks in" the tendon tissue and makes for a smoother external surface'. (Matthews 1989)

In practice, there probably *is* a higher level of surgical skill because, in the late twentieth century in developed countries, it became possible to bring to the patient on the day of injury a surgeon who had been trained specifically in hand surgery.

It is important to grasp that none of the above mobilisation programmes includes the normal use of the hand: very precise and controlled exercises must be carried out and are the only movements allowed. The therapist plays a crucial role in this: it was a therapist, Pam Gratton, who worked out the Belfast regimen in collaboration with the plastic surgeons. Success requires a good surgeon, a good therapist and a good patient – all working together.

Indeed, therapy is a very important part of hand surgery, and requires the skills of both physiotherapists and occupational therapists. In other countries they are hand therapists, but the rather rigid structure in the UK impedes this so, in practice, they work together on patients with hand problems – just as orthopaedic and plastic surgeons do.

The rehabilitation of the injured hand owes a great deal to Kit Wynn-Parry, a physician who in 1982 was President of the British Society for Surgery of the Hand! His *Rehabilitation of the Hand*, based on his experience in the Medical Service of the Royal Air Force and first published in 1958, was the first on this subject.

NERVE INJURIES

Here a unique situation exists. The function to be restored is not mechanical strength or a waterproof tube, but the ability to conduct electrical impulses normally. The anatomy is also unique, since the lower motor neurone has its motor nuclei in the anterior horn of grey matter in the spinal cord and its sensory nuclei in the dorsal root ganglion; from these, immensely long, thin cell bodies (whose length/width ratio is comparable to the M1 motorway) extend down to the end-organ. When repairing a cut peripheral nerve, therefore, we are actually sewing together two halves of the same cells!

'Galen believed the peripheral nerve to be incapable of regeneration and this view dictated therapy into the Middle Ages' (Brushart 1999). However, nerve suture was practised by William of Saliceto (1210–77) (Bishop 1960) and by Guy de Chauliac (1300–70) of Montpellier, 'who observed in young patients that "cut nerves and tendons have been so well restored by suture and other remedies that afterward one could not believe that they had been cut." In spite of these early observations, nerve suture again fell into disrepute, and by the late 18th century it was commonly believed that nerves did not regenerate' (Brushart 1999).

In the early nineteenth century, the first experimental work on nerve injuries was done by Joseph Swan (1791–1824). His forebears had been doctors in Lincoln for several generations and, after apprenticeship to his father, he was sent to study in London at the United Borough Hospitals (Guy's and St Thomas's) in 1810. Four years later he was appointed Surgeon to the Lincoln County Hospital (Boyes 1976). According to the *Dictionary of National Biography*, he was 'a born anatomist, with a native genius for dissection', though it was difficult for him to obtain cadavers to study. It is said that Sir Astley Cooper sent him each year a Christmas present of 'a large hamper labelled "Glass, with care", containing a well-selected human subject'.

He won the Jacksonian prize of the Royal College of Surgeons of England in 1817 with an essay on 'Deafness' and won it again two years later with a dissertation 'On the Treatment of Morbid Affections of Nerves'. This is preserved at the College. It is written in beautiful copper-plate script and describes a series of studies on animals which, sometimes as treatment by vets, had been subjected to various types of nerve injury: ligature, puncture or partial division, complete division, and excision. In most of the animals 'the skin about the os calcis became ulcerated'. As he says, 'It is difficult to determine from an experiment on the limb of an animal the exact time at which the nerve again performs its functions', but he was able to show that the nerves could reconstitute, even after neurectomy, as the following case shows. 'A horse had been lame for five years, at the end of which an inch of each nerve going to the foot was cut out. After this he went very well for six months, when he again became lame and continued so five months. At the end of this time he appeared to suffer such dreadful pain that he was killed … On examination the nerves were found to have reunited'. However 'when a large portion of a nerve has been removed it is seldom restored'. If the nerve was ligated, changes took place which reversed if the ligature was removed soon.

In 1827 he 'moved to London and took a house at 6 Tavistock Square, where he converted the billiard-room into a dissecting room. Here he continued his labours at leisure till the end of his life, never attaining any practice as a surgeon, but doing much for the science of anatomy'. His chief work was, *A Demonstration of the Nerves of the Human Body* (1830). A year later he was elected a life member of the Royal College of Surgeons of England and he served on the council of the College from 1843 to 1869.

Swan should not be confused with F. T. Schwann, originally from Germany but who could not get an academic job there and became a Professor of Anatomy in Belgium in the nineteenth century. He was the first to describe the sheath of the axis cylinder of nerves. (He also was one of the first to show that fermentation is associated with living organisms, an idea later developed by Pasteur.) Together with a botanist, he developed the concept of cells being the structural units of living organisms.

Sir James Paget (1814–99), who as a young man had studied the blood supply of tendons, described a child of eleven whose cut median nerve was accurately repaired and was said to have made a complete recovery within a month. It may be that, in common with one-fifth of the population, this child had anomalous innervation of the thenar muscles and in any case his age is important: children recover much better than adults. From this, Paget postulated that immediate union of nerve fibres could occur if the cut ends were apposed: this was not correct but encouraged the idea of suture.

Paget did not know about Wallerian degeneration.

'Augustus Waller (1816–1870) was a busy general practitioner at St. Mary Abbott's Terrace in Kensington, London, where he carried out the research on degeneration of nerves in frogs with which his name is associated and for which he was elected a Fellow of the Royal Society at the age of 35. This shows that one need not be prevented from doing research by shortage of time or facilities: the real impediment is the lack of will to do it. Waller was also interested in the ability of white blood corpuscles to escape from capillaries and such was his dedication that he courageously attempted to study the microcirculation in his own prepuce, though after a few attempts he changed to the frog's tongue and was

able to demonstrate that pus contained extravasated leucocytes. In the same period he also published papers on the physiology of vision, the microscopy of hailstones and the formation of coloured films by the action of halogens on metals. After 10 years in practice, he moved first to Bonn and then to Paris to obtain more favourable opportunities for carrying out his scientific work, and returned to England in 1858 as Professor of Physiology in Queens College, Birmingham (which has since become the University) and Consultant Physician to the Queen's Hospital in Bath Row' (Marsh & Barton 1996),

whose buildings later housed the Birmingham Accident Hospital and are now a student hostel.

As regards nerves, he showed that the distal part of the cut neurone died and degenerated, so that function could only be restored by a slow process of regeneration. However, surgeons were still afraid to suture cut nerves for fear of tetanus.

In the 1870s J. W. Hulke, then surgeon to the Middlesex Hospital, repaired the cut median and ulnar nerves of a woman. This was the first successful secondary suture of a divided nerve in London (Birch et al 1998).

Surgical repair of nerves, like many aspects of trauma, has advanced as a result of war. The first organised clinical observation of nerve injuries was directed by Weir Mitchell during the American Civil War. He coined the term 'causalgia' for the dreadful pain which may follow nerve injuries. Even as late as 1915 when Inspector-General E. Delormé, in an address to the Académie de Medicine, recommended surgical repair of nerves injured in gunshot wounds, he was 'sharply criticised by the great and the good of French neurology' (Birch et al 1998). It was Tinel's experience of treating nerve injuries in the First World War that led him to describe his tingling sign which shows the progress of regeneration. In the Second World War he worked with the French Resistance in hiding Allied airmen who had been shot down, for which he was imprisoned for two years; his son, who had led the airmen over the Spanish border, died in Buchenvald.

Nerve injuries sustained during the latter conflict were studied by Professor Sir Herbert Seddon (1903–77) in England: first at Oxford and later in London. He accumulated a vast fund of knowledge and concluded that delayed repair was best (Le Vay 1990). This was doubtless true of wounds sustained on the battlefield, but did not necessarily apply to the clean cuts more likely to occur in civilian life. It took some years for the authority of Seddon's pronouncements to be overcome and primary repair resumed. However, his classification of nerve injuries into neurapraxia (meaning nerve not working), axonotmesis and neurotmesis remains fundamental. (Seddon gave credit for these three 'Greek' names to Sir Henry Cohen, later Lord Cohen.)

Brooks recalls that, for an international meeting after the War, Seddon arranged a clinical demonstration 'of what we regarded as some of the more spectacular results of nerve repair and nerve grafting. You can imagine Seddon's irritation when Sterling Bunnell, surrounded by a coterie of his "boys", marched around the patients describing to his audience what ought to have been done!' (Brooks 1991).

Sir Sidney Sunderland in Australia described the internal architecture of the major peripheral nerves, which led to the concept of repairing groups of fascicles instead of just the epineurium around the whole nerve. With the advent of the operating microscope this became practical, but unfortunately it has not been shown to improve the results.

To determine the best method of treatment, one must have a reliable way of measuring the results. The Medical Research Council five-grade scale of muscle power, evolved during the Second World War, has proved a satisfactory system for motor function – but only in flaccid paralysis (it does not apply to spastic muscles) – and has been universally adopted. However, their sensory scale is less satisfactory and there is still no really good method of measuring sensory recovery. The problem is that patients do not recover 40 or 70% of normal sensation: they develop a different kind of sensation and sometimes an unpleasant one. Erik Moberg (1905–93) of Gothenburg, Sweden (Fig. 9.5), pointed out that digits without sensation are 'blind' and will not be used much, if at all (Lundborg 1993). He stressed the importance of functional tests, such as picking up small objects, in measuring sensory recovery.

It was the need to bridge gaps caused by gunshot wounds in the Second World War that led to the development of nerve grafting, although it had been tried in 1916. This method was taken up by Hanno Millesi in Vienna who has shown that a graft gives a better result than a repair done under tension. Nerve grafting made it possible to look again at brachial plexus injuries. Algy Narakas (Bonney 1994), at Lausanne in Switzerland, showed that surgery could help, at least in the upper trunks, but made no extravagant claims for recovery in adults. However, it is now clear that obstetric brachial plexus injuries (which are surprisingly common even in advanced countries) do benefit from early surgery. Where the nerve root has been avulsed, it is possible to transfer another nerve, whose function is not essential, to the distal end of the avulsed one, using a graft if necessary to bridge a gap: this is called neurotisation. An obvious donor is an intercostal nerve; more startling are the phrenic nerve or even the intact contralateral C7 nerve root! (Gu et al 1992).

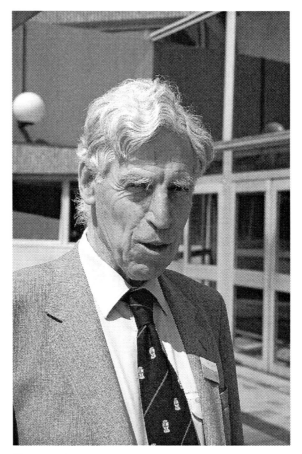

Fig. 9.5 Erik Moberg, the founder of hand surgery in Scandinavia

Moberg, after his retirement as professor, took up the cause of tetraplegics, many of whom consider the limited use of their arms to be the worst aspect of their disability. He established that carefully planned surgery with clearly defined aims, which are not over-ambitious, can make life easier for these unfortunate patients.

Finally, one must mention the pain that sometimes follows severe nerve injuries and can be even worse to bear than the paralysis. There are no easy answers, but Kit Wynn-Parry and others have evolved methods of treatment that can afford some relief.

DUPUYTREN'S CONTRACTURE

'Given an eponym, one may be sure that: (1) the man so honoured was not the first to describe the disease ...; or (2) he misunderstood the situation; or (3) he is generally misquoted; or (4) 1, 2 and 3 are all simultaneously true' (Ravitch 1979).

The early history of the condition called Dupuytren's contracture has been comprehensively told by Elliot (1989) in a fascinating series of three papers. Its distribution suggests that the disease originated in Northern Europe. 'In Great Britain this view is supported by the apparently high incidence of the condition today in those parts of the country which faced the Norsemen, namely north-east England and the north and west of Scotland' (Elliot 1989). This probably accounts for the curse of the MacCrimmons. That Scottish clan was recognised as producing the best players of the bagpipes and, at the end of the fifteenth century, a college of piping, under the tutelage of MacCrimmons, was established on the island of Skye. James Boswell in his *Journal of a Tour to the Hebrides with Samuel Johnson* in 1773 says of this college that 'it subsisted in a certain degree until last year'. The curse was a condition that bent the little finger and made it impossible to play the pipes properly.

The first written description was probably by Felix Platter, a disciple of Vesalius, working at Basle, Switzerland, in 1614. (Vesalius taught in Padua but his famous *De Humani Corporis Fabrica* was published in Basle. This, too, challenged some accepted teachings of Galen). 'A certain well-known master mason, on rolling a large stone, caused the tendons to the ring and little fingers in the palm of the left hand to cease to function. They contracted and in so doing were loosed from the bonds by which they are held and became raised up, as two cords forming a ridge under the skin. These two fingers will remain contracted and drawn in forever' (Anonymous Editorial 1968). Elliot considers this description to be pathognomonic, though Boyes (1976) interpreted it as rupture of the pulleys over the flexor tendons. Either way, it was one of John Hunter's pupils, Henry Cline Senior of St Thomas's Hospital in London, who first dissected a hand with what is now called Dupuytren's contracture and soon afterwards, in 1777, described its treatment by palmar fasciotomy. (Perhaps the name 'clinodactyly' should have been applied to this disease instead of the congenital lateral deviation of the finger!)

Cline, in turn, taught Astley Cooper (1768–1841) who gave an account of the contracture in his *Treatise on Dislocations and Fractures of the Joints*. Cooper and Dupuytren 'visited each other on several occasions during the period which preceded the latter's famous lecture of 5 December 1831' (Elliot 1989), so it is strange that Dupuytren was apparently unaware of the contributions from London on this subject (Fig. 9.6). Cooper 'was made a baronet by George IV for removing a wen from the royal scalp' (Boyes 1976).

Guillaume Dupuytren (1777–1835), whose family originated in the hamlet of Le Puytren near Limoges in central France (Barsky 1984), was sent to school in Paris

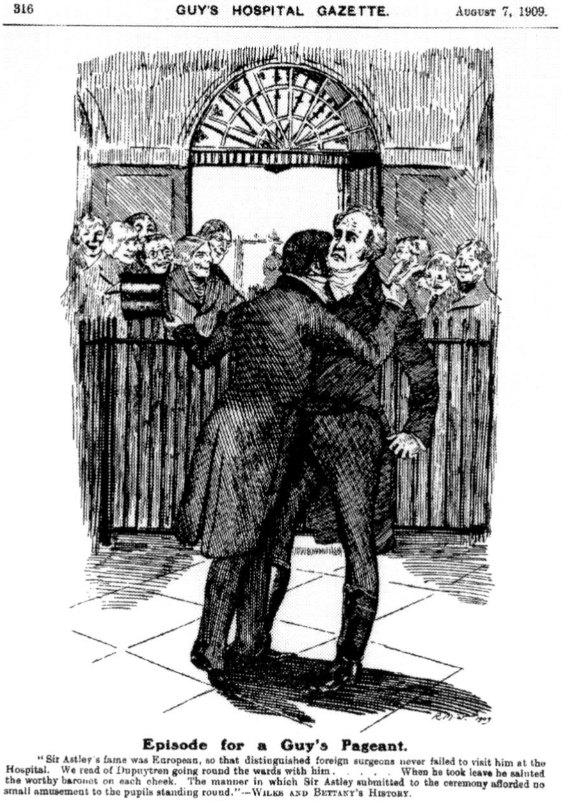

Episode for a Guy's Pageant.
" Sir Astley's fame was European, so that distinguished foreign surgeons never failed to visit him at the Hospital. We read of Dupuytren going round the wards with him . When he took leave he saluted the worthy baronet on each cheek. The manner in which Sir Astley submitted to the ceremony afforded no small amusement to the pupils standing round."—WILKS AND BETTANY'S HISTORY.

Fig. 9.6 Dupuytren's farewell to Sir Astley Cooper. Courtesy of the Editor of *Guy's Hospital Gazette* and of David Elliot

in 1789, the year in which the French Revolution shattered the order of the old world, so he lived through it. His biographer Hannah Barsky (1984), herself the wife of a hand surgeon, does not accept the traditional tale (Rang 1966) of his being abducted by a rich lady on account of his good looks. Subsequently he worked as a prosector and lived above the cloister of the Convent des Cordeliers on the Rue de l'École de Médicine, of which the refectory survives at No. 15 and can be visited. This had been the meeting place of one of the revolutionary clubs whose members included Dr Jean-Paul Marat, who lived at No. 20 in the same street and was there stabbed to death in the bath by Charlotte Corday in 1793, as depicted in the famous painting by Jacques-Louis David. Marat had lived in Britain for twelve years and in 1775 received the degree of Doctor of Medicine from St Andrew's University. On his return to Paris two years later, he became a fashionable and expensive physician to the wealthy aristocracy, despite his own egalitarian opinions. When his scientific works were ignored by the French Academy of Sciences, he became completely paranoid and set out to destroy that aristo-cratic society whom he had previously treated (Appleyard 1971). 'The Cordeliers District was a filthy warren of alleys and narrow streets where savagery and murder were commonplace' (Appleyard 1971). Dupuytren was then very poor and at one stage lived for six weeks on bread and cheese alone; it is said that he read books by the light of oil from the cadavers he dissected. Later he became rich and powerful as the *chirurgien-en-chef* at the Hôtel-Dieu, a hospital founded in the Middle Ages on the Ile de la Cité, where Ambroise Paré had worked. It stood on the river side of what is now the square in front of Nôtre-Dame and, according to a local saying, there was a sick person, a dying person and a corpse in every bed. (About 1860 it was demolished, the square created and the present elegant Hôtel-Dieu built on the opposite side of the square.)

In 1831 Dupuytren said that he had seen thirty or forty cases of the contracture over the previous twenty years but not operated on one until 12 June 1831, when he carried out multiple fasciotomies on the hand of a wine merchant, after which the hand was splinted in extension and the gap which had been opened up in the skin left to heal by secondary intention (anticipating the McCash technique).

This child of the Revolution is often characterised as a tyrant but was probably misrepresented by his enemies, such as Lisfranc who called him 'the brigand of the Hôtel-Dieu'. Dupuytren made an enormous contribution to the golden age of surgery in Paris in the wake of the Revolution. Perhaps he does not deserve to be credited with the contracture, but he was the first to describe 'Madelung's' deformity of the wrist, 'Langer's' lines in the skin and 'Gillies'' method of reducing zygomatic fractures (Elliot 1989), as well as many other original contributions, large and small, the latter including a description of subungual exostosis in 1817 – but this was in the big toe, not the hand (Rang 1966). He is also remembered in the Rue Dupuytren, a small side-road off the other end of the Rue de l'École-de-Médicine, close to where he lived when he was an impoverished prosector.

According to McGrouther (1988), 'The next development in surgical technique was the actual removal of the contracted tissue'. In those days surgery had to be done without anaesthetic and was frequently followed by infection, so it was not until much later that more extensive operations were invented for Dupuytren's contracture. This approach was carried to its extreme by Lexer who, *c.*1900, excised most of the palm of the hand and split-skin-grafted it.

A slightly less radical operation was favoured by Sir Archibald McIndoe (1900–60), the plastic surgeon who became famous for his treatment of burnt airmen in the Second World War (Mosley 1962, Barron 1990). He did what he called a total fasciectomy, though in fact the palmar fascia ramifies so widely throughout the hand and digits that it is impossible to excise it completely: what McIndoe did was to excise the whole of the palmar aponeurosis, which is the most obvious part of the palmar fascia. Later, he developed the disease himself:

'In 1943, he noticed a contracture appearing in the fingers of his left hand. There was no doubt about the diagnosis; he was hatching a Dupuytren's contracture. Like many others before him, he fought against the increasing disability but it soon became obvious that he should submit to surgery. He consulted his friend and colleague, Rainsford Mowlem, who agreed to take the responsibility of operating on this very special hand. It is typical that, far too early in his convalescence, he returned to his beloved airmen at East Grinstead'. (Barron 1990)

However, the 'total' fasciectomy was often followed by complications and follow-up showed that recurrence was not diminished, so in the last fifty years the extent of surgery has been shrinking. Most surgeons now excise only the abnormal tissue and a surrounding margin of normal aponeurosis and fascia ('partial' or 'limited' fasciectomy). There is even a trend to excision of just 1 cm of diseased cord, following which it is claimed that the remaining cord regresses (McGrouther 1988, Moermans 1991). This is not much more than a fasciotomy, so brings us back almost to the original operation of Cline and Dupuytren.

As regards the skin, Hueston of Melbourne (where Rank and Wakefield established an important group of hand surgeons) considered that the disease *starts* in the skin and that excision of the involved skin prevents recurrence. This latter is probably true, but dermatofasciectomy is a major undertaking and is usually reserved for recurrent cases. If an ordinary fasciectomy is done through a transverse (or partly transverse) incision, then the release of the contracture allows the fingers to extend and creates a wide gap between the skin edges. However, there is no skin missing and McCash (1964) advised that the wound be left open to heal gradually: this it does in a few weeks, leaving a linear scar and abolishing the complications of haematoma (as it can get out) and skin necrosis (as it is under no tension).

Our knowledge of pathological anatomy has increased. Graham Stack (1915–92), while a busy surgeon in London and Essex (Fisk & Barton 1992, Bolton & Robins 1993), flew to the Netherlands at the weekends to study the unique collection of foetal hands in Professor Landsmeer's Anatomy Department. The result was his book on *The Palmar Fascia*, though even this did not include the fascia on the ulnar side of the hand which was studied later by White (1984). An important advance in our understanding was made by MacFarlane of Ontario, Canada, who showed that the disease does not develop randomly but follows preordained pathways of palmar fascia which may originally spiral around the digital nerve and can, when contracted to a tight cord, straighten out so that the nerve now spirals around the cord and is in danger during an operation (McFarlane 1974).

As to the cause of the disease, much research has been done but in truth we still do not know. Bunker has pointed to some interesting pathological similarities with frozen shoulder, but the natural histories of the two conditions are different.

Most of the modern surgeons mentioned above were plastic surgeons. This illustrates that hand surgery is not just a branch of orthopaedics, but contains a large element of plastic surgery.

THE ARTHRITIC HAND

Osteoarthritis, such a common surgical problem in the lower limbs, seldom requires operation in the upper limbs.

'What are those hard little knobs, about the size of a small pea, which are frequently seen upon the fingers, particularly a little below the top, near the joint? They have no connection with the gout, being found in persons who never had it; they continue for life and, being hardly ever attended with pain, or disposed to become sores, are rather unsightly than inconvenient, though they must be some little hindrance to the free use of the fingers.' So wrote William Heberden (1710–1801), a London physician (Major 1948). He actually wrote it in Latin: the volume in which this short description occurs was published in 1802 and was probably the last medical textbook in Latin. The answer to his question is that they are a manifestation of osteoarthritis of the DIP joints and are now called Heberden's nodes. As he said, they seldom need treatment.

The carpometacarpal joint of the thumb, in contrast, quite often requires an operation. All three of the classic operations of orthopaedics have been used: arthrodesis, osteotomy and arthroplasty. Arthrodesis gives a strong grip and may be best in men, but they rarely need such an operation as the condition is much more common in women. Osteotomy near the base of the first metacarpal can relieve pain (as at the hip) and correct the adduction deformity. Arthroplasty is the operation most often used, in all three types: excision, interposition and replacement.

Excision of the trapezium was first reported by W. Harvey Gervis of Tunbridge Wells who, at the British Orthopaedic Association meeting in 1948, 'said that he had performed this operation on eighteen occasions. One

patient was able to milk cows for many hours a day' (Gervis 1949). By 1973 he had done over a hundred cases, of which he reported a twenty-five-year follow up (Gervis 1973). Like McIndoe, he showed his faith in his operation by having it done on himself. 'When the author developed pain in his own right trapeziometacarpal joint, which gradually got worse and made operating tiring and hobbies distasteful, he had no doubts and had his own trapezium excised two years ago. He can now operate and indulge in hobbies in comfort. At that time he was just starting to remake the back wheel of a gypsy caravan, more than 1½ metres in diameter. Shaping the curve of the felloes to the rim of the wheel with chisel, spokeshave and plane was excellent therapy' (Gervis 1973). He stressed that it takes up to a year to recover.

Surgeons in Denmark and the USA added soft-tissue reconstructions, using spare bits of tendon both as check-reins to prevent subluxation and as interposition material. These have become *de rigueur* in America where, in 1991, I was told that 'nobody just excises the trapezium any more', though I still did. A recent prospective randomised controlled study (Davis et al 1997) showed that there is in fact little or no benefit from these more complicated procedures.

Total replacement of the joint can be done, the best known being that of de la Caffinière from Luxemburg which resembles a miniature Charnley hip (de la Caffinière & Aucouturier 1979). It gives superb results at first, but most surgeons have found that the prosthesis soon becomes loose; however, this is not a disaster as removing it leaves an excision arthroplasty which, at this site, is very acceptable (in contrast to a Girdlestone). Al Swanson devised a silastic trapezial prosthesis with a stem going up the first metacarpal, but this had a tendency to sublux and silastic replacements for the carpal bones often produce a particulate synovitis so are no longer available. This is a pity, because silastic replacement of the lunate was a good treatment for Kienbock's disease. The prostheses for the MP joints are fortunately not subject to the same problem.

'*Rheumatoid* hand surgery, child of the fifties, adolescent of the sixties, has now come of age', wrote Ed Nalebuff (who contributed greatly to this development) in 1971. The 1956 edition of Bunnell's book had no chapter on the rheumatoid hand, whereas the 1999 edition of Green's book has five. Before 1950, surgeons did not bother much about the rheumatoid hand, but in the next twenty-five years there was an explosion of operations for this disabling and distressing condition, since when there has been surprisingly little further progress.

This sprint forwards was not the work of one man (though it was much encouraged by the publication of Adrian Flatt's book in 1963) but of many from all over the world, especially Kauko Vainio from Finland, Mack Clayton of Denver, Colorado, Norbert Gschwend in Zurich and Brookes Heywood at Cape Town. Space does not allow me to mention all the others, but only to pick out a few highlights.

One of these was the realisation that the problem lay as often in the tendons as in the joints. It was Oliver Vaughan Jackson in London who first realised that rupture of the extensor tendons of the fingers was usually due to attrition over a sharp spike of bone between two erosions on the lower end of the ulna: essential knowledge because, if this is not dealt with, the tendons will remain at risk. Lennart Mannerfelt, originally from Sweden but later working in Germany, showed that in the same way the radial digital flexor tendons may rupture over a rugosity on the front of the scaphoid.

Excision and interposition arthroplasties of the finger-joints having proved rather unsatisfactory, prosthetic replacement was attempted by Brannon, whose device was modified by Flatt but still did not work well. With all prostheses and orthoses, the problem is the fixation to the patient's tissues. In large joint replacement, this was largely solved by using acrylic cement which spreads out between the trabeculae and distributes the load over their wide surface area. There is a fundamental problem in applying this to the small cylindrical bones of the hand: once they have been reamed, there is virtually no cancellous bone left: just a cortical tube in which a cylinder of cement can rotate (Lee & Ling 1977). This difficulty was successfully evaded by Al Swanson's silicone-rubber ('silastic') implants, for the MP joint (Swanson 1973), originally intended as temporary spacers, which make no attempt at fixation but are allowed to piston up and down. These were introduced over thirty years ago (I took part in the original field trials, while working in the USA) and have still not been bettered. By the time rheumatoid patients come to hand surgery, the pain has usually stopped troubling them, but they cannot open their hands widely to grasp large objects and they are distressed by the deformed appearance of their hands, which are constantly on show. Swanson's implants improve both, and that is why the patients are always so grateful, even though the range of flexion is limited. Swanson (Fig. 9.7), who works in Grand Rapids, Michigan, became a very active Secretary and later President of the International Federation of the Society for Surgery of the Hand.

In the wrist, pain *is* the symptom. Where this arises at the inferior radio-ulnar joint, excision of the lower end of the ulna will usually abolish it. (I was told by one of Darrach's former residents that he preserved the medial cortex and styloid, with the ulnar collateral ligament. Similar modifications have been recommended by

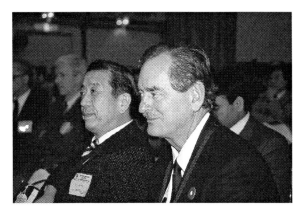

Fig. 9.7 Al Swanson (right) and Tatsuya Tajima (left)

Bowers and Kirk Watson.) At the carpal joints, arthrodesis has long been known to be a good operation and is easy to achieve in rheumatoid patients, who have a tendency to ankylosis. Various types of prosthetic replacement have been used, but none seems reliable enough to supersede arthrodesis: a contrast to the larger joints where fusion causes major disability.

REPLANTATION AND FREE TISSUE TRANSFER

In 1894 the President of the French Republic was assassinated by an anarchist whose knife had severed the main vein from the liver. A French surgeon, Alexis Carrell from Lyons (1873–1948), realised that the President's death from internal haemorrhage might have been prevented if it had been possible to repair the damaged blood vessels. By 1902 he had worked out a method and 'first performed the vascular end-to-end anastomosis by hand with a 3-stay suture technique, which has been a fundamental technique of vascular surgery up to now' (Tamai 1993). For this he received a Nobel Prize in 1912. Thus the foundation stone of vascular surgery was laid early in the twentieth century.

The first reattachment of a completely amputated limb with vascular anastomosis seems to have been that done by Malt and McKhann (who were general surgeons in Boston, Massachusetts) on 23 May 1962 (Malt & McKhann 1964). The patient was a twelve-year-old boy whose arm had been run over by a train. The success of this procedure was shown when, in his twenties, he used his replanted hand to steal something from a shop; a policeman caught him. Malt and McKhann did another replant on 5 September 1963 and I was introduced to this patient five years later; his arm was of limited functional value, but he did use it to give me a religious tract!

The first replantation of the hand was done in China. The circumstances were unusual. A surgeon called Zhong-Wei Chen (Fig. 9.8) had, like many professional people during Mao's Cultural Revolution, been sent to work in a factory. Here, on 2 January 1963, another workman cut off his hand through the forearm. The foreman was aware of Chen's previous occupation and instructed him to put the hand back on. Chen did not know if this was possible, but plated the radius and sutured the vessels (without benefit of microsurgery) and other soft tissues. The hand survived, and so did Chen.

Within the next twenty years there were 1131 replantations of limbs and 2604 of digits in China, mostly successful. The reason for this probably lies in the Chinese attitude to bodily deficiencies, inherited from Confucius 'who considered the human body to be a gift from the parents which should never be damaged in any way. When it did get damaged, the victim was responsible for the silly act. Thus he had failed to honour his parents by failing to protect what had been handed down to him. The disgrace involved meant tremendous dishonour' (Leung 1989). Moreover, for many centuries criminals in China had been punished by amputation (as still happens in parts of Arabia) so lack of a limb or digit was doubly shameful.

Technically the repair of the larger arteries and veins in the proximal and central part of a limb is relatively easy: repair of the large nerves is also not too difficult but unlikely to be followed by good recovery of distal function. Distally, the nerves are more likely to make a useful recovery but the vessels were considered too small to repair. Sir Harold Gillies (1882–1960), the pioneer of British plastic surgery, was born on the same day as Bunnell and was a friend of his but, being (like his successor and distant cousin McIndoe) originally from New Zealand, he claimed seniority on account of the International Date Line! (Campbell Reid 1981). In 1940 he published a paper in *The Lancet* proposing a possible operation to autograft an amputated digit. 'The suggestion was to remove carefully the skin envelope from the amputated digit, preserving the tendons, joints and nerves together with the bone. Bone would then be joined to bone, tendons and nerves sutured and the whole inserted into a tubed flap' (Campbell Reid 1981). Stuart Gordon in Canada first did this in 1942.

When the binocular-operating microscope, made by the German optical company Zeiss, became available in 1953, it was realised that if you could see it, you could sew it. Magnification was first used surgically in 1921 for operations on the ear by Nylen in Stockholm. It has since become a routine tool in every surgical speciality except general surgery and orthopaedics.

In the 1950s a young American called Harry Buncke spent some time with Tom Gibson, a distinguished plastic surgeon in Glasgow who predicted that large blocks of tissue would be transferred on their own blood supply and encouraged Buncke to develop microvascular techniques for the extremities. (Jacobson and Suarez, neurosurgeons from Vermont, reported experimental anastomosis of vessels 1 or 2 mm in diameter to the American College of Surgeons in 1960 and coined the term 'microsurgery'. They later applied this clinically to intracranial thrombosis and aneurysms.)

On his return to California, Buncke began amputating and replanting the ears of rabbits. At first he 'tried to develop some kind of mechanical vascular suturing machine, but without success. Later he

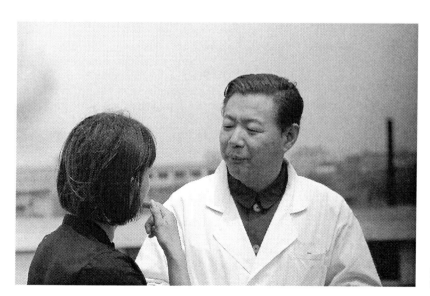

Fig. 9.8 Zhong-Wei Chen, a pioneer of replantation. Courtesy of David M. Evans

decided to try small vessel anastomosis by hand under a microscope. In order to perform his experiments, he remodelled a garage in his home to a laboratory and his wife, who is a dermatologist, sometimes assisted him'. Over and over again, the ear died. After fifty-three failures, he was at last successful! 'In the following 20 years he trained a number of microsurgeons from all over the world, and has been called "the father of microsurgery"' (Tamai 1993).

Probably the first surgeon to carry out successful human microvascular repair of a digital vessel (in a nearly amputated thumb) was Harold Kleinert, who was originally a cardiovascular surgeon. This was in the early 1960s. Kleinert was already in such trouble with the American Hand Society about his flexor tendon repairs that he kept very quiet about it at first! (His original application to join the Society in 1960 had been rejected; in 1976 he became its President.) The earliest microsurgical replantation of a completely amputated thumb was by Tamai and Kamatzu in Japan on 27 July 1965: this remains a prime indication, because no reconstruction of the thumb is ever as good as the original (Tamai 1993). (Japanese surgeons, notably Tatsuya Tajima (Fig. 9.7) and Kenya Tsuge, have made important contributions to other aspects of hand surgery.)

The ability to carry out reliably successful microvascular anastomosis opened a whole new era of surgery in which it became possible to transfer almost any part of the body to almost any other part.

Skin cover in the hand had long posed problems. Split skin grafting was first done by Jaques Louis Reverdin (1842–1929) of Geneva. (It was Reverdin who noticed that after thyroidectomy some patients developed myxoedema, from which it was realised that myxoedema is due to thyroid deficiency). Split skin grafting is simple, reliable and can be applied on most surfaces but it is not very suitable for the hand. It is not elastic enough for the back of the hand and not tough enough for the grasping surface; worse still, it lacks sensation. Full-thickness skin grafting was introduced by an ophthalmic surgeon called Wolfe 'of Hungarian-Jewish ancestry' (Boyes 1976) but who worked in Glasgow (easily confused with the Prussian named Wolff, who originated the law about bone growth, as they both had the initial J. and were almost contemporary). The Wolfe graft provides better quality of skin and is now preferred in operations for syndactyly or recurrent Dupuytren's contracture. Local flaps have limited usefulness, though neurovascular island flaps did give some sensation.

Pedicled distant flaps (the tubed pedicle was developed by Gillies), and especially the groin flap devised by Ian McGregor of Glasgow in 1972 (McGregor & Jackson 1972), provided good safe cover for large skin defects on the hand but, even after later thinning, were still rather too bulky. The 'Chinese' flap of skin from the forearm on a distally based vascular pedicle established a new principle: where there is a rich vascular anastomosis, this can be used to send blood in the reverse direction to usual. Thus the Chinese flap is based retrogradely on the radial artery, now supplied through the palmar arterial arches from the ulnar artery and the carpal arches. Similar flaps have been devised within the fingers to replace the skin of the fingertip.

However it is now possible (as Gibson predicted) to apply free flaps of skin, plus whatever other tissues are needed, to any defect on the hand or elsewhere. Moreover, these are sometimes done as emergency procedures: part of a trend in the treatment of all trauma to do the definitive surgery straight away, which is replacing the earlier policy of stabilising the situation (e.g. with a split-skin graft) and doing a final procedure later.

In elective surgery, an absent thumb or finger could now be replaced by a toe. (This had actually been done in 1898, by Carl Nicoladoni (1847–1902), Professor of Surgery at Innsbruck in Austria, in two stages as a form of pedicle graft: first the big toe was applied to the hand while still also attached to the foot, and three weeks later – when it had acquired a new blood supply – it was detached. However, this was unreliable and extremely uncomfortable.) The first human vascularised free toe-to-thumb transfers were done in 1968 by John Cobbett, who had spent some months with Buncke, at East Grinstead in England (Cobbett 1969) and also by Yao and colleagues in Japan (Tamai 1993). These restored the ability to pinch but did not look good: the big toe is too big and the lesser toes too small. The result is a 'thoe', looking like neither. By 1980 Wayne Morrison in Melbourne, working in Professor Bernard O'Brien's department, had evolved the 'wrap-around' procedure in which the soft tissues and nail of the big toe are transferred but the osseous support is provided by an iliac bone graft which is thinner than the phalanges of the big toe (Morrison et al 1980). To replace fingers, the second or third toe is a reasonable size but many patients (including the Chinese, for the reason stated) are reluctant to sacrifice a toe and may be wise in their caution as the loss of a toe is not wholly harmless and not to be undertaken unless absolutely necessary.

Fully vascularised composite tissue grafts, including skin, bone, muscle, tendon and nerve as required, are now routine procedures. On a more modest scale, local vascularised free transfers can be used to provide reasonable replacement for the unique skin of the fingertips or even for the growing nail.

All these are autografts, as usually the patient has enough spare tissue elsewhere to fill a defect. What about homografts, from other individuals?

John Hunter 'made many attempts at tissue grafting, notably by implanting a human tooth into a cock's comb', but was 'frustrated by sepsis' (Le Vay 1990). Peter Medawar was a lecturer in zoology at Oxford in 1941 when a large bomber 'crashed into the garden of a house about 200 yards away and immediately exploded with a fearful whomp!' The pilot survived but with 60% burns, and his plastic surgeon suggested that Medawar should investigate how to provide skin cover in this situation. 'I guessed that if one could use a graft transfer of skin from a donor the treatment of war wounds would be transformed' (Le Fanu 1999). In the years to come, Medawar did much experimental work and discovered the immunological basis of rejection, though when asked after a lecture by a young surgeon called Roy Calne whether he could see any clinical application of his studies, he replied 'Absolutely none.'

What made it possible was the development by Calne of the immunosuppressive drug aziothioprine, which, when combined with steroids, was really effective. This led in the 1960s to successful transplants (from unrelated individuals) of kidney, liver and heart.

The first hand transplant was performed as early as 1964 in Ecuador, but 'resulted in loss of the transplant at two weeks, perhaps not surprising in view of the primitive immunosuppressive regime used' (Kay 2000). Over thirty years passed before the second hand transplant was carried out on 23 September 1998 at Lyons in France by an international team, and was soon followed by a third at Louisville, Kentucky. In both these cases the hand survived, with some long tendon function and early signs of nerve recovery. However the first patient suffered chronic rejection consistent with non-compliance in taking the immunosuppressive drugs; in addition he never really accepted the transplant psychologically and after two years it was amputated at his request. The second patient remains happy with his new hand. Several more hand transplants have been carried out since, but it is too early to determine their outcomes. Technically these are little different to replants, but the patient has to continue taking immunosuppressive drugs for the rest of his life and this raises ethical questions. These drugs have complications that can even be lethal and many surgeons feel that it is not justifiable to take that risk to treat a problem which, though seriously disabling, is not in itself fatal. The French medical authorities shared this fear and the team at Lyons was allowed to continue this work only on patients who had lost *both* hands which is, of course, dreadfully

disabling. It carried out its first double hand transplant in January 2000. Another double transplant has been done in Innsbruck and more are planned in various centres.

It may in future be possible to control rejection by a single course of drugs, in which case their danger would be lessened. (There is an alternative: Simo Vilkki in Finland has reshaped the stumps and transplanted a toe, providing a surprisingly strong pinch.)

Thus there has been an explosive and world-wide development in microvascular operations, like that in rheumatoid surgery but starting more or less when that petered out and continuing until now. In Britain it has largely become the province of plastic surgeons due to the insatiable demands of fractures and joint replacements, but this is a pity. Young orthopaedic surgeons can learn microsurgical techniques as quickly as any other specialist and in France, for example, the leading exponents of microsurgery to the hand are orthopaedic surgeons.

SOME OTHER DISORDERS

Fractures

Many fractures of the hand do best with little or no treatment. This led to a rather *laissez-faire* attitude that failed to pick out those which do need immobilisation and those few which need an operation.

Strapping the injured finger to the adjoining intact finger was recommended by Alexander Munro Tertius (1773–1859) who in 1800 was appointed Conjoint Professor (with his father!) of Medicine, Surgery and Anatomy at Edinburgh; from 1817 to 1846 he was sole professor. From 1808 he delivered the whole course of lectures and, according to the notebook of one of his students said 'We first treat the fracture and then tie it to its neighbour.' (The notebook is kept at the Royal College of Physicians of Edinburgh. It is now thought that this lecture should be attributed to Alexander Munro Secundus in the late eighteenth century, though Tertius was still giving his father's lectures in the early nineteenth century. Alexander Munro Primus, the father of Secundus, had preceded him as professor and is regarded as the father of the Edinburgh Medical School). When splintage is required, a major contribution was the insistence of J. I. P. James that the hand must be splinted in the safe position (see p.123).

Internal fixation of hand fractures was introduced by Albin Lambotte (1866–1955), the Belgian pioneer of osteosynthesis, who stabilised Bennett's fractures with thin carpenter's nails. 'In 1924, Tennant reported fixing fragments of metacarpal fractures with steel phonograph needles … while a German surgeon was developing a system that used piano strings' (Meals & Meuli 1985).

This was Martin Kirschner (1879–1942) who 'was in a very real sense a general surgeon, his day-to-day work and his special interests encompassing the full spectrum of contemporary surgery' (Wilton 1988). He studied under Trendelenberg and in 1924 was the first surgeon to perform successfully a Trendelenberg operation for the removal of an embolus from the pulmonary artery. He gave credit to his old teacher 'who, in return, credited Kirschner with being able to set up such an efficient system that the operation could be carried out in time to be successful'. Indeed Kirschner's greatest ability seems to have been in organising departments (like James in our own day): he was successively Professor at Königsberg, Tubingen and Heidelberg. In 1909 he described the use of what we call Steinmann's pins (though Steinmann used broad-headed steel nails) 'to transfix a tibia or femur above and below a fracture, to provide traction and counter-traction through a form of external fixator. He was unhappy with the soft-tissue damage that might be caused by those large pins and worked on reducing their diameter, by 1927 settling on chrome-plated piano wires between 0.7 mm. and 1.5 mm. in diameter' (Meals & Meuli 1985). He also did experimental work that was the basis of later tendon grafting in humans (Boyes 1976).

One of the first papers reporting internal fixation of phalangeal fractures was by Frederick Vom Saal of New York in 1953. Like Bunnell's classic paper on flexor tendon injuries, this was at first rejected by the *Journal of Bone and Joint Surgery* in a letter which implied that it was tantamount to malpractice. Vom Saal later gave a paper about it at a meeting and was invited to submit it for publication in that journal! 'Send them a copy of their original letter', said Mrs Vom Saal. Her husband sent them the article instead.

In 1979 the first of many papers on the biomechanics of internal fixation in the hand showed that plates on the back or side of a phalanx gave less rigid fixation than Kirschner wires (Fyfe & Mason 1979). Biomechanically, it would be best to put a plate on the flat front of the phalanx, but the flexor tendon is there; moreover there is a tendency for the tendons to adhere and make the finger stiff. (As with cement fixation of prostheses but for different reasons, the solutions worked out for larger bones are seldom applicable to the phalanges.) There is, however, some place for plates on the metacarpals, where they can be placed dorsally to prevent the usual angulation into flexion.

In the 1970s I used to lecture about internal fixation of hand fractures, which was seldom done. However, the growing popularity of AO techniques generally and the seductive appeal of sets of tiny plates and screws led to increasing attempts to apply them to the phalanges, often resulting in stiff fingers. By the 1990s my lectures were advocating conservative treatment, which was in danger of being forgotten.

Scaphoid fractures have an interesting history. Destot of Lyons, France, writing in the early twentieth century, said 'osseous consolidation between the fragments is exceptional. Pseudo-arthrosis is the rule' (Destot 1925). It seems, however, that he only immobilised them for a week or two, so his poor results are hardly surprising. A longer period in plaster became the rule and in 1955 Watson Jones wrote that, if necessary, the immobilisation should be continued for ten months! In Continental Europe and North America, an above-elbow cast is usually employed, but in Britain a below-elbow cast, including the proximal phalanx of the thumb, was favoured, so much so that it became known as a 'scaphoid cast'. Geoffrey Fisk's Hunterian Lecture entitled 'Carpal Instability and the Scaphoid Fracture' (Fisk 1970) stimulated a renewal of interest which has called into question many previously accepted tenets, both as to the best method of conservative treatment (Clay et al 1991) and the indications for internal fixation. The screw devised for the latter by Tim Herbert in Sydney, Australia, embodied an entirely original concept, having two threads of different pitches so that tightening it up compresses the fracture (Barton 1996).

I have written elsewhere how Bennett described his fracture of the base of the first metacarpal; also of the fractures of Colles and Smith, though these may be regarded a part of the common currency of orthopaedics rather than hand surgery (Barton 2000).

Carpal tunnel syndrome

In 1853 Sir James Paget (1814–99) said that Mr Hilton had told him of a patient at Guy's Hospital

'who, in consequence of a fracture at the lower end of the radius, repaired by an excessive quantity of new bone, suffered compression of the median nerve. He had ulceration of the thumb and fore and middle fingers, which resisted various treatments and was only cured by so binding the wrist that the parts on the palmar aspect being relaxed, the pressure on the nerve was removed' (Rang 1966).

Thirty years later Joseph Ormerod (1848–1925), an aspiring neurologist at St Bartholomew's Hospital, described in the reports of that hospital the syndrome so familiar to us. 'The symptoms occur in women, usually about the climacteric age, and begin on the right. On waking, the patient has a feeling in the hands of numbness, deadness, pins-and-needles; sometimes there is actual pain, severe enough to wake her' (Rang 1966). However, Ormerod did not realise the cause of the syndrome or how it could be cured.

James Learmonth first performed surgical decompression in 1933 when he was working at the Mayo Clinic. (Some American authors who refer to this seem unaware that he soon returned to Scotland where he became Professor of Surgery at Edinburgh and was knighted.) However, the key paper was that by Brain (what a wonderful name for a neurologist!) and colleagues who, in 1947, recognised the cause of the nocturnal acroparaesthesiae and advocated the simple operation to cure them. I recommend reading this paper and also the spirited – sometimes heated – correspondence that followed the publication of the paper in *The Lancet*. My late colleague Professor William Waugh remembered reading it when he was a medical student: this shows how recent is the proper understanding of what is probably the commonest condition requiring hand surgery.

Ligamentous injuries of the wrist

In the 1970s, surgeons in the USA began to study the joints of the wrist and to realise how complicated they are (Taliesnik 1976). The anatomy of the ligaments (best seen from inside the joint; now by arthroscopy) was worked out and various forms of carpal instability – hitherto unrecognised, as in the knee – were described. Unfortunately, the nomenclature used was and is hard to understand (and its abbreviations are even worse), which has added unnecessary difficulty to an already difficult subject (Larsen et al 1995). In clinical practice, some of these faults are intermittent and therefore particularly difficult to diagnose. Even with arthroscopy and MRI, it is not always easy to relate observed abnormalities to symptoms. Moreover, ligamentous reconstruction operations have not proved very satisfactory. The alternative is a limited carpal fusion of only one or two joints within the wrist complex. The conventional orthopaedic doctrine that, if one is going to fuse anything in the wrist, one must fuse everything is challenged by Kirk Watson of Connecticut, an original thinker about the wrist, who advocates various types of limited carpal fusion. In the first edition of David Green's *Operative Hand Surgery* (1982) only two pages were devoted to such operations: in the fourth edition they fill a chapter of twenty-two pages. It is now clear that there is a place for some of these intercarpal fusions, but unfortunately most surgeons have not found them reliable in relieving pain attributed to carpal instability.

Watson also recognised the characteristic sequence in which osteoarthritis develops in the wrist (excluding the trapezial joints), which allows a rational approach to management (Watson & Baker 1984).

De Quervain's stenosing tenovaginitis

This condition was described in 1895 by Fritz de Quervain, who succeeded Kocher as Professor of Surgery at Bern in Switzerland. He was a general surgeon with a special interest in goitre: he had assisted Kocher at the first thyroidectomy and was himself instrumental in introducing iodised salt into Switzerland. The building that housed his operating theatre is now the Physiotherapy Department of the University Hospital at Bern. Grey Turner visited his clinic in 1908 and was vividly struck by de Quervain's resource and imagination:

'It was a badly united fracture of the femur and he was finding difficulty in getting correct alignment and in fixing the fragments. In the middle of the operation, and apparently without premeditation, he sent for an old-fashioned vulcanite pessary. This he heated and moulded into a sort of angulated peg which fitted into the medullary cavities of the bone ends and served to give stability to the fragments while the wound was closed and the limb put up in a fixation apparatus' (Rang 1966).

When describing the condition affecting the thumb tendons, de Quervain was stressing that this was not due to tuberculosis. He added that 'the outer surface of the synovium showed not the slightest change', which is why he did *not* call it tenosynovitis, although this has crept in as a modern misnomer. In Continental Europe, his name is also applied to trans-scaphoid perilunar dislocation.

Ganglia

Heister, who was mentioned on p.124 in connection with tendon repair, described in his textbook of 1718 a variety of traditional treatments for ganglia:

'The inspissated matter of a recent ganglion may often be happily dispersed by rubbing the tumour well each morning with the fasting saliva and binding on a plate of lead upon it afterwards for several weeks successively. Many attribute a stronger discutient virtue to the lead when it has first had some mercury rubbed upon it, and others, with less reason, prefer a bullet that has killed some wild creature, especially a stag. Sometimes indeed a recent ganglion will speedily vanish ... by adding a repeated pressure with all one's might by the thumb ... or a wooden mallet armed with lead. If none of these means prove effectual ... they may be safely removed by incision provided you are careful to avoid the adjacent tendons and ligaments. But as for rubbing them with the hand of a dead man and the like superstitious ceremonies, they are of so little consequence and founded on so weak a basis, that, I presume, my reader will readily excuse me from insisting on them' (Clay & Clement 1988).

Of these, only surgical excision has stood the test of time, and its results are improved by attention to the paper by Angelides and Wallace (1976) showing that ganglia on the back of the wrist always arise, wherever they may present on the dorsal surface, from the scapho-lunate joint. The pedicle must therefore be traced down to this joint and excised.

Paralysis

Tendon transfers for paralysis were first carried out in 1881 by Carl Nicoladoni (already mentioned on p.135 as carrying out two-stage toe-to-thumb transfers), who transferred the peronei to the Achilles tendon of a boy whose calf muscles had been paralysed by *polio* (Le Vay 1990). In the arm, Sir Robert Jones (1858–1933) is credited with having worked out the transfers for radial nerve palsy which, slightly modified so that a wrist flexor is preserved, are still used. Leo Mayer (1884–1972) in New York carried out important studies of the anatomy and physiology of tendons, with a view to improving the effects of tendon transfers.

In the hand itself, polio, which tends to pick out certain groups of muscles, most often affects the thenar muscles and Arthur Steindler (1878–1959), who in 1907 emigrated from Vienna to the USA where he worked in Iowa and wrote *Reconstructive Surgery of the Upper Extremity*, is credited with the first opponensplasty in 1917 for which he used a radial slip of the tendon of flexor pollicis longus. Bunnell experimented with various techniques for opponensplasty (including that later attributed to Camitz) and favoured transfer of the flexor digitorum superficialis tendon from the ring finger. Unfortunately, this requires some sort of pulley, and many variations of transfer and pulley have been devised. More recently extensor tendons have been used, the best being probably extensor indicis proprius, which can be brought round the ulnar side of the wrist whence it runs in a straight line to the thenar area: this was devised by Burkhalter of Florida (Burkhalter et al 1973). An alternative principle was employed by Huber's (1921) transfer of abductor digiti minimi: a muscle transfer rather than a tendon transfer. This also supplies some bulk in the thenar region.

In contrast, *leprosy* most often affects the muscles supplied by the ulnar nerve and Paul Brand, an Englishman working at Vellore in India, worked out ingenious transfers for the resultant intrinsic paralysis. These use one of the radial wrist extensors as the motor, brought round to the front of the hand and lengthened by slips of palmaris longus which pass back through the lumbrical tunnels to the extensor surface. They have not proved so useful in the West, where intrinsic paralysis is rare anyway. This may be because Brand was a specially good surgeon, or because the Asian hand is more supple that the Caucasian one (but that sounds suspiciously like Bunnell saying that English hands were limber than American hands!)

While in India, it is right to mention the contributions made there to hand surgery by B. B. Joshi of Mumbai (formerly Bombay) on the orthopaedic side and R. Venkataswami in Madras from the plastic side.

Spastic paralysis is a much more difficult problem, partly because the strength varies and is hard to measure but even more because there may be an associated sensory deficit. Edwardo Zancolli of Buenos Aires has made thoughtful studies and has also written two important books on the hand: one on surgery and one on anatomy.

Congenital abnormalities

These present a bewildering variety and a wide range of complexity. An important step forward was the general acceptance of a classification commissioned by the American Society for Surgery of the Hand and later adopted by the International Federation of Societies for Surgery of the Hand (Entin et al 1972). It comprises seven main categories and avoids pseudo-Greek words:

1. Failure of formation of parts – subdivided into longitudinal and transverse deficiencies.
2. Failure of differentiation (or separation) of parts.
3. Duplication.
4. Overgrowth (gigantism).
5. Congenital constriction band syndrome.
6. Miscellaneous.
7. Generalised skeletal abnormalities.

This classification is not perfect, but is the best workable one available. Although paediatricians have identified many syndromes that include anomalies of the hand, in my practice as a hand surgeon most patients presented isolated hand problems.

As a sweeping generalisation, one may divide congenital abnormalities of the hand into two grades: minor and major. By minor I mean those which are really only cosmetic problems, such as syndactyly and extra digits: Anne Boleyn is said to have had six fingers and been extremely sensitive about this. Major abnormalities are those that impair function, usually because of absent digits. The most important single digit is, of course, the thumb and a finger can replace an absent thumb. This operation of pollicisation was devised by Gosset in France for treating patients injured during the Second World War, but was developed and improved by J. William Littler of New York, one of Bunnell's young men (see below) and one of the founder members of the American Hand

Society. Congenital absence of the thumb is, however, more difficult because structures may never have developed which are at least partly present in the injured thumb (and there is often also a radial club hand deformity). Pollicisation for this purpose was introduced by Zancolli, developed by Bob Carroll in New York and refined by Dieter Buck-Gramcko of Hamburg (Fig. 9.9) who acquired an enormous and unique experience (Buck-Gramcko 1971) of treating babies deformed by thalidomide: he has now done over five hundred pollicisations, a record unlikely to be beaten.

Buck-Gramcko, incidentally, was the founder of hand surgery in Germany. He started its journal in 1969 and has been its Editor ever since. In addition, he has been Secretary of the German Hand Society for thirty-three years. These are two more records unlikely to be broken! He is greatly respected all over the world.

If only one or two digits are present, some pinch can now be provided by toe transfer.

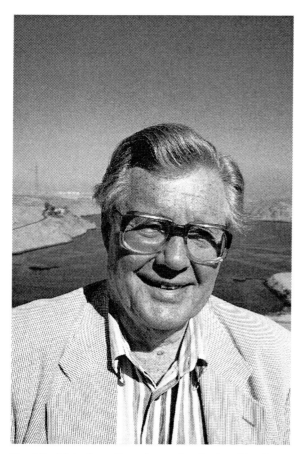

Fig. 9.9 Dieter Buck-Gramcko, another leader of hand surgery in our own time

SURGERY UNDER TOURNIQUET

Sterling Bunnell said, 'You can't mend a watch in an inkwell' and delicate hand surgery requires a bloodless field. It is therefore appropriate to consider the history of deliberate exsanguination.

The history of this has been well described by Klenerman (1962), who says, 'The early development of the tourniquet is bound up with the operation of amputation' for which it was used from the Roman period. Jean Louis Petit (whom we have already met repairing tendons and who began as an army surgeon) invented a screw tourniquet, which had the advantages of not needing an assistant to hold it in place and of being readily released. He called it a 'tourniquet' from the French *tourner* meaning 'to turn'. 'It was only about a hundred [and forty] years ago that the tourniquet was first used in other operations on the limbs' (Klenerman 1962). This was by no less a figure than Joseph Lister (1827–1912). He 'came from a well-off Yorkshire Quaker background. After studying at University College he became assistant surgeon in Edinburgh under Syme in 1854. (On marrying Syme's daughter, he was compelled to leave the Society of Friends, who did not accept "marrying out".) After six years, he gained the Regius chair of Surgery in Glasgow' (Porter 1997), where his development of antiseptic surgery has overshadowed his other contributions.

He used a tourniquet for excision of the wrist joint in tuberculosis.

'And I found that when the hand was raised to the utmost degree and kept so for a few minutes and then, while the elevated position was still maintained, a common tourniquet was applied to the arm being screwed up as rapidly as possible, so as to arrest all circulation in the limb and at the same time avoid venous turgescence, I had practically a bloodless field to operate on and thus gained the double advantage of avoiding haemorrhage and inspecting precisely the part with which I was dealing' (Klenerman 1962).

Johann Esmarch (1823–1908), from Schleswig-Holstein (now part of Germany, but then the southern part of Denmark from which it was struggling for freedom),

'studied at Gottingen and Kiel, becoming an assistant to Langenbeck [who also trained Billroth and Trendelenberg]. It was during the insurrection against Denmark in 1848–50 that he began surgery – he also organised the resistance movement. In 1857 he became Professor of Surgery at Kiel, succeeding Stromeyer, the tenotomist, and marrying his daughter. He was engaged in military surgery again between 1866 and 1871 in the wars with Austria and France; in 1871 he became Surgeon General of the army [when Prussia, which had its eye on the naval port of Kiel, occupied Holstein and later Schleswig. In 1920 the former became part of Germany and the latter of

Denmark, which still applies. Lord Palmerston once said that only three people had understood Schleswig-Holstein: the Prince Consort, who was dead, a German professor, who had gone mad, and himself, who had forgotten all about it]. Soon after he married again – this time a Princess of Schleswig-Holstein. In the same year he published his description of the bandage that bears his name. He used this to produce a clear bloodless field for surgery and to diminish the blood loss during amputations in particular. His contributions to medicine were mainly derived from his battlefield experience' Rang 1996).

In a lecture in 1876, later published in a book, he said 'Gentlemen – You all witnessed yesterday a difficult and tedious operation, in which the patient lost a very large quantity of blood, in spite of all the care that was taken to prevent it. … I shall perform an operation today in which the loss of blood would be still greater, if I did not adopt a procedure before commencing it which enables us to prevent the haemorrhage entirely'. He then described the application of 'elastic bandages, which were made of woven indiarubber, the uniform compression of which drove the blood out of the vessels of the limb' ['As he acknowledged, others including Sir Charles Bell, had used similar methods earlier'; Klenerman 1962.] 'Immediately above the knee, where the bandage ends, we now apply this indiarubber tubing, well drawn out, four or five times round the thigh, and connect the end with the other by means of a hook and brass chain. …We now remove the bandages and you see that both legs below the tubing resemble completely those of a corpse. … We operate precisely *as in the dead subject*' (Rang 1996). This last shows that, although Esmarch used his bandage mainly to conserve blood, it was also to see better what he was operating on. His description reveals the same wonder at the bloodless field as Lister, who changed from the screw tourniquet to Esmarch's version but continued to use elevation for exsanguination.

Note that the actual tourniquet was a rubber tube, not a flat bandage. The flat red rubber bandage used both to exsanguinate and as a tourniquet, which we call the Esmarch bandage, was actually devised later by Langenbeck (Fletcher & Healy 1983). Both methods had two disadvantages: there was no control over the pressure and the tourniquet could be forgotten and left in place when the operation had ended. Bunnell 'insisted that it was the surgeon's responsibility to see to it that the tourniquet was deflated and completely removed from the arm. Often he would say "the tourniquet is not off unless it is across the room"' (Brown 1989).

Both these problems were largely eliminated by the introduction of the pneumatic tourniquet by Harvey Cushing, the famous American pioneer of brain surgery, in 1904. He realised the need for rapid inflation, which

was done by 'one or two quick strokes of the piston' of a bicycle pump. He also suggested a manometer to keep the pressure slightly above systolic. He used his tourniquet mainly around the head to control bleeding from the scalp at craniotomy. It is no longer used for that purpose but has come into its own on the limbs.

Nowadays the pressure is applied from a cylinder of compressed gas mounted on a mobile stand: taking this out of the operating theatre with the patient would not pass unnoticed. The gauge measures the pressure in the box rather than the cuff itself and must be checked monthly against a mercury manometer: Hallett checked tourniquets at seventeen hospitals in London in 1982 and found that 30% of the gauges were inaccurate (Hallett 1983). In practice, this is more likely to cause later problems than keeping the tourniquet on for too long. Bunnell in his book said that when the tourniquet time 'exceeded two hours there is a degree of tissue reaction in the form of local induration at the site of operation'. He advised a 10-minute 'breathing-spell' after 1½ hours; this has now been shown to be of little or no benefit, but the limit of 2 hours remains generally correct, assuming that the pressure is also correct (Fletcher & Healy 1983).

It is possible to do small operations under local anaesthetic using a tourniquet, provided you can be quick. Most patients can tolerate the tourniquet for 15–20 minutes, with increasing discomfort. (An anaesthetic colleague who tried it on himself could not bear it longer than 28 minutes and by then was pacing up and down to try and distract himself.)

The process of exsanguination was simplified by Noel Rhys-Davies, first a naval doctor and then a GP who became a full-time Clinical Assistant in Orthopaedics at Yeovil in Somerset. In the 1970s he devised and used an inflated elastic cylinder that could be rolled onto a limb to exsanguinate it quickly and comfortably. This was published in 1985 (Rhys-Davies & Stotter 1985) and the Rhys-Davies exsanguinator is now widely employed. (It is not effective on the digits, whose diameters are too small.)

August Bier (1861–1949) was Esmarch's assistant and later became Professor of Surgery in Berlin (Van Zundert & Goerig 2000). He gave the first spinal anaesthetic and introduced the 'tin hat' to the German army during the First World War. Our concern here is with his innovation of injecting the congested veins distal to the tourniquet with local anaesthetic. His purpose was to produce local anaesthesia for operations on the elbow but it is now widely used for hand surgery although it is difficult (even using two cuffs) to get a really bloodless field. It is also very well suited to manipulation of Colles' fractures.

Dr J. Hannington-Kiff, an anaesthetist at Frimley in Surrey, 'hit upon the idea of using guanethidine in a kind of Bier block, when faced with the need to produce sympathetic (anti-noradrenergic to be more precise) block in the causalgic hand of a patient whose general health was very poor' (Hannington-Kiff 1984). This has proved a useful tool in the treatment of reflex sympathetic dystrophy and some other pain syndromes in the arm and hand.

HAND SURGERY AS A SPECIALITY

In October 1944 the US Army Surgeon General 'requested that Sterling Bunnell be designated as special civilian consultant to the Secretary of War' because, having been stationed at the Presidio in San Francisco, he knew of Bunnell's 'interest and expertise in hand surgery'. Bunnell's appointment 'coincided with the publication of his *Surgery of the Hand*, which became not only the official text on the subject by the Army, but also the key text in establishing the speciality of hand surgery' (Newmeyer 1995).

Bunnell (Fig. 9.2) was based in San Francisco, where his father had worked for the Wells Fargo Company. He had begun to concentrate on hand surgery in the 1930s and had trained a number of hand surgeons. Now

'Bunnell's charge was to organise, energise, supervise and educate hand surgery services at nine Army hospitals scattered throughout the USA. Between 1944 and 1947, with indefatigable energy, he made eight tours of these hand centres. No one seems to remember how he travelled to the centres, but he was in his early 60s at the time and had a stiff hip from a fractured femur (and subsequent bone graft) sustained when a small plane he was piloting crashed on landing near Yosemite National Park in 1927. He was described as 'portly'. Despite all this, each recollection of him at every center he visited is of a man with tremendous energy, drive and enthusiasm' (Newmeyer 1995).

The surgeons he trained there became the first generation of American hand surgeons, in a way reminiscent of Robert Jones and his young orthopaedic assistants in Britain during the First World War (Bunnell, 1955).

It was Bunnell who conceived the American Society for Surgery of the Hand, which came into being in 1946, with thirty-five founder members. Bunnell was the first President and Joe Boyes was first Secretary/Treasurer, an office he held for seven years. Fifty years later it had grown to over 1300 members (Newmeyer 1995) and it remains the leading Hand Society in the world. It consists of about two-thirds orthopaedic surgeons and one-third plastic and succeeded, after many political difficulties, in establishing an examination providing a

qualification in hand surgery, which first took place in 1990 (Omer 1995).

The second Hand Society was the Scandinavian one, created in 1987 under the leadership of Erik Moberg (Fig. 9.5) of Gothenburg, Sweden, who was an immensely influential figure in Europe (Carstam & Stack, 1990). In a letter dated 5 July 1987 Bunnell wrote to Moberg to congratulate him on this achievement. He added, 'Nothing could please me more. For several years I have tried to induce the surgeons of England to form such a society but they have never done so. Eventually, of course, they will' (Hagert 2001).

Eventually they did. Julius Bruner, from Iowa, who had trained alongside McIndoe at the Mayo Clinic in 1927, said 'Archie [McIndoe] had told me in 1950 of his plans for a hand society in Great Britain' (Bruner 1973). The first step, a year after Bunnell's letter, was the creation of the Hand Club, but after a few years it became 'a dining club with hand surgery as gossip' (James, quoted by Barton 1998). A group of younger surgeons led by Graham Stack (1915–92; Fig. 9.10; Fisk & Barton 1992, Bolton & Robins 1993) who were mostly senior registrars at the time, founded the Second Hand Club in 1956 and this went from strength to strength (Campbell Reid 1981, Fisk 1990). In 1964 the two clubs merged to become the British Club for Surgery of the Hand, still joined by invitation only, but in 1969 it was reconvened as the British Society for Surgery of the Hand (BSSH). I have described its subsequent progress elsewhere (Barton 1998).

Guy Pulvertaft of Derby (Robins 1987, Varian 1992), a member of the original Hand Club, became also a member and father-figure of the Second Hand Club and first President of BSSH (Fig. 9.3). The second President was John Barron of Salisbury, another plastic surgeon who came from New Zealand (Lamb 1992); he did much to create the close and happy relationship between plastic and orthopaedic surgeons in BSSH. Its first Secretary was Douglas Lamb from Edinburgh, who held the post for seven years (like Joe Boyes at the ASSH; both much longer than any of their successors) and created the structure and pattern of activities of BSSH.

Other nations also formed Hand Societies and in 1966 an International Federation of Societies for Surgery of the Hand was formed with eight member societies (those of the USA, UK, France, Germany, Scandinavia, Japan, Italy and Brazil), though it was at first only a co-ordinating body and did not start holding meetings until 1978. The Presidents have been Moberg (Sweden), Pulvertaft (UK), Tubiana (France), Buck-Gramcko (Germany), Tajima (Japan), Stack (UK), O'Brien (Australia), Swanson (USA), Lamb (UK), MacFarlane (Canada),

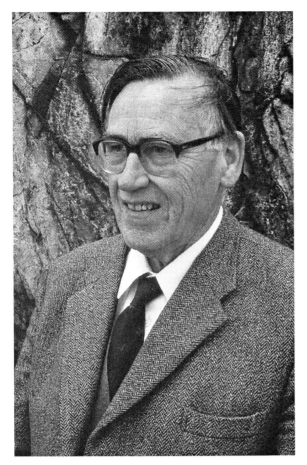

Fig. 9.10   Graham Stack, who created the British volume of *Journal of Hand Surgery* and who more than any other individual was responsible for establishing the Second Hand Club and then the British Society for Surgery of the Hand

comprehensive. The best of all, in my view, is Green's *Operative Hand Surgery*; when the first edition appeared in 1982 I wrote in a review that it was one of the three books I would take to a desert island. It was hard to imagine how it could be improved. The original edition was almost all by American contributors, but authors from other countries have since been drawn in, especially in the 4th edition of 1999.

The first journal devoted to hand surgery was Italian, *Revista de Chirurgia della Mano*, appearing in 1964. Five years later, by pure coincidence, the German journal *Handchirurgie*, edited by Buck-Gramcko (Fig. 9.9), appeared in the same month as the British journal *The Hand*, edited (and virtually published) by Graham Stack (Fig. 9.10; Pulvertaft & Robins 1987, Fisk & Barton 1992, Bolton & Robins 1993). The American *Journal of Hand Surgery* appeared in 1976. This was edited by Joe Boyes of Los Angeles, who had taken over the authorship of Bunnell's book while Lot Howard continued Bunnell's practice in San Francisco (James 1990). Boyes also wrote a book on notable names in hand surgery called (in the words of Isaac Newton) *On the Shoulders of Giants* (Boyes 1976). It is not really a history of hand surgery, but brief biographies of surgeons whose names have become eponyms in surgery of the upper limb. Boyes had the most complete mastery of hand surgery, in theory and in practice, of anyone I have met.

It was obvious that it would be beneficial to have the American and British journal linked, like the *Journal of Bone and Joint Surgery*. Unfortunately Boyes did not like Stack, but eventually he was out-manoeuvred by younger Americans and *The Hand* became the British volume of *Journal of Hand Surgery*. In 1992 this was accepted as the official publication of FESSH and became the British and European volume, the name British being retained because it is still produced in Britain and owned by the BSSH. There are also hand surgery journals from France, Japan, Scandinavia and the Pacific countries and a *Journal of Hand Therapy*.

What lies ahead in hand surgery? Simon Kay (2000) has discussed some of the technical advances that may be anticipated.

Should hand surgery become a separate speciality, with its own training programme and no necessity to go through a full orthopaedic or plastic training first as at present? In the past, orthopaedic and plastic surgery had to fight to get out from under general surgery. Now they are reluctant to allow subspecialities to split off from them; understandably, but using just the same arguments as were once used by the general surgeons. These were vividly expressed in a telegram from Sir Reginald Watson-Jones to Guy Pulvertaft on 26 July 1952:

Brunelli (Italy) and Yamauchi (Japan). There are now forty-six member societies representing eighty-three countries, with a total membership of over eight thousand practising hand surgeons.

A Federation of European Societies for Surgery of the Hand (FESSH) came into being in 1990 and has established an examination leading to the award of a voluntary Diploma in Hand Surgery. This is the only qualification in Hand Surgery open to British surgeons and a number of young British consultants have taken and passed it (Nachemson, 2000).

Hundreds of books have been published on aspects of hand surgery. The French have been notable in this field, the book in 1928 by Marc Iselin (1898–1987), who was the founder of Hand Surgery in France (Loda 1991), being one of the first on the hand and the multi-volume tome by Raoul Tubiana being one of the most

YOU MUST THINK LONG CAREFULLY AND BROADLY BEFORE SUPPORTING SOCIETY FOR SURGERY OF HAND WITH CLINICAL MEETINGS WHICH WOULD MEAN ALSO SOCIETY FOR SURGERY OF SPINE WITH NEURO SURGEONS SOCIETY FOR SURGERY OF PELVIS WITH EURO-LOGICAL SURGEONS SOCIETY FOR SURGERY OF STERNUM WITH THYMUS SURGEONS AND SO AD ABSURDAM WILL WRITE AS SOON AS POSSIBLE = REGINALD.

This telegram was reproduced showing the telegraphist's spelling mistakes) by Chapman C W (1987). Two of Sir Reginald's dire predictions have already come to pass (three if 'Eurological' was a foretaste of EFORT!) and orthopaedic and urological surgeons do work together in treating patients with pelvic fractures.

However, Bunnell said in 1955, 'The hand surgeon must work from the elbow down in three overlapping specialities: plastic, orthopaedic and neurosurgery. The hand is so intricate in structure that if dissected in turn by three different specialists it is likely to be wrecked beyond repair. The bones, joints, muscles, tendons, nerves and skin are all parts of a composite mechanism in the function of the hand and they can best be repaired by the surgeon who assumes responsibility for the whole. Hand surgery is an area speciality, not a tissue speciality'. His contemporary Gillies wrote in 1957, 'As there are few orthopaedic surgeons with a plastic outlook and possibly fewer plastic surgeons with orthopaedic skill, it was natural for a new group of hand specialists to develop' (Campbell Reid 1983).

Note that Bunnell defined the hand as 'from the elbow down', because the muscles of the forearm work the hand. He had earlier said that it extends to the opposite cerebral cortex. Nobody now suggests quite such a wide definition for hand surgery but since, in practice, hand surgeons have the most experience of peripheral nerve surgery, it does usually extend up to the brachial plexus. Sir Charles Bell (see page 122) wrote: 'With the possession of an instrument like the hand, there must be a great part of the organisation which strictly belongs to it, concealed. The hand is not a thing appended, or put on, like an additional movement in a watch, but a thousand intricate relations must be established throughout the body in connection with it' (Boyes 1976). There is a current vogue for 'upper limb surgeons', but I think that is inappropriate: the techniques for replacing the shoulder and elbow joint have nothing in common with those for hand surgery and belong either with replacement of the hip and knee or as a separate speciality on their own.

Hand surgery, however, is *not* a subspeciality of orthopaedic surgery: it is a fusion of elements from orthopaedic and from plastic surgery for which we coined the term 'interface speciality' (which has now been taken up by other groups). A fusion bomb is more powerful than a fission bomb! Hand surgery is already a separate speciality in many countries, the greatest number of such specialists being in the USA. In Europe, Sweden and Switzerland regard hand surgery as a speciality on its own. It is clear that in due course this will happen in the UK, and the present 'interface committee' with members from the Plastic and Orthopaedic SAC's (Speciality Advisory Committees) will become a separate SAC. King Canute knew that he could not hold back the tide: it was his less intelligent courtiers who thought he could.

Nevertheless, it must be accepted that this does pose problems. It is no longer acceptable to have a lone specialist and in the foreseeable future it is unlikely that every DGH will have two or more hand specialists though if they treated all the hands, including the many injuries now treated (often rather badly) in A&E departments, there would certainly be enough work. A careful analysis of workload in a large DGH has shown that every 100,000 people generate 475 hand injuries and 289 elective hand disorders per annum, the injuries requiring 139 in-patient days and 1723 out-patient visits while the elective cases need 221 days in hospital (including day-case surgery) and 1039 visits to the out-patient clinic (Burke et al 1991).

In practice, it is likely that at the average hospital minor hand injuries will continue to be treated in A&E departments, hand fractures in the general fracture clinic and patients with carpal tunnel syndrome and ganglia by orthopaedic and plastic surgeons who will, therefore, continue to need some training in hand surgery. This postulates two levels of training: ordinary level for plastic and orthopaedic surgeons and advanced level for hand specialists working in larger referral centres and taking on the more complex problems. That happens now, but the difference would be that a young surgeon who has chosen to become a hand surgeon would not need to spend time learning hip replacement or facial surgery which are not relevant to what he will do for the rest of his life, though it would be beneficial for him to spend a year doing appropriate work in a plastic unit and another year in an orthopaedic department, followed by two years in pure hand surgery. However, this could sow a legal minefield and it would be essential to establish that orthopaedic and plastic surgeons without advanced training in hands are nevertheless qualified to undertake the smaller and more routine hand operations until the time comes, as it must in the end, that hand surgery becomes a completely separate speciality.

ACKNOWLEDGEMENTS

I am grateful to the following colleagues who have supplied information: Dieter Buck-Gramcko, Bruce Conolly, John Curran, Tim Davis, David Elliot, David M. Evans, Simon Kay, Harold Kleinert, Douglas Lamb, P. C. Leung, Hugh McKim Thomas and John Tricker. The librarians at the Royal College of Surgeons of England, the Royal College of Physicians of Edinburgh and the Royal College of Veterinary Surgeons were also very helpful. The first section is adapted from a chapter by the author in Hughes S P F, Benson M K d'A, Colton C L (eds) 1987 *Orthopaedics: The Principles and Practice of Musculoskeletal Surgery and Fractures;* Churchill Livingstone, Edinburgh. Perhaps fortunately, I was not able to track down a copy of Boyes' book (1976) until after I had written this chapter, but it covers different ground and the two complement each other. I have borrowed some useful snippets from it and here make general acknowledgement. All photographs were taken by the author unless otherwise indicated.

REFERENCES

It is not practical to give references for every surgeon or operation mentioned. I have mostly chosen ones that give additional historical or biographical information; these often include the details of that surgeon's original article. The date for books is that of the first edition.

Adamson J E, Wilson J N 1961 The history of flexor-tendon grafting. J Bone Joint Surg 43A: 709–716

Angelides A C, Wallace P F 1976 The dorsal ganglion of the wrist: its pathogenesis, gross and microscopic anatomy, and surgical treatment. J Hand Surg 1: 228–235

Anonymous Editorial 1968 Felix Platter (1536–1614). Basle physician. J Am Med Assoc 203: 119–120

Appleyard O B 1971 Jean-Paul Marat. Revolutionary and doctor of medicine. Practitioner 206: 826–835

Barron J N 1990 Recollections of Archibald McIndoe. J Hand Surg 15B: 381–385

Barsky H K 1984 Guillaume Dupuytren. A Surgeon in His Place and Time. Vantage, New York

Barton N J 1996 The Herbert screw for fractures of the scaphoid. J Bone Joint Surg 78B: 517–518

Barton N J 1998 The first 30 years of the British Society for Surgery of the Hand. J Hand Surg 23B: 711–723

Barton N J 2000 The growth of orthopaedics in Great Britain. Current Orthopaedics 14: 61–72, 133–140

Birch R, Bonney G, Wynn Parry C B 1998 Surgical Disorders of the Peripheral Nerves. Churchill Livingstone, Edinburgh

Bishop W J 1960 The Early History of Surgery. Robert Hale, London

Bolton H 1991 The Chicago school of hand surgery. J Hand Surg 16B: 116–117

Bolton H, Robins R H C 1993 Obituary: Hugh Graham Stack. J Hand Surg 18B: 270–271

Bonney G 1994 Obituary: Professor Algimantas Otonas Narakas. J Hand Surg 19B: 401–402

Boyes J H 1976 On the Shoulders of Giants. Notable Names in Hand Surgery. J B Lippincott, Philadelphia

Brain W R, Wright A D, Wilkinson M 1947 Spontaneous compression of both median nerves in the carpal tunnel. Lancet i: 277

Brooks D 1991 Sir Herbert Seddon. J Hand Surg 16B: 223–224

Brown P W 1989 Recollections of Sterling Bunnell. J Hand Surg 14B: 355–356

Bruner J M 1973 The contributions of Sir Archibald McIndoe to surgery of the hand. Ann Roy Coll Surg Engl 53: 1–12

Brushart T M 1999 Nerve repair and grafting. In: Green D P, Hotchkiss R N, Pederson W C (eds) Green's Operative Hand Surgery, 4th edn. Churchill Livingstone, New York, p 1381

Buck-Gramcko D 1971 Pollicisation of the index finger. Methods and results in aplasia and hypoplasia of the thumb. J Bone Joint Surg 53A: 1605–1617

Bunnell S 1918 Repair of tendons in the fingers and description of two new instruments. Surg Gyn Obstet 26: 103–110

Bunnell S (ed) 1955 Surgery in World War II: Hand Surgery. Department of the Army, Washington, DC

Bunnell S 1944 Surgery of the Hand, Lippincott, Philadelphia

Burke F D, Dias J J, Lunn P E, Bradley M 1991 Providing care for hand disorders: trauma and elective. The Derby Hand Unit experience (1989–1990). J Hand Surg 16B: 13–18

Burkhalter W, Christensen R C, Brown P 1973 Extensor indicis proprius opponensplasty. J Bone Joint Surg 55A: 725–732

Caffinière J Y de la, Aucouturier P 1979 Trapezio-metacarpal arthroplasty by total prosthesis. Hand 11: 41–46

Campbell Reid D A 1983 The emergence of hand surgery in the United Kingdom: the Gillies Memorial Lecture 1981. Br J Plast Surg 36: 278–290

Capener N 1959 Fingers, compensation and King Canute. In: Proceedings of the Second Hand Club, BSSH, 1975, p 47

Carstam N, Stack H G 1990 Erik Moberg. J Hand Surg 15B: 3–4

Chamay A 1997 L'histoire de la chirurgie des tendons fléchisseurs. Annales de Chirurgie de la Main 16: 9–13

Chapman C W 1987 The British Society for Surgery of the Hand. In: Wallace A F (ed) The History of the British Association of Plastic Surgeons. Churchill Livingstone, Edinburgh

Clay N R, Clement D A 1988 The treatment of dorsal wrist ganglia by radical excision. J Hand Surg 13B: 187–191

Clay N R, Dias J J, Costigan P S, Gregg P J, Barton N J 1991 Need the thumb be immobilised in scaphoid fractures? A randomised prospective trial. J Bone Joint Surg 73B: 828–832

Cobbett J R 1969 Free digital transfer: report of a case of transfer of great toe to replace an amputated thumb. J Bone Joint Surg 51B: 677–679

Cooper, Sir A 1822 Treatise on Dislocations and Fractures of the Joints, Longmans, London

Davis T R C, Brady O, Barton N J, Lunn P G, Burke F D 1997 Trapeziectomy alone, with tendon interposition or with ligament reconstruction? A randomised prospective study. J Hand Surg 22B: 689–694

Destot E 1925 Injuries of the Wrist: A Radiological Study, trans. Atkinson F B R. Ernest Benn, London

Duran R J, Houser R G 1975 Controlled passive motion following flexor tendon repair in zones II and III. In

American Academy of Orthopedic Surgeons Symposium on Tendon Surgery in the Hand. C V Mosby, St Louis

Elliot D 1999 The early history of contracture of the palmar fascia [in three parts]. J Hand Surg 13B: 246–253, 371–378; 14B: 25–31

Entin M, Barsky A, Swanson A 1972 Classification of congenital malformations of the hand and upper extremities. Hand 4: 215–219

Fisk G R 1970 Carpal instability and the fractured scaphoid. Ann Roy Coll Surg Engl 46: 63–76

Fisk G R 1990 The development of hand surgery in Great Britain. J Hand Surg 15B: 139–146

Fisk G, Barton N J 1992 Obituary: Hugh Graham Stack. J Hand Surg 17B: 595–596

Flatt A E 1963 The Care of the Rheumatoid Hand. C V Mosby, St Louis

Fletcher I R, Healy T E J 1983 The arterial tourniquet. Ann Roy Coll Surg Engl 65: 409–417

Fyfe I S, Mason S 1979 The mechanical stability of internal fixation of fractured phalanges. Hand 11: 50–54

Gervis W H 1949 Excision of the trapezium for osteo-arthritis of the trapezio-metacarpal joint. J Bone Joint Surg 31B: 134

Gervis W H 1973 A review of excision of the trapezium for osteoarthritis after 25 years. J Bone Joint Surg 55B: 56–57

Green D P 1982 Operative Hand Surgery, Churchill Livingstone, New York

Gu Y-D, Zhang G-M, Chen J-G, Yan X-M Cheng, Chen L 1992 Seventh cervical nerve root transfer from the contralateral healthy side for treatment of brachial plexus root avulsion. J Hand Surg 17B: 518–521

Hagert C-G 2001 The history of hand surgery in Sweden. J Hand Surg 26B: 78–83

Hallett J 1983 Inaccuracies in measuring tourniquet pressures. Br Med J 286: 1267–1268

Hannington-Kiff J 1984 Pharmacological target blocks in hand surgery and rehabilitation. J Hand Surg 9B: 29–36

Heister L 1718 Chirugie, Nuremberg

James J I P 1990 L. D. Howard. J Hand Surg 15B: 271–272

Kanavel A B 1916 Infections of the Hand. Lea & Febiger, Philadelphia.

Kay S 2000 The challenge of hand surgery. Current Orthopaedics 14: 47–51

Kleinert H E, Spokevicius S, Papas N H 1995 History of flexor tendon repair J Hand Surg 20A: S46–52

Klenerman L 1962 The tourniquet in surgery. J Bone Joint Surg 44B: 937–943

Lamb D 1992 Obituary: John Barron. J Hand Surg 17B: 704

Lamb D W 1994 Development of hand surgery in Britain. (Unpublished document prepared for BSSH and kept in their archives)

Larsen C, Amadio P, Gilula L, Hodge J 1995 Analysis of carpal instability: 1: Description of the scheme. J Hand Surg 20A: 757–764

Le Fanu J 1999 The Rise and Fall of Modern Medicine. Little, Brown, London

Le Vay D 1990 The History of Orthopaedics. Parthenon, Carnforth, pp 563–566, 672–674

Learmonth J R 1933 The principle of decompression in the treatment of certain diseases of peripheral nerves. Surg Clin N Am 13: 905

Lee A S C, Ling R S M 1977 The optimised use of PNMA bone cement and some limitations of its use in the fixation of upper limb prostheses. In: Institute of Mechanical Engineering and British Orthopaedic Association: joint replacement in the upper limb: Proceedings of conference. Mechanical Engineering Publications, Bury St Edmunds, pp 41–44

Leung P C 1989 The Chinese culture and hand reconstruction. In: Landi A (ed) Reconstruction of the Thumb. Chapman & Hall, London, pp 11–16

Lister G D, Kleinert H E, Kutz J E, Atasoy E 1977 Primary flexor tendon repair followed by immediate controlled mobilisation. J Hand Surg 2: 441–457

Loda G 1991 Marc Iselin. J Hand Surg 16B: 350–351

Lundborg G 1993 Obituary: Erik Moberg. J Hand Surg 18B: 407

Major R H 1948 Classic Descriptions of Disease, 3rd edn. C C Thomas, Springfield

Malt R A, McKhann C F 1964 Replantation of severed arms. J Am Med Assoc 189: 716–222

Marsh D, Barton N J 1996 Musculo-skeletal trauma: nerve. In: Yeoman P M, Spengler D M (eds) Orthopaedic Practice. Butterworth-Heinemann, Oxford

Matthews J P 1989 Early mobilisation after flexor tendon repair. J Hand Surg 14B: 363–367

McCash C R 1964 The open palm technique in Dupuytren's contracture. Br J Plast Surg 17: 271–280

McFarlane R M 1974 Patterns of the diseased fascia in the fingers in Dupuytren's contracture and displacement of the neurovascular bundle. Plast Reconst Surg 54: 31–44

McGregor I A, Jackson I T 1972 The groin flap. Br J Plastic Surg 25: 3

McGrouther D A 1988 La maladie de Dupuytren. To incise or excise? J Hand Surg 13B: 368–370

Meals R A, Meuli H C 1985 Carpenter's nails, phonograph needles, piano wires, and safety pins: the history of operative fixation of metacarpal and phalangeal fractures. J Hand Surg 10A: 144–150

Moermans J P 1991 Segmental aponeureotomy in Dupuytren's disease. J Hand Surg 16B: 243–254

Mooney E E, Prendiville J B 1991 The hand in Irish legend and folklore. Plast Reconstr Surg 87: 1131–1133

Morrison W A, O'Brien B M, MacLeod A M 1980 Thumb reconstruction with a free neurovascular wrap-around flap from the big toe. J Hand Surg 5: 575–583

Mosley L 1962 Faces From the Fire. Weidenfeld & Nicholson, London

Nachemson A K 2000 The FESSH diploma examination in hand surgery. J Hand Surg 25B: 235–6.

Nalebuff E A 1971 Present state of rheumatoid hand surgery. Am J Surg 122: 304–318

Newmeyer W L 1995 In: American Society for Surgery of the Hand: The First Fifty Years. Churchill Livingstone, New York

Nigst H 1997 Medizinhistorischer Beitrag: Handchirurgie bei Lorenz Heister. Handchir Microchir Plast Chir 29: 114–123

Omer G 1955 In: American Society for Surgery of the Hand: The First Fifty Years. Churchill Livingstone, New York

Porter R 1997 The Greatest Benefit to Mankind. HarperCollins, London

Pulvertaft G, Robins R 1987 Graham Stack. J Hand Surg 12B: 3–4

Rang M 1966 Anthology of Orthopaedics. Churchill Livingstone, Edinburgh

Ravitch M M 1979 Dupuytren's invention of the Mikulicz enterotome with a note on eponyms. Perspectives Biol Med 22: 170–184

Rhys-Davies N C, Stotter A T 1985 The Rhys-Davies exsanguinator. Ann Roy Coll Surg Engl 67: 193–195

Robins R H C 1987 Robert Guy Pulvertaft. J Hand Surg 12B: 144–145

Small J O, Brennen M D, Colville J 1989 Early active mobilisation after flexor tendon repair in zone 2. J Hand Surg 14B: 383–391

Stack H G 1973 The Palmar Fascia. Churchill Livingstone, Edinburgh & London

Steindler A 1923 Reconstructive Surgery of the Upper Extremity, New York

Swan J 1830 A Demonstration of the Nerves of the Human Body, London

Swanson A B 1973 Flexible Implant Resection Arthroplasty in the Hand and Extremities. C V Mosby, St Louis

Taliesnik J 1976 The ligaments of the wrist. J Hand Surg 1: 110–118

Tamai S 1993 History of microsurgery – from the beginning until the end of the 1970s. Microsurgery 14: 6–13

Van Zundert A, Goerig M 2000 August Bier 1861–1949. Reg Anaesth Pain Med 25: 26–33

Varian J 1992 Guy Pulvertaft. J Hand Surg 17B: 118–119

Vaughan Jackson O J 1962 Rheumatoid hand deformities considered in the light of tendon imbalance. J Bone Joint Surg 44B: 764–775

Verdan C 1980 Evolution historique de la chirugie des tendons fléchisseurs. Rev Méd Suisse Romande 100: 639–652

Verdan C 2000 The history of hand surgery in Europe. J Hand Surg 25B: 238–41

Vom Saal F H 1953 Intramedullary fixation in fractures of the hand and fingers. J Bone Joint Surg 35A: 5

Watson H K, Baker F L 1984 The SLAC wrist: scapho-lunate advanced collapse pattern of degenerative arthritis. J Hand Surg 9A: 358–365

White S 1984 Anatomy of the palmar fascia on the ulnar border of the hand. J Hand Surg 9B: 50–56

Wilton T J 1988 Kirschner wires. In: Barton N J (ed) Fractures of the Hand and Wrist. Churchill Livingstone, Edinburgh

Wynn-Parry C B 1958 Rehabilitation of the Hand Butterworth, London

Young R E S, Harmon J M 1960 Repair of tendon injuries of the hand. Ann Surg 151: 562–566

10

Children's orthopaedic Surgery

John A. Fixsen

The term 'children's orthopaedics' is really a misnomer as the word 'orthopaedia' coined by Nicholas Andry in 1741 from the Greek *Orthos* meaning straight or without deformity and *Pais* or *Paidon*, a child, implies the treatment of children. Andry, who was Professor of Medicine at the University of Paris, championed the cause of conservative non-surgical treatment of children's deformities. He advocated what might be thought a modern concept that parents should take an active part in the treatment of their child's deformity from as early as possible.

Certain children's deformities such as club foot and spinal deformity have been recognised since antiquity. Elliot Smith in his studies of the Royal Egyptian mummies from 1912 to 1924 described a number of club feet and equinus deformities (Smith & Dawson 1924). These may well have been acquired from trauma or poliomyelitis rather than being truly congenital. Beasley, in his paper on Homer and orthopaedics, wrote about club feet in ancient Greece (Beasley 1972). Hippocrates (460–370 BC) was familiar with club foot and advised manipulative correction as soon as possible after birth, using bandages and splints, very similar to those used today.

Jean André Venel (1740–91) was born in Geneva and in 1780 founded what is considered the first orthopaedic hospital at Orbe in the Canton of Vaud in Switzerland. The hospital contained what he considered 'the essentials for orthopaedic management', i.e. a separate hospital on one site dedicated to the treatment of orthopaedic problems. Within the hospital there should be facilities for the production of all special apparatus and appliances required for the treatment of patients. Education should be available for children and vocational training for adolescents and young adults. Venel treated conditions such as club foot, scoliosis and tuberculosis. The so-called 'sabot de Venel' club foot

splint devised by him was still in use in a modified form in some centres in Switzerland until 1955. Venel was also unusual in that at a time when many practitioners were often jealous and secretive about their methods of treatment. He recorded and published with drawings and plaster moulds the results of his treatment and encouraged others to do likewise.

The second specialist orthopaedic institution in Europe based on similar lines was founded by Johann Georg von Heine in 1812 in Würzburg. In 1817 the first orthopaedic hospital in Britain was founded in New Street, Birmingham, called the General Institution for the Relief of Persons Labouring under Bodily Deformity. Its main initial function was to supply trusses and surgical appliances to the poor and needy. It subsequently became known as the Orthopaedic and Spinal hospital and was given the title of Royal by Queen Victoria in 1888. The Birmingham Cripples' Union was started in 1898 and George Cadbury donated a house called 'Woodlands' which opened in 1909 as an orthopaedic hospital with thirty-seven beds. In 1913 Naughton Dunn (1884–1939) was appointed as the first orthopaedic surgeon. This hospital united with the Royal Orthopaedic and Spinal Hospital in 1925 to form the Royal Cripples' Hospital, which finally became the Royal Orthopaedic Hospital in 1949.

One of the earliest forms of surgery for the treatment of orthopaedic deformity in childhood was tendo achillis tenotomy. Thilenius, a physician in Germany who did not undertake surgery himself, in 1784 arranged for an open transection of the Achilles' tendon to be performed on a seventeen-year-old girl for probably a paralytic club foot deformity by the then conventionally subordinate surgeon, a gentleman called Lorenz, with outstanding success. Brockman (1930) states that the second such operation was performed by Petit in 1799 but gives no details of this operation in his monograph on club foot.

Sartorius in 1806 and Michaelis in 1809 undertook open tendo achillis tenotomy for equinus deformity. In general, at this time surgery was considered to be dangerous, particularly as in many anatomical texts there was no distinction between tendon and nerves. Hippocrates in considering the dangers of open tendo achillis tenotomy stated:'This tendon, if bruised or cut, causes most acute fevers, produces choking, deranges the mind and at length brings death.' Presumably this very pessimistic attitude was due to infection following such open tenotomies. Delpech in Montpellier advocated subcutaneous tenotomy and operated on a nine-year-old child with club foot in 1816. The operation is reported as successful but this method of treatment was opposed by his surgical colleagues in Paris. Georg Louis Stromeyer in Hanover performed his first subcutaneous tenotomy in 1831 and was also prepared to divide both the tibialis posterior and the flexor hallucis longus in the correction of club foot.

W. J. Little (1810–94) graduated at The London Hospital, now The Royal London Hospital. He suffered from poliomyelitis at the age of two and developed a paralytic equinus. He was unable to obtain surgical treatment in Britain and was operated on by Stromeyer in Hanover in 1836. He subsequently returned to England in 1837, an ardent advocate of subcutaneous tenotomy for the correction of limb deformities. He founded The Infirmary for the Cure of Club Foot and Other Contractures in Bloomsbury Square in 1838 (see Chapter 1), which subsequently became the Royal Orthopaedic Hospital in 1845. Initially Little thought he was the first person to perform tenotomy of the tendo achillis in England but in fact a Mr Whipple of Plymouth performed either an open or a subcutaneous tenotomy of the tendo achillis in 1836 before Little returned from Hanover. Little wrote a treatise on the *Nature of Club Foot* in 1839 and his famous treatise on *The Nature and Treatment of Deformities of the Human Frame* in 1853, in which he described the relationship between problems at birth and the later development of spastic deformities. He enlarged on this in his famous paper on Congenital Spastic Palsy in the Transactions of the Obstetric Society of London in 1862.

In 1851, a second orthopaedic hospital, the City Orthopaedic Hospital, was founded in London, mainly because of the long waiting lists at the Royal Orthopaedic Hospital. The third orthopaedic hospital in London, which became the National Orthopaedic Hospital in 1863, started as 'A society for the treatment in their own homes of poor persons afflicted with diseases and distortions of the spine, chest, hip, etc.' in 1836. In 1850 the Society moved to 84 Northold Street, which later became Bolsover Street adjacent to Great

Portland Street. In 1856 this became the Spinal Hospital for the Cure of Deformities, with ten beds, and was finally renamed the National Orthopaedic Hospital in 1863. Henry Dick who excised the cuboid for club foot was one of the surgeons at the hospital and Little's son, Louis Stromeyer Little, performed there the first osteotomy for knock knees (genu valgum) in Britain in 1865. By the 1890s the National Orthopaedic Hospital had expanded considerably into Great Portland Street and ultimately the Royal Orthopaedic Hospital and the National Orthopaedic Hospital merged in 1905 and the City Hospital joined in 1907. The amalgamated institution became known as the Royal National Orthopaedic Hospital and was based in Great Portland Street with a country branch at Stanmore in Middlesex.

It is important to return to the development of children's hospitals at this stage. The City Orthopaedic Hospital in 1859 had thirty-six beds and mothers were admitted with their children. This was most unusual as most doctors at that time felt that children in hospital were dangerous to adults and should be nursed at home. The first children's hospital in Europe was the Hôpital des Enfants Malades in Paris, which was founded in 1802. In 1834 hospitals for children were opened in St Petersburg in Russia and Berlin and Dresden in Germany. The Hospital for Sick Children, Great Ormond Street in London opened as the first children's hospital in the country in 1852 followed shortly afterwards by the Jenny Lind Children's Hospital in Norwich in 1853 and the Manchester Children's Hospital in 1855. The need for such hospitals is starkly highlighted by the census of 1843 that showed that there were fifty thousand deaths annually in London of which nearly half were of children.

There was a strong orthopaedic influence at Great Ormond Street in the latter half of the nineteenth century. Sir Thomas Smith, who was surgeon to the hospital from 1854 to 1910, wrote his famous paper 'On the acute arthritis of infants' in 1874. Howard Marsh, another early surgeon on the staff of Great Ormond Street, specialised in orthopaedics and subsequently became Professor of Surgery at Cambridge. Sir William Arbuthnot Lane described screw fixation for tibial fractures in 1894 and introduced plates for internal fixation in 1905. Sir Thomas Fairbank (1876–1961) was appointed visiting surgeon to the hospital in 1906 and developed a lifelong interest in skeletal dysplasias culminating in the publication of his *Atlas of General Affections of the Skeleton* in 1951. Mr E. I. Lloyd (1892–1954) took over in 1928 with a major interest in children and orthopaedics, having trained in both specialties at St Bartholomew's Hospital and Great Ormond Street. He was President of the Orthopaedic section of the Royal

Society of Medicine and a quiet, hard-working Quaker. He tends to be overshadowed by his house surgeon in 1928, Sir Denis Browne (1892–1967), who came from Melbourne and championed the cause of the specialty of paediatric surgery. He made significant contributions to children's orthopaedics with his splints for club foot and congenital dislocation of the hip (CDH). He believed that club foot was largely due to intrauterine moulding. He published his well known paper on the subject in *The Lancet* in 1934. He felt that all surgery in children should be under the care of specialised paediatric surgeons. However, at Great Ormond Street and in Britain in general it is the specialist surgeons in orthopaedics, plastics, neurosurgery, etc. who have taken over the management of these specialties in children. In France, by contrast, a significant number of paediatric orthopaedic surgeons have trained primarily in paediatric surgery and subsequently specialised in orthopaedic surgery. Until quite recently, children's fractures at The Royal Sick Children's Hospital in Edinburgh were primarily treated by paediatric surgeons. Following Lloyd's death in 1954, he was succeeded in 1955 by Mr G. C. Lloyd-Roberts (1914–86), who, in the words of Professor James, was 'a great surgeon and teacher and an unceasing source of stimulation and clarity of thought who influenced a whole generation of trainee orthopaedic surgeons who had the good fortune to work for him at Great Ormond Street', many of whom developed a major interest in the practice of children's orthopaedics.

To return to the second half of the nineteenth century, Sir Robert Jones, who is considered the father of British orthopaedic surgery, was born in 1857. He was the nephew of Hugh Owen Thomas (1834–91) who can be considered the grandfather of British orthopaedics. Owen-Thomas came from the fourth generation of a family of Welsh bone setters. However, he qualified in medicine in Edinburgh and subsequently studied both in London and Paris. He never had a hospital appointment, but practised from 11 Nelson Street in Liverpool. He had a major interest in children's orthopaedics, developing his so-called Thomas wrench for, among other things, the forceful manipulation of club foot and also the famous Thomas splint for the treatment of fractures of the femur. Sir Robert Jones was apprenticed to his uncle at 11 Nelson Street and worked there from 1873 until his death in 1933. He qualified in medicine in 1878 at Liverpool and his first hospital appointment was as honorary assistant surgeon at the Stanley Hospital, Liverpool, in 1881. He was always very interested in the care of children at a time when many children's diseases resulted from poor housing, malnutrition and a lack of hygiene. He was a strong advocate of special facilities for the care of children. He believed that 'few children are so incurable that they could not become well if placed in proper circumstances for treatment'. He therefore set out to promote proper hospitals for children. In 1898 a ward was provided specifically for children in the West Kirby Convalescent Home and in 1900 the Royal Liverpool Country Hospital was founded at Heswall. This was in the same year as Agnes Hunt opened the Baschurch Home for Children, with four boys and four girls 'who needed country air and good food'. In 1903 she had consulted Jones for 'something the matter with her leg' and subsequently would take children to see him at the Royal Southern Hospital. Jones visited Baschurch every third Sunday of the month where he would examine up to fifty patients and subsequently operate on fifteen or more. In 1920 with financial help from The British Red Cross Society, the Baschurch Home moved to the military hospital at Gobowen near Oswestry and later became the Robert Jones and Agnes Hunt Orthopaedic Hospital after Sir Robert's death in 1933. In October 1919, Jones with Girdlestone, who worked with him at Oswestry, published a paper on 'The cure of crippled children', a proposed national scheme, in the *British Medical Journal*. This set out to establish country hospitals with their own peripheral clinics. The country would be divided up into regions as it is under the present National Health Service. Within each region there would be country hospitals with operating theatres, gymnasia, work shops for handicrafts, school and playrooms. By 1935 some forty hospitals with six thousand beds had been set up, servicing about four hundred peripheral orthopaedic clinics. Until very recently the management of major long-term children's orthopaedic problems such as congenital dislocation of the hip (developmental dysplasia of the hip), club foot, Perthes' disease, scoliosis and other spinal deformity, was centred in these hospitals. To some extent even today there are major children's departments at the Royal National Orthopaedic Hospital, Stanmore, the Nuffield Orthopaedic Hospital, Oxford, and the Robert Jones and Agnes Hunt Orthopaedic Hospital, Oswestry.

The concentration of children's orthopaedic problems in orthopaedic and children's hospitals led to specialisation amongst orthopaedic consultants. Until very recently there have been no purely children's orthopaedic surgeons in the UK and even today the majority of consultants with a major interest in children's orthopaedics continue to undertake some adult practice, unlike paediatric orthopaedic surgeons in North America and some parts of Europe. Within the specialised orthopaedic hospitals, orthopaedic surgeons with an interest in children would tend to take a major interest in a particular condition; for instance at the Royal National Orthopaedic Hospital Sir Herbert Seddon and David Trevor had a major interest in congenital dislocation of the hip, as it was then called. Similarly, Edgar Sommerville at Oxford, John Wilkinson at Southampton, Rowland Hughes at Oswestry and George Mitchell at Edinburgh also had a major interest in this condition, to mention just a few of the famous names in this field. In the management of club foot, Dillwyn Evans at the Prince of Wales Hospital, Cardiff, made major contributions, but other surgeons working in general hospitals or children's hospitals such as Attenborough in Bromley, Kent, Denham in Portsmouth, Professor Clark in Leeds, Dwyer in Liverpool, Lloyd-Roberts at Great Ormond Street Hospital for Sick Children, London, were also active in this field. Conditions such as Perthes' disease, which in the past were treated by long-term bed rest, were particularly treated in the specialised orthopaedic hospitals such as the Royal Orthopaedic Hospital, Birmingham, where Harrison developed his special splint and the Robert Jones and Agnes Hunt Orthopaedic Hospital, where Rowland Hughes did some interesting early work on the use of femoral osteotomy in this condition. W. J. W. Sharrard, working in the Children's Hospital in Sheffield with his paediatric surgical colleagues, made major contributions to the orthopaedic treatment of meningomyelocele and cerebral palsy. In the upper limb, Douglas Lamb at the Princess Margaret Rose Orthopaedic Hospital, Edinburgh, contributed to the management of upper limb deficiency, and particularly radial club hand. Ruth Wynne-Davis, also in Edinburgh, was a pioneer in the genetics of many orthopaedic conditions.

Bone and joint infection, which was the scourge of children in the late nineteenth and early twentieth centuries, has been greatly affected by the development of antibiotics, improved hygiene and better nutrition. Trueta and Morgan (1954) reported remarkable results with only one patient showing resistance to penicillin and no deaths or amputations. They advocated open surgery and antibiotics. Subsequently Blockey and Watson (1970) from Glasgow advocated a much less invasive approach, provided the infection was seen early enough. Today, although bone and joint infection is much less common in the so-called developed countries than in the past, certain groups are particularly vulnerable, such as children in the intensive care unit, children undergoing chemotherapy and other treatments in which immunosuppression is necessary, and children suffering from AIDS and other immune deficiency conditions. In all these situations, the orthopaedic surgeon can be deceived as the classical

presentation of acute infection may be masked by the underlying condition or situation.

Children's orthopaedics as a separate subspecialty has really only evolved over the last fifteen to twenty years in the UK. There are a number of factors responsible for this. The Paediatric Orthopaedic Society (POS) was founded in the USA in 1970 under the Chairmanship of W. G. Green. Some orthopaedic surgeons from the group were involved with Dr Tachdjian's famous paediatric orthopaedic seminars held alternately in San Francisco and Chicago which attracted an international faculty and a large number of trainees from throughout North America and beyond. In 1971 meetings were held in Chicago and Newington under the presidency of Burr Curtis. A second group called the Paediatric Orthopaedic Study Group (POSG) was founded in 1974 under the Co-Chairmanship of Harry Cowell, Hamlet Peterson and Lynn Staheli. In 1983 the groups merged and held their first combined meeting in Charlottesville, Virginia. Subsequently this became the Paediatric Orthopaedic Society of North America (POSNA). The society has had an important influence not only on the evolution of paediatric orthopaedics in North America, but also in the rest of the world, organising a prestigious annual meeting and having close links with other paediatric orthopaedic societies around the world. The *Journal of Pediatric Orthopaedics*, first published in 1980 from America under the Editorship of R Hensinger and L Staheli, has become a major journal for the subspecialty of paediatric orthopaedics. In 1992 the European volume was published as *Journal of Pediatric Orthopaedics* Part B under the Editorship of Henri Bensahel in Paris. The American Board Examinations considered paediatric orthopaedics a subspecialty and from this arose the concept of an orthopaedic surgeon who practised only on children and not on adults. In Britain, this situation is still very rare. The majority of consultants with a major interest in children still retain some adult interest, which is of particular value when dealing with chronic, disabling disorders such as meningomyelocele, cerebral palsy, the late effects of DDH, club foot and Perthes' disease that continue to raise problems for the patient in adult life. There are distinct advantages to being able to follow up patients into adult life having seen them throughout their childhood.

The British Society for Children's Orthopaedic Surgery (BSCOS) was founded in 1984, with Mr A. Catterall as Secretary. The first meeting was held at Charing Cross Hospital in London and the second at The Hospital for Sick Children, Great Ormond Street. Mr J. A. Wilkinson was the first President and subsequently the society has flourished and now has over one hundred members. It organises a one-day meeting in January and June/July. The first combined meeting with the French paediatric orthopaedic society (Group Etude Orthopaedic Paediatrique, GEOP) was held in London on 28–29 January 2000. Two other major pressures have led to the evolution of children's orthopaedics as a subspecialty. The development of Specialist Advisory Committees (SACs) for surgical training in the specialties has led to the evolution of initially the Intercollegiate Fellowship of the Royal College of Surgeons in Orthopaedics (FRCS[Orth]). The first examination took place in Edinburgh in November 1990. Subsequently it has become known as the Intercollegiate Fellowship of the Royal College of Surgeons in Trauma and Orthopaedics (FRCS[Tr&Orth]). Before this there were specialist examinations in Orthopaedics in Liverpool, the MCh(Orth) for many years, and for a period the FRCS(Orth) of the Royal College of Surgeons of Edinburgh. In the Intercollegiate FRCS(Tr&Orth) there is a separate viva for the subspecialties of hand surgery and paediatric orthopaedics. The SAC stipulates that in four years of specialised training in orthopaedics, six months should be spent in children's orthopaedics. This has led to every orthopaedic trainee spending some time in children's orthopaedics and trauma. The teaching of children's orthopaedics and trauma forms part of the postgraduate orthopaedic training programme of all the training rotations in the UK.

The other major influence on the evolution of the subspecialty is the increasing specialisation of paediatricians and anaesthetists. Within paediatrics, paediatricians have divided themselves into those who deal with intensive and neonatal care, leading to the paediatric intensivist. There are those who deal with general paediatrics and others who deal with paediatrics in the community, particularly the problems of disability, i.e. the consultant in community paediatrics. The increasing subdivision and complexity of the treatment of children has meant that many children can only be treated, particularly when surgery and anaesthetics are required, in specialised children's units of a general hospital or in specialised children's hospitals. This creates a problem for major orthopaedic hospitals that treat children in that they now have to have very sophisticated children's care within the hospital. At the beginning of the twentieth century Jones and Girdlestone advocated the treatment of children with orthopaedic conditions in specialised hospitals which formed a very successful network of such hospitals and peripheral clinics throughout the UK. Now at the beginning of the twenty-first century the increasing specialisation and complexity of children's treatment is leading to the concentration of children's care in specialised children's hospitals such as Great Ormond Street Hospital for Sick Children, Alder Hey Children's Hospital, Liverpool, etc. or in major children's departments in large University General Hospitals because the District Hospital cannot provide the intensive care and in particular the paediatric anaesthetic care now considered necessary for the management of orthopaedic problems, particularly of young children in hospital.

CLUB FOOT

Club foot (congenital talipes equinovarus, CTEV) is one of the earliest known orthopaedic deformities. It is depicted on the pyramids and found in Egyptian mummies. The principles of conservative management of manipulation and bandaging started as soon as possible after birth were laid down by Hippocrates in the fourth century BC and are still the basis of modern conservative treatment today. There was little change in the Middle Ages apart from the use of different materials for splintage such as the iron splint introduced by Francisco Archaeus (c.1493–1573). The management of deformities such as club foot was in the hands of barber surgeons and bone setters until the end of the eighteenth century. William Cheseldon, a famous surgeon and anatomist, wrote in 1740 about club foot: 'The first knowledge I had of a cure for this disease was from a Mr Presgrove, a professed bone setter. I recommended the patient to him, not knowing how to cure him myself.' Jean André Venel developed his special club foot boot at his orthopaedic hospital founded in Switzerland in 1780. Antonio Scarpa (1752–1832) published his famous study of the anatomy of club foot in 1803 that recognised the displacement of the navicular on the talus. He incorporated a dynamic component in his club foot splint by using a spring in Venel's boot. He is said to have borrowed or stolen the idea from two truss-makers, Sheldrake in London and Typhesne in Paris.

Plaster of Paris was introduced by Dieffenbach in Germany and first used for club foot in 1834. Julius Wolff (1836–1902), famous for Wolff's law, introduced serial plasters and wedging for progressive correction of club foot. This method was strongly advocated by Hiram Kite in America in the 1930s. With regard to manipulation, there have been two main schools: those that preferred repeated, gentle manipulation and those which preferred forceful manipulation or osteoclasis. Hugh Owen Thomas used his Thomas wrench, which was a form of osteoclast, among other things, for the management of club foot. Osteoclasis was also practised by Gratton in

Cork, Ireland, Bradford in Boston, Massachusetts, USA and Lorenz in Vienna, Austria.

The early history of club foot surgery in Europe has already been described. The development of more extensive open surgery had to await advances in the management of surgical infection, particularly the work of Joseph Lister (1827–1912) in the latter half of the nineteenth century. Phelp (1851–1902) in New York introduced extensive open release of the tendons and ligaments on the medial side of the foot and reported his results at the International Congress in 1888 in Copenhagen. Codivilla (1861–1912) working at the Rizzoli Institute in Bologna in Italy from 1899 did much to popularise this type of posteromedial surgery for club foot in Europe. Bony surgery in the form of excision of the cuboid was introduced by Solly at St Thomas's Hospital, London, in 1857, but apparently with little success. Astragalectomy (talectomy) for club foot was practised extensively in the first decade of the twentieth century and popularised by Royal Whitman in the USA. It was largely superseded by triple arthrodesis in its various forms described by Hoke in 1921, Naughton Dunn in 1922 and Ryerson in 1923. More recently, Dillwyn Evans in 1961 introduced the concept of collateral release combining a medial soft tissue release with a lateral calcaneo cuboid fusion. Brockman in 1930, in his famous monograph *Congenital Club Foot*, stated that surgery in those under the age of three years was too dangerous because of the anaesthetic problems in young children. With the evolution of modern anaesthetics after the Second World War, the safety of operations in the first year of life or shortly after birth greatly improved, and in the 1960s and 1970s it was felt that early surgery under the age of six months was important for those children who failed conservative treatment. Posterior release was popularised by Attenborough (1966). More extensive forms of posteromedial soft tissue release were developed particularly by Clark (1968) in Leeds and Turco (1971) in the USA who strongly advocated internal fixation with Kirschner wires to hold the corrected deformity. The beginning of the twenty-first century is seeing a return to a more conservative approach sometimes with the use of continuous passive motion as advocated by Dimeglio et al (1996). Very early surgery has not produced the hoped for benefits. Very extensive surgery has not prevented relapse and is producing an increasing number of cases with the difficult problem of over-correction of the foot. The Ilizarov apparatus is another powerful new tool that may have a useful place in the management of the difficult relapsed foot.

MANAGEMENT OF CONGENITAL DISLOCATION OF THE HIP (CDH), NOW KNOWN AS DEVELOPMENTAL DYSPLASIA OF THE HIP (DDH)

Congenital dislocation of the hip (CDH) was recognised by Hippocrates. Although the ancient Greeks are reported to have reduced traumatic hip dislocation successfully, there is no record that they treated congenital hip dislocation. Ambroise Paré in the sixteenth century stated that reduction was frequently impossible because the joint cavity (acetabulum) was too shallow and that the ligaments which hold the bones in a joint were too soft and relaxed.

In 1879, Roser in Germany believed that many cases would be curable if the diagnosis was made as soon as possible after birth and a simple abduction splint applied. This remarkably modern view was ignored as operative treatment was being developed at that time. Humbert and Jacquier in France in 1853 reported they had successfully reduced a congenital dislocation of the hip in an eleven-year-old girl by a single session of forced traction on a machine in under an hour. They probably reduced the femoral head into the obturator foramen or the sciatic notch and not the true acetabulum. However, Pravaz in Lyon in 1847 reported nineteen cases in which after nine months of traction the femoral head was brought down to the acetabulum and reduced by abduction in extension. The child spent the next two years in a special self-propelled chair with gears and cranks which moved the child's legs so 'grinding out' the socket, a very early form of a continuous passive motion (CPM) machine. Buckminster Brown in Boston is thought to be the first to apply the Pravaz method in America in 1885. In England, Bernard Brodhurst used the Pravaz method in 1866 on a twelve-year-old boy combined with a section of the trochanteric muscles.

As far as surgery was concerned, Guerin in 1848 in Paris tried to deepen the posterosuperior rim of the acetabulum by scarification of the ilium in an early form of shelf operation. Hueger in 1877 described a turn down osteoperiosteal flap, fastening it to the capsule as was popularised by Wainwright (1976) in the UK. Dupuytren in 1826 wrote a classical treatise on 'original or congenital displacement of the heads of the thigh bones'. This was a remarkably accurate description of the long-standing congenital deformity. As a result, he argued very strongly that all forms of treatment were useless and liable to cause damage. A major step forwards in the non-operative treatment of the condition was made by Agostino Paci (1845–1902), an Italian working in Pisa who demonstrated manipulative reduction in 1886. Lorenz from Vienna subsequently reported 450 cases reduced by his so-called 'bloodless' manipulative reduction in 1900. He admitted to three deaths, thirteen fractures, twelve major nerve palsies and one total gangrene of the limb as well as stiffness and anterior transposition. He claimed good results in 52.6% of cases. Röntgen's discovery of X-rays in 1895 meant that by this time such claims had to be confirmed by radiography. The term 'bloodless method' took on a new meaning when Lorenz's cases were followed up and a very high incidence of avascular necrosis reported. This was probably the result of a combination of forceful manipulation and the position of 90° flexion, 90° abduction (the 90/90 position) in which the hips were immobilised following reduction.

Schede in 1892 recognised femoral neck anteversion as a common cause of redislocation. He tried to correct this by a subcutaneous subtrochanteric external rotation osteotomy, but this was difficult to control as metal fixation was only just beginning to be developed at the time. Some surgeons performed a distal supracondylar femoral osteotomy as a preliminary to reduction such as Reiner in Germany in 1910 and Russell Hibbs in New York in 1915. Poggi in 1880 in Italy described surgical deepening of the socket and remodelling of the femoral head. This approach was taken up enthusiastically by Lorenz and Hoffa in Germany in the 1890s.

In 1923 an American commission consisting of Goldthwaite, Adams and De Forest Willard reported on a large number of cases treated in the USA and Canada. They noted a high incidence of late destructive changes or deformity of the femoral head, which would now be called avascular necrosis (AVN), that they attributed to forceful manipulative reduction.

To return to early screening and diagnosis, as suggested by Roser (1879), Le Damany in Brittany first instituted large-scale screening of the newborn population and developed a simple triangular abduction pillow in the first ten years of the twentieth century. He also did fundamental research work that showed that the acetabulum was at its shallowest at birth, making displacement particularly likely at and around birth (Le Damany 1912). This was taken up by Vittorio Putti from The Rizzoli Institute in Bologna where he started a similar screening programme following the First World War, also using a simple abduction pillow. Ortolani in 1937 described his well-known test for dislocation and relocation of the hip in the newborn. This was popularised in 1962 by von Rosen in Malmo, Sweden, and Barlow in Salford, England, where it became known as the 'clicking hip' test. Unfortunately, many minor largely benign ligamentous clicks can be elicited very easily from the hips in the newborn and this led to much

confusion and over-treatment. More recently ultrasound screening has been popularised in Europe by Graf (1983) and in America and the UK by Harcke et al (1984). This has proved to be more accurate than clinical screening but it is also liable to produce overtreatment. Unfortunately abduction splintage is not entirely benign and cases of avascular necrosis have been reported, both in the normal and abnormal hip from all forms of abduction splintage.

In the UK, Somerville (1957) working in Oxford developed a protocol for the management of CDH based on conservative treatment on an abduction frame followed by arthrography. If the femoral head was satisfactorily reduced, a plaster was applied, but if there was obstruction to reduction of the femoral head in the form of a limbus, then limbectomy followed six weeks later by a femoral derotation osteotomy was performed. Limbectomy has fallen into disfavour as it can damage the growth cartilage of the acetabular rim and lead to acetabular dysplasia, particularly in early adolescence. Pelvic surgery to reorientate the acetabulum was popularised by Salter (1961) when he described innominate osteotomy. Later it became clear that in older patients double or triple osteotomy, dividing the innominate bone not only above, but also below the acetabulum, was necessary to obtain satisfactory reorientation of the acetabulum over the femoral head. If there is gross deformity of the acetabulum or the femoral head, then acetabuloplasty is indicated. The so-called capsular acetabuloplasty was described by Hey Groves (1927) in Bristol and Colonna (1932) in Canada. In this radical operation the acetabulum is deepened by reaming and the femoral head covered with capsule, which is interposed between the acetabulum and femoral head. Pemberton's pericapsular osteotomy (1965) combines redirection of the acetabulum with some alteration of its shape by hinging the acetabulum on the Y cartilage.

Augmentation acetabuloplasty is indicated when the femoral head is basically too big for the acetabulum. Producing a bony shelf or buttress over the enlarged femoral head was first described in the late nineteenth century. A modern and more stable form, the so-called tectoplasty, was described by Saito et al (1986). Chiari's pelvic osteotomy was a method of producing a bony buttress over the femoral head and also displacing the acetabulum medially, thereby altering the stress on the hip.

In those countries with well-organised screening programmes, late presenting cases of CDH or rather developmental dysplasia of the hip (DDH) as it is now called are rare. Avascular necrosis (AVN), which leads to deformity and growth disturbance of the femoral head, remains one of the major unsolved problems and always has a deleterious effect on the result of treatment. It can be caused by both conservative and operative treatment. The blood supply to the femoral head appears particularly susceptible to damage in the first year of life. The adoption of the so-called 'human' position of immobilisation, i.e. flexion above 90° and abduction of no more than 45°, as the position of immobilisation for the hip has helped considerably. Recent Doppler studies by Robinson et al (1997) of the blood supply to the femoral head suggest that some femoral heads are much more susceptible to the range of abduction than others. In patients not identified by an early screening programme, the adoption of femoral osteotomy with shortening, as described by Klisic, has led to much better results in the stable reduction of late DDH and in reducing the incidence of avascular necrosis.

LEGG–CALVÉ–PERTHES' DISEASE (LCPD COXA PLANA)

Waldenström in Sweden in 1909 described a number of children with a hip disease showing flattening of the femoral head (coxa plana) which he thought was an atypical form of tuberculosis of the hip in children. In 1910 Legg in America, Calvé in France and Perthes in Germany all independently described a similar disorder with flattening of the femoral head as described by Waldenström, but they did not believe it was due to tuberculosis. Legg described five patients with the condition and postulated that it was secondary to pressure following injury. Calvé described ten patients and called it a self-limiting non-inflammatory condition which he thought was due to abnormal or delayed osteogenesis. Perthes reported six patients and believed it was an inflammatory joint disease. In 1913 Perthes published a second paper in which he called the condition 'osteochondritis deformans juvenilis'. In one of these patients a biopsy of the femoral head had been obtained and based on the pathological and histological appearances Perthes suggested that the disease might be due to interference with the blood supply to the femoral head. Sundt (1920) published a monograph based on a study of sixty-six cases. He thought it was a form of osteodystrophy following an infection or trauma in a susceptible patient and was the first to suggest the modern concept of the 'susceptible child' in this condition. Phemister in 1921 published the results of an operation on the femoral head in one case. He noted evidence of bone necrosis, granulation tissue, and old and new bone formation. He suggested that this type of osteonecrosis was probably inflammatory in origin and was an essential part of the histology of Legg–Calvé–Perthes' disease (LCPD).

Waldenström in 1922 described his classification into four different stages or phases. He used both terms

in his original paper, which was based on a study of twenty-two cases from the onset of the disease until growth was complete. He noted that there was a typical pattern to the course of the disease and described four stages or phases; the initial stage, the reparative stage, the growing stage and the definitive or final stage. More recently this staging has been modified so stage 1 is the so-called incipient or synovitis stage where soft tissue changes in the hip joint are associated with effusion and widening of the joint space on X-ray. This very early stage is often not seen as it only lasts about one to three weeks. The second stage of aseptic necrosis or avascular stage corresponds to Waldenström's initial stage. The third stage is known as the regenerative or fragmentation stage and corresponds to Waldenström's reparative stage and lasts one to three years, and the final stage is known as the residual stage and corresponds to the growing and definitive stages of Waldenström. Sundt, in 1949, published a follow up of 153 cases with a detailed radiological classification. Based on this, he described four groups of patients based on the shape of the femoral head, namely spherical, ovoid, cylindrical or quadrangular. This is a precursor of the classification published later by Stulberg et al in 1981 on the natural history of Legg–Calvé–Perthes' disease describing the appearance of the hip at maturity in five groups (1, normal hip; 2, spherical femoral head with abnormalities to the head, neck/acetabulum; 3, non-spherical but not flat femoral head, with abnormalities of the head, neck/acetabulum; 4, flat head with abnormalities of the head, neck/acetabulum; 5, flat head in a normal acetabulum) and relating this to the subsequent prognosis in adult life. Groups 1 and 2 show spherical congruence and the risk of osteoarthritis is not increased in adult life; groups 3 and 4 show aspherical congruence and are likely to develop osteoarthritis over forty to fifty years of age, and group 5 has aspherical incongruence and is likely to get osteoarthritis in early adult life.

Soeur and DeRacker in 1952 were the first to suggest femoral osteotomy as a suitable operative treatment for Legg–Calvé–Perthes' disease. Prior to this, conservative methods either resting the hip in bed, with or without traction, or in some sort of weight-relieving calliper or splint had been the recommended treatment. However, there have always been surgeons such as Legg in 1927, Sundt in 1949 and Stulberg et al in 1981 who have questioned whether any form of treatment really alters the natural history of this disease. Axer in 1965 reported the results of twelve femoral osteotomies. He thought that the femoral head was being extruded from the acetabulum and that by femoral osteotomy he could contain the femoral head and thereby achieve better remodelling of the femoral head at maturity. This concept of containment had already been suggested using conservative means by Parker in Cardiff and Eyre Brook in Bristol. Subsequently, Harrison in Birmingham produced his Birmingham splint holding the hip in abduction and internal rotation to obtain containment conservatively. Petrie and Bitenc (1971) reported excellent results using an abduction 'broomstick' long leg plaster. To avoid the problems of long-term plaster immobilisation, various abduction braces developed, the most popular being the Atlanta Scottish Rite orthosis. More recently this has been shown to be effective in younger children but over the age of seven or eight or in the heavy overweight child it is unlikely that such a brace does produce containment of the hip.

In 1959, O'Garra, in an important study based on the radiological appearance of the femoral head in the early stages of the disease and the ultimate prognosis, noted that in those patients in whom only the anterior half of the femoral head was involved the prognosis was nearly always good with excellent reformation of the femoral head. Alternatively, those with whole head involvement tended to have a slower recovery and often a poor final result, particularly if the patient was over the age of seven or eight at the time of presentation. In 1971 Catterall, stimulated by the work of O'Garra and Lloyd-Roberts, produced his well-known classification of the disorder based on the radiological appearances on the anteroposterior (AP) and lateral radiograph into four groups. Although there has been some criticism of inter- and intra-observer error with this classification, it has been generally accepted, although the lateral pillar classification of Herring can be used on an AP X-ray film only and is somewhat easier to apply.

One of the problems with all these classifications is that they concentrate on the radiological appearance of the hip. Clinical signs and particularly loss of movement are now recognised as being extremely important. Catterall not only described radiographic signs of the patient 'at risk', but also subsequently emphasised clinical 'at risk' signs, namely the heavy patient, the patient with progressive limitation of movement and the patient presenting for the first time with the disorder over the age of eight.

Although very considerable progress has been made in our thinking about this disease over the last century, at the beginning of the twenty-first century we still fail to understand this disorder. It is important that orthopaedic surgeons remember that at least 50–60% of patients will do well without any intervention apart from symptomatic treatment when the hip is painful in the early stages of the disease. In the remaining patients it is suggested that containment may improve head remoulding leading to a more spherical contained hip at maturity. Containment is always a relative term, as the surface area of the femoral head is greater than the acetabulum so true containment within the mould of the acetabulum can never be achieved. Perhaps one of the most important features that has become clear is that retaining movement and particularly abduction is very important in this disease. Treatments that maintain movement are probably more important than strict containment. So-called containment can be achieved by non-operative or operative means, but the older and heavier the child the less likely non-operative containment will work. The child over the age of seven or eight appears more likely to have a poor result for a number of reasons. One of which is almost certainly the fact that the time left for remodelling both on the femoral and acetabular side is less. A recent paper pointed out that in the older child those hips that do very badly are within six months of closure of the acetabular Y cartilage, i.e. they have little or no acetabular growth left. They are likely to develop a Stulberg type V hip, i.e. a flat head in a normal acetabulum as the acetabulum does not have the ability to grow and remodel in relation to the deformed femoral head. This disorder continues to fascinate and frustrate orthopaedic surgeons as we still do not understand the underlying aetiology properly and real hard proof that treatment does affect the natural history of the disease remains elusive.

REFERENCES

Attenborough C G 1966 Severe congenital talipes equinovarus. J Bone Joint Surg 48B: 31

Axer A 1965 Subtrochanteric osteotomy in the treatment of Perthes' disease. J Bone Joint Surg 47B: 489

Barlow T G 1962 Early diagnosis and treatment of congenital dislocation of the hip. J Bone Joint Surg 44B: 292

Beasley A W 1972 Homer and orthopaedics. Clin Orthop 89: 10

Blockey N J, Watson J T 1970 Acute osteomyelitis in children. J Bone Joint Surg 52B: 77

Brockman E P 1930 Congenital Club Foot. A Wright & Sons, Bristol

Browne D 1934 Talipes equinovarus. Lancet ii: 909

Calvé J 1910 Sur une forme particuliére de pseudo coxalgie. Rev Chir 42: 54

Catterall A 1971 The natural history of Perthes' disease. J Bone Joint Surg 53B: 37

Clark J N P 1968 Treatment of club foot. Early detection and management of the unreduced club foot. Proc Roy Soc Med 61: 779

Colonna P C 1932 Congenital dislocation of the hip in older subjects. J Bone Joint Surg 14: 277

Dimeglio A, Bonnet F, Nazeau Ph, De Rosa V 1996 Orthopaedic treatment and passive motion machine: consequences for the surgical treatment of club foot. J Paediatr Ortho Part B: 5: 173

Fairbank Sir H A T 1951 An Atlas of General Affections of the Skeleton E & S Livingstone, Edinburgh and London

Graf R 1983 New possibilities for the diagnosis of congenital dislocation by ultrasonography. J Paediatr Ortho 3: 354

Harcke H T, Clarke N M P, Lee M S, Bourne P F, MacEwen P D 1984 Examination of the infant hip with real time ultrasonography. Ultrasound Med 3: 131

Hey Groves E W 1927 Reconstructive surgery of the hip. Br J Surg 14: 486

Jones R, Girdlestone 1919 The cure of crippled children. British Medical Journal ii 457

Le Damany P 1912 La luxation congenitale de la hanche. Felix Alcan, Paris

Legg A T 1910 An obscure affection of the hip. Boston Med Surg J 162: 202–204

Little W J 1839 A Treatise on the nature of clubfoot and analogous distortions. W Jeffs & S Highley, London

Little W J 1853 On the Nature and Treatment of Deformities of the Human Frame. Longman Green, London

Little W J 1862 On the influence of abnormal parturition, difficult labours, premature birth and asphyxzia neonatorum on the mental and physical condition of the child especially in relation to deformities. Trans. Obstet. Soc. London 3: 283

O'Garra J A 1959 The radiographic changes in Perthes' disease. J Bone Joint Surg 41B: 465

Pemberton P A 1965 Capsular arthroplasty for congenital dislocation of the hip – indications and techniques. J Bone Joint Surg 47A: 437

Perthes G C 1910 Uber Arthritis Deformans Juvenilis. Deutsch Z Chir 107: 111

Petrie J G, Bitenc I 1971 The abduction weight bearing treatment in Legg–Perthes' disease. J Bone Joint Surg 53B: 54

Robinson A H N, Bearcoft P W, Butler G J, Bernam L H 1997 Power Doppler demonstration of vascular flow in the neonatal proximal femoral epiphysis *in vivo*. J Bone Joint Surg 79B (suppl. 1): 107

Roser W 1879 Über Angeborene Hüftverrenkung Verm. Dtsch. Ges. Chir., 8th Congress. Arch. Klin. Chir. 24: 309

Saito S, Pakaoka K, Ono K 1986 Tectoplasty for painful dislocation or subluxation of the hip. J Bone Joint Surg 68B: 55

Salter R B 1961 Innominate osteotomy in the treatment of congenital dislocation and subluxation of the hip. J Bone Joint Surg 43B: 518

Scarpa A 1803 Memoir on Congenital Clubfoot (Translated from Italian) A Constable, Edinburgh 1818

Smith G E, Dawson W R 1924 Egyptian Mummies. Allen & Unwin, London

Smith Sir T 1874 On the acute arthritis of infants,. St. Barts. Hosp. Ref. 10: 189

Soeur R, DeRacker C 1952 L'aspect anatomopathologique de l'ostèochondrique a les theories pathogèniques qui s'y rapportent. Acta Orthop Belge 18: 57

Somerville B W, Scott J C 1957 The direct approach to congenital dislocation of the hip. J Bone Joint Surg 39B: 623

Stulberg S D, Cooperman D R, Wallenstein R 1981 The natural history of Legg–Calvé–Perthes' disease. J Bone Joint Surg 63A: 1095

Sundt H 1920 Udersökelser Over Malum Coxae Calvé– Legg–Perthes. Thesis Kristiania Norge

Trueta J, Morgan J D 1954 Late results in 100 cases of acute osteomyelitis. Br J Surg 41: 449

Turco V J 1971 Surgical correction of the resistant club foot, one stage posterio medial release with internal fixation: a preliminary report. J Bone Joint Surg 53A: 447

Von Rosen S 1962 Diagnosis and treatment of congenital dislocation of the hip joint in the new born. J Bone Joint Surg 44B: 284

Wainwright D 1976 The shelf operation for hip dysplasia in adolescents. J Bone Joint Surg 58B: 159

Waldenström H 1922 The definite form of coxa plana. Acta Radiol 1: 384

11

Evolution of spinal surgery

John Dove

The evolution of operative spinal surgery proper begins with the dawn of the nineteenth century. Prior to that there was a long and fascinating background to the non-operative management of spinal deformity, the literature being adorned with numerous illustrations of gruesome traction devices beginning with those of Hippocrates and followed by some of the most illustrious names in the history of medicine such as Galen, Paul of Aegina, Ambroise Paré and André. For a description of the management of spinal disorders prior to the beginning of operative surgery, see, for example, Moe (1987).

The evolution of operative spinal surgery will be considered in three parts: first, the nineteenth century when spinal surgery was just beginning to become a realistic possibility; second, the twentieth century at the end of which a multiplicity of new techniques together with an abundance of different types of internal fixation systems has led to subspecialisation within spinal surgery; and finally the twenty-first century and the new millennium when the author will indulge in speculation about the future of spinal surgery.

The author will concentrate on what he sees as the main developments in spinal surgery. He does not intend to provide an exhaustive catalogue but the reader's attention will be directed to the appropriate literature for more extensive reviews.

THE NINETEENTH CENTURY: THE EMERGENCE OF SPINAL SURGERY AND INTERNAL FIXATION

Acknowledgement is made here to the excellent publications of Thomas Keller (1996) and Martin Holland (1997) in relation to the early history of spinal surgery. The first specific record of a spinal operation is that of a laminectomy in 1829 by Smith. However, posterior decompressions had clearly been practised well before that because in Britain in 1816 Sir Charles Bell denounced laminectomy because of the terrible operative pain, inevitable infection and poor results. However, a few years later in 1832 an equally distinguished British surgeon, Astley Cooper, was arguing in favour of laminectomy. It is against this background that in 1829 Alban Gilbin Smith of Danville, Kentucky, reported the first successful lumbar laminectomy. The patient was a young man who developed progressive paraparesis after a fall from a horse two years before. The operation involved the removal of the posterior elements of three thoracic vertebrae following which the patient experienced a return of sensation in the lower limbs.

Just a few years later in France in 1839 Guérin was describing surgical myotomies for the correction of scoliosis (Guérin 1839, 1842).

Following these early ventures the development of spinal surgery as a surgical speciality had to wait for other important medical advances in the second half of the nineteenth century, those being in particular the antiseptic principles developed by Joseph Lister (1867), the development of general anaesthesia (Bigelow 1846), the advances made in the diagnostic localisation of spinal pathology by the German physician Ernst von Leyden (1874) and the French neurologist Jean Charcot (1876), and finally the introduction of radiographic investigation (Röentgen 1895).

Although internal fixation of the spine did not become commonplace until the second half of the twentieth century, the first attempts at stabilising the spine with metalwork were made in the later nineteenth century. For a detailed description of the history of the development of the internal fixation of the spine, see Wiltse (1992). The author is particularly grateful to Dr Wiltse not only for making his review available to him, but also for bringing to his attention the first description from the USA of metallic internal fixation of the spine

(Wilkins 1888). The surgery was carried out by Capt. William F. Wilkins who was described rather magnificently as scholar, soldier, lawyer, doctor, author, orator, civic leader, clinical researcher, master surgeon and Professor of Medicine at the College of Physicians in Kansas City, Kansas. He operated on a six-day-old child with a fractured dislocation of T12 on L1 and stabilised the spine with carbolised silver wire (Fig. 11.1).

The years 1887 and 1888 were landmark years in terms of spinal surgery becoming a respectable speciality. In 1887 Horsley in England and in 1888 Abbe in the USA performed the first successful laminectomies for the removal of spinal tumours (Gowers and Horsley 1888, Abbe 1890). In relation to Horsley's work in developing spinal surgery due credit must be given to his co-author, William Gowers. Gowers was a neurologist at the National Hospital, Queen's Square, London. He recognised the role that surgery might have to play in spinal disorders and it was he who in 1887 referred to Horsley the patient with a spinal tumour and who encouraged Horsley's further development of spinal surgery thereafter. The importance of this encouragement from a pillar of the medical establishment cannot be underestimated in terms of the development of spinal surgery as a respectable speciality.

In 1891 Berthold Hadra, who emigrated from Germany to Texas, described a case in which he stabilised a fracture dislocation of the cervical spine by wiring of the spinous processes. He generously gave full credit to Wilkins's pioneering work.

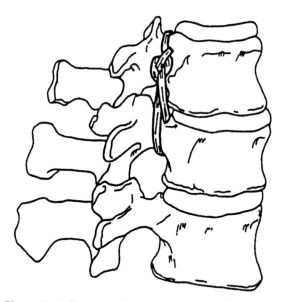

Figure 11.1   First operative drawing of internal fixation of the spine by Capt. William F. Wilkins in Kansas in 1887

The last important development in the nineteenth century was the description in France by Ménard (1895) of costotransversectomy for the evacuation of a tuberculous abscess.

Thus, by the end of the nineteenth century as the result of developments primarily in Britain, France, Germany and the USA, operative spinal surgery had become a realistic consideration in the management of spinal disorders.

THE TWENTIETH CENTURY: NEW TECHNIQUES, INTERNAL FIXATION SYSTEMS AND SUBSPECIALISATION

In 1910 Lange in Germany further developed the ideas of Wilkins and Hadra and was the first to use rods to stabilise the spine. In 1910 he reported the use of steel rods fixed to the spinous processes with silk and then later with carbolised silver wire.

A year later there were two reports from the USA that were important in the development of posterior fusion of the spine. These accounts were by Hibbs (1911) and Albee (1911) who worked independently at two different hospitals in New York to develop a technique for spinal fusion. That of Albee involved using a strut of tibial bone whereas Hibbs's technique involved a meticulous subperiosteal dissection and the splitting of the spinous processes to form a continuous bony ridge. It was this latter technique which became standard in the surgical management of scoliosis.

The next few years were relatively quiet in terms of advances in spinal surgery. There were isolated reports of new techniques such as that of an anterior spinal epiphysiodesis (MacClennan 1922) and, from Australia, the first account of the removal of a hemivertebra (Royle 1928). However, although Capener reported lumbar interbody fusion for spondylolisthesis in 1932, a damper had been put on the enthusiasm for spinal fusions created by publications of Albee and Hibbs, when Steindler reported his results in 1929. His results of surgical fusion for scoliosis were so poor that he gave up the technique and returned to a programme of exercises and bracing. This despondency was confirmed in 1941 by a report from the American Orthopaedic Association after studying 214 cases of idiopathic scoliosis treated by fusion which found that only thirty-one had a good or excellent result.

The next major advance was in the field of low back problems with the understanding of lumbar disc protrusions consequent upon the publication by Mixter and Barr in 1934. It is true that in 1857 Virchow in Germany had described what is now known to have been a lumbar disc prolapse, but its significance in relationship to back and leg pain was not recognised at the time. Furthermore in the USA in 1911 Goldthwaite postulated that a rupture of the annulus fibrosus might be the cause of back and leg pain but never applied his ideas to treatment. Thereafter in 1916 Elsberg described the appearance and operative excision of 'enchodromata' that were causing nerve root compressions but recognition of the true nature of disc protrusions and their relevance to leg pain had to wait for Mixter and Barr, who in 1934 in addition showed the effectiveness of surgery in fifty-eight cases. Thereafter in the subsequent decades there was a worldwide explosion in surgery of the lumbar disc referred to dramatically by Macnab (1977) as the 'dynasty of the disc'.

Meanwhile efforts were being made by surgeons to improve the results of lumbar fusions by supplementing them with internal fixation. King in the USA in 1944 described the technique of screw fusion of the

facets and then in 1959 Boucher in Canada reported an improvement on King's technique with the first description of the use of pedicle screws.

In England in the 1950s early attempts were being made to use metalwork for the correction of scoliosis by Allan (1955) with his jack and Roaf (1966) with his detorsion bar (Fig. 11.2). The next big step forward, however, came in the USA at the beginning of the 1960s as the result of two important advances which have to be considered together. First, Moe (1958) introduced a greatly improved bony fusion technique combining a meticulous subperiosteal dissection with facet joint excision and thorough decortication and, second, Harrington (1960) introduced his hook and rod fixation system. This combination of effective instrumentation and bony fusion dramatically reduced the incidence of pseudarthroses and greatly improved the results, making this the standard method for scoliosis correction

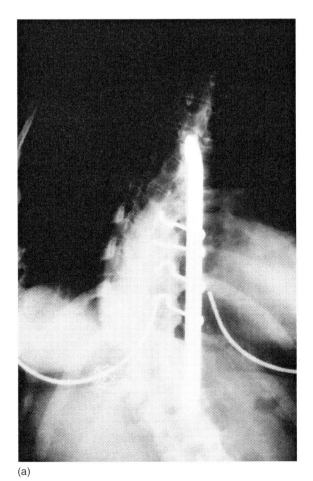

(a)

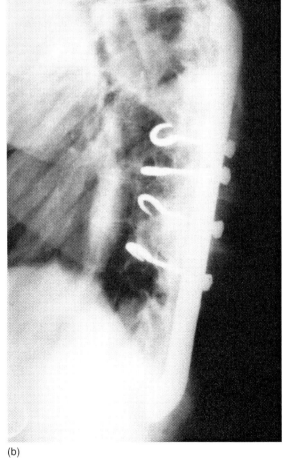

(b)

Figure 11.2 Example of Professor Robert Roaf's detorsion bar for the correction of scoliosis: (a) anteroposterior, (b) lateral

and fusion throughout the world for more than a quarter of a century. Also in the 1960s in the USA in the field of fusions for low back pain results were improved by the introduction by Wiltse (1968) of a bilateral muscle splitting approach and the laying on of cortico-cancellous graft on a decorticated intertransverse bed.

Nonetheless, rather as in the nineteenth century the flowering of spinal surgery in the latter half of that century had depended on advances in other medical fields, so in the latter half of the twentieth century the burgeoning of spinal surgery depended on advances in other medical specialities. In particular there were dramatic advances in the field of imaging beginning at the time of the Second World War with myelography (Knuttson 1942). The limitations and complications of the initial oil-based media were overcome later by the introduction of water-soluble contrast media (Grainger et al 1976). Key steps forward in imaging came in Britain in the 1960s and 1970s with the introduction of CT scanning (Hounsfield 1973) and magnetic resonance imaging (Mansfield & Maudsley 1977). At the same time important developments in the field of anaesthesia together with the creation of high dependency and intensive care units meant that surgeons could safely be much more aggressive in the scale of their operative procedures (Ben-David et al 1987). Equally important, especially in the correction of spinal deformity, was the development of spinal cord monitoring initially in France with the wake-up test (Vauzelle et al 1973) and then by electrical spinal cord monitoring (Nash et al 1974).

In the early part of the second half of the twentieth century there was an important conceptual advance in the development of internal fixation systems for the spine. Although the Harrington system had been a major step forward, it did have important disadvantages in that the rod was too straight and that fixation depended on security of the hooks at each end of the rod. A number of surgeons recognised that the spine is a segmental structure and that therefore effective internal fixation should also be segmental. The development of segmental systems not only allowed much more secure fixation and much better correction of spinal deformity, but also at the same time allowed the surgeon to reproduce the normal sagittal curves of the spine.

The earliest forms of segmental fixation for spinal deformity were developed in the 1950s in Spain and Portugal. In Spain, Hernandez-Ros (1965) used a tibial strut fixed by segmental wires to the bases of the spinous processes, whilst in Portugal Resina (1963) and Resina and Ferreira Alves (1977) also used segmental spinous process wires but with a malleable metal rod rather than a bone strut. Segmental wiring of

the spine did not, however, attract widespread interest until Luque (1974, 1984) in Mexico City developed the system of double rods secured by sublaminar wires. Thereafter Luque's system was modified in England by Dove (1987) still using sublaminar wires but combining the two rods to form a single construct known as the Hartshill rectangle.

At the same time that segmental wiring was being developed in Portugal, Roy-Camille in Paris was tackling segmental fixation in a different way by using a plate and pedicle screws (Roy-Camille et al 1970). During the same decade segmental spinal fixation was being approached from a different angle in Australia by fixing the front of the spine. The concept of fixing the spine from the front was possible as the result of the development of the anterior approaches to the spine in Hong Kong in the 1950s. Although in the earlier twentieth century there were sporadic reports of anterior spinal surgery, it was not until Hodgson and Stock (1960) in Hong Kong developed a system of surgical approaches to the whole of the front of the spine that anterior spinal surgery became commonplace. It was thus in the 1960s in Australia that Dwyer was enabled to develop his anterior segmental spinal fixation system which involved the correction of scoliosis using vertebral body screws and a flexible cable (Dwyer et al 1969). The Dwyer system was then modified and improved with the use of a threaded rod by Zielke in Germany (Zielke & Pellin 1976).

The last major development in segmental instrumentation came from Cotrel and Dubousset (1985) in Paris who developed a double-rod system using a combination of hooks and pedicle screws. Since then there has been a bewildering explosion in the commercial development of spinal internal fixation systems but what they all have in common is that they are segmental and fixed to the spine by wires, hooks, screws, or a combination of all three.

Whilst the result of advances in imaging, anaesthesia, spinal cord monitoring and segmental fixation systems surgery for spinal deformity in the latter half of the twentieth century have moved on to a grand scale, at the same time surgery for lumbar disc problems has moved in the opposite direction towards the minimally invasive. The first step was to preserve rather than remove the lamina (Love 1939). It then became possible to carry out lumbar disc surgery through a tiny incision with the assistance of a microscope (Williams 1977). Thereafter, percutaneous techniques were developed (Kambin & Gellmann 1983). There is now a variety of such techniques available, and for a comprehensive review of these, see Kahanovitz et al (1996).

STATE OF SPINAL SURGERY AT THE END OF THE TWENTIETH CENTURY

Whereas to begin with spinal surgery was just part of the armamentarium of a surgeon, in the latter half of the twentieth century as the result of the development of the multiplicity of new approaches and techniques not only is it commonplace for surgeons to specialise purely in the surgery of spinal disorders, but also there has been some specialisation within spinal surgery so that there are now different professional societies for spinal deformity, the cervical spine, the lumbar spine, minimally invasive techniques, etc. At the end of the twentieth century current practice in the different fields of spinal surgery is as given below.

Spinal deformity

Standard practice for the posterior correction of a thoracic scoliosis is to use a posterior segmental correction system in conjunction with spinal cord monitoring. In the skeletally immature this is combined with a preliminary anterior epiphysiodesis or growth arrest procedure with the dual purpose of allowing increased mobility of the spine and preventing continuing anterior growth thereby avoiding late recurrence of the rib hump by what is known as the crankshaft phenomenon (Dubousset et al 1989). Either the anterior or posterior procedure is commonly combined with a costoplasty to improve cosmesis and provide an additional rich source of bone graft. Although scoliosis surgery is a very major operative undertaking, minimally invasive techniques are beginning to play their part with the development of video-assisted thoracic techniques (Mehlman et al 1997).

For the correction of thoracolumbar and lumbar curves standard surgical practice is through an anterior approach to correct the curve with one of the many available segmental systems.

For major scoliosis and in particular long neuromuscular curves, a combination of anterior and posterior approaches is used when either the anterior procedure will be used to perform an extensive release, which is then combined with a posterior correction and stabilisation, or internal fixation may be used for both the anterior and posterior procedures.

Explorations have been made into early, preventative surgery for spinal deformity but to date this has only really proved successful in deformity secondary to hemivertebrae (Marks et al 1995).

Spinal fractures

Stabilisation of injuries of the cervical spine is frequently required. With the development of locking plate systems for the front of the neck and effective segmental fixation systems for the back of the neck, open surgical stabilisation of these injuries is now more common than external fixation with devices such as a halo-vest.

In order to try to address the mechanics of injuries at the thoracolumbar junction, specific instrumentation systems such as the 'fixateur interne' have been developed (Magerl 1981). The management of thoracolumbar fractures remains, however, highly controversial with, on the one hand, the proponents of surgery claiming that operative stabilisation allows early mobilisation and discharge from hospital, prevention of painful, late post-traumatic kyphosis and improved results in relation to neurological function, whereas, on the other hand, the advocates of conservative management point to the complications from failure of internal fixation systems and claim that the neurological outcome is not influenced by surgery.

Spinal tumours

Primary tumours are rare and are dealt with on an individual basis, but the principles are radical excision and stabilisation by bone grafting and internal fixation. In recent years there has been increasing recognition of the value of operative stabilisation in metastatic disease affecting the spine. Working in conjunction with the oncologist to understand the natural history of the underlying disease better, the spinal surgeon can stabilise the spine to relieve pain and protect the spinal cord (Taneichi et al 1997).

Lumbar spine

The management of lumbar disc protrusions is, as described above, becoming increasingly less invasive (Williams 1977, Kaublin & Gellmann 1983, Kahonovitz et al 1996). Less invasive techniques are also being introduced for stabilisation of the lumbar spine with laparoscopic techniques being introduced for interbody fusions (Mathews et al 1995). After the initial enthusiasm that followed the introduction of the various internal fixation devices the place of lumbar fusions for the management of back pain is under critical examination. What prospective studies there are have failed to confirm the validity of fusions for low back pain and the management of the 'failed back' has become a subspecialty in its own right (Zdeblick 1993). It has become recognised that too much reliance has been placed on the appearances on imaging and that in the selection of patients for low back pain surgery a proper understanding of non-physical factors is crucial (Fairbank et al 1980, Waddell et al 1980, Main et al 1992).

THE TWENTY-FIRST CENTURY

Thus, in both the nineteenth and twentieth centuries developments in spinal surgery in the first half of those centuries were slow and then blossomed following important developments in other fields of medicine. What then does the author envisage about the future of spinal surgery in the twenty-first century and further in the new millennium?

Spinal deformity

Although in specialised units front and back scoliosis surgery has become a standard procedure and is very rewarding both for the surgeon and patient, nonetheless it is a very major and destructive surgical undertaking, but there is light at the end of the tunnel in the search for a more logical basis to the management of spinal deformity as basic scientific studies begin to identify the genetic basis for certain types of scoliosis (Child et al 1996, Inoue et al 1998). Once we have a proper understanding of the cause of scoliosis then it is not too fanciful to suppose that genetic engineering might prevent spinal deformity. Genetic engineering might prevent spinal deformity and avoid the need for surgery.

Spinal injuries

The major catastrophes complicating spinal injuries are paraplegia and tetraplegia. Realistic advances will need to be made on two broad fronts. First, a greater understanding of the epidemiology of spinal injuries must lead to safety measures and regulations preventing the injuries in the first place. Second, current basic scientific work on practical electrical stimulation for restoring neurological function will become a realistic possibility (Marsolais and Kobetic 1988) and at the same time current research using embryonic material will lead to effective repair of the spinal cord.

Spinal tumours

Basic studies into the understanding of the cause of malignant disease will lead to prevention and solution of the current epidemic so that end-stage surgery for metastatic disease will become a rare necessity.

Lumbar spine and back pain

Current laser techniques will become refined so that the management of lumbar disc protrusions and nerve root compression will be carried out completely non-invasively by automated laser methods (Quigley & Maroon 1994).

The current epidemic of back pain will be solved by a better understanding of the health and function of the lumbar spine together with sensible exercise regimens both at home and in the work place. For those cases where surgery is still necessary the placement of internal fixation devices will become less invasive, much more accurate and safer by the development of robotic computer-assisted systems (Nolte et al 1995).

Organisation and training

At present the organisation of spinal surgery is fragmented, the centres throughout the world having developed as the result of the pioneering efforts of various spinal specialists. There are still large areas of the world where patients do not have access to the benefits of modern surgical treatment of the spine so that a fairer distribution of spinal services will need to be developed. Furthermore, the basic training of spinal surgeons is different depending on historical factors and which country is concerned. In some countries spinal surgery is primarily the province of orthopaedic surgeons, in some of neurosurgeons and elsewhere of trauma surgeons. The bony and neurological elements of the spine are intimately related and it is clear that a specialist training in spinal surgery should have training in both orthopaedic surgery and neurosurgery. This must become the norm for all spinal surgical training.

The author envisages that developments in spinal surgery in the twenty-first century will be the reverse of what happened in the two preceding centuries. Whereas the previous two centuries consisted in the first half of tentative attempts to develop new surgical techniques followed in the latter half by an explosion in operative surgery, in the twenty-first century during the first half of the century the number of open surgical operations will gradually level off and then in the second half of the century surgery will become much less necessary; firstly as the result of better understanding of the natural history from epidemiological studies and secondly as the result of prevention of disease and trauma. This should not, however, cause the surgeons of the future to be despondent. Major spinal surgery as well as being a tremendous undertaking for the patient is physically demanding for the surgeon. The newer, computer-guided, automated techniques will need to be directed by those trained in open surgery and with a proper understanding of the anatomy and pathology of spinal disorders. The development of automated, robotic techniques that the surgeon can direct from the comfort of an armchair (given, of course, frequent breaks for an exercise regimen for the surgeon's own low back) is an exciting prospect for the spinal surgeon of the future!

REFERENCES

Abbe R 1890 Spinal surgery. A report of eight cases. Medical Record 33: 85–92

Albee F A 1911 Transplantation of a portion of the tibia into the spine for Pott's disease J Am Med Assoc 57: 885–886

Allan F G 1955 Scoliosis: operative correction of fixed curves. J Bone Joint Surg 37B: 92–96

American Orthopaedic Association Research Committee 1941 End result of the treatment of idiopathic scoliosis. J Bone J Surg 23A: 963

Bell C 1816 A System of Operative Surgery, 2 vols, 2nd American edn. George Goodwin & Son, II, pp 255–259

Ben-David B, Haller G S, Taylor P 1987 Anaesthesia for surgery of the spine. In: Bradford D S, Lonstein J E, Moe J H, Ogilvie J W, Winter R B (eds) Moe's Textbook of Scoliosis, 2nd edn. W B Saunders, Philadelphia, pp 607–628.

Bigelow H J 1846 Insensibility during surgical operations produced by inhalation. Boston Med Surg J 35: 309–317, 379–382

Boucher H H 1959. A method of spinal fusion. J Bone Joint Surg 41B: 248

Capener N 1932 Spondylolisthesis. Br J Surg 19: 374

Charcot J M 1876 Leçons des localisations dans les maladies du cerveau at de la moelle épinière. V. A. Delahaye, Paris

Child A H et al 1996 The role of fibrillin deficiency: Marfan syndrome and adolescent idiopathic scoliosis. J Bone Joint Surg 78B: 159

Cooper A 1832 A Treatise on Dislocation and Fractures of the Joints, 2nd American edn. Lilly & Wait, Boston

Cotrel Y, Dubousset J 1985 New segmental posterior instrumentation of the spine. Orthop Trans 9: 118

Dove J 1987 Luque segmental spinal instrumentation: the use of the Hartshill rectangle. Orthopedics 10: 955–961

Dubousset J, Herring J A, Shufflebarger H 1989 The crankshaft phenomenon. J Pediatr Orthop 9: 541–550

Dwyer A F, Newton N C, Sherwood A A 1969 An anterior approach to scoliosis: a preliminary approach. Clin Orthop 62: 192–202.

Elsberg C A 1916 Diagnosis and Treatment of Surgical Diseases of the Spinal Cord and its Membranes. W B Saunders, Philadelphia

Fairbank J C T et al 1980 Oswestry disability questionnaire. Physiotherapy 66: 271–273.

Goldthwaite J G 1911 The lumbosacral articulation. An explanation of many cases of 'lumbago', sciatica and paraplegia. Boston Med Surg J 164: 365–372

Gowers W R, Horsley V 1888 A case of tumour of the spinal cord. Medico-Chirurgical Trans 71: 377–428

Grainger R et al 1976 Lumbar myelography with metrizamide. Br J Rad 49: 996–1003

Guérin J 1839 Mémoire sur les déviations simulées de l'épine et les moyens. Gaz Méd de Paris 7: 241–247

Guérin J 1842 Remarques préliminaires sur le traitement des déviations de l'épine par la section des muscles du dos. Gaz Méd de Paris 10: 1–6

Hadra B E 1891 Wiring of the vertebrae as a means of immobilisation in fractures and Pott's disease. Medical Times and Register 22: 1–8

Harrington P R 1960 Surgical instrumentation for management of scoliosis. J Bone Joint Surg 42A: 1448

Hernandez-Ros A 1965 Nuevas tacticas, tecnicas operationias en el tratamiento del escoliosis. In Scritti medici en onore de P sel torto. Saveriu Pipola, Naples, pp 71–97

Hibbs R A 1911 An operation for progressive spinal deformities. NY Med J 93: 1013

Hodgson A R, Stock F E 1960 Anterior spine fusion. Br J Surg 48: 172

Hounsfield G N 1973 Computerised transverse axial scanning (tomography). Br J Rad 46: 1016–1022

Inoue M et al 1998 Idiopathic scoliosis in twins studied by DNA fingerprinting. J Bone Joint Surg 80B: 212–217

Kahanovitz V V, Benoist M, Osti O L 1996 In: Wiesel S W et al (eds) Alternative Techniques for Disc Decompression in the Lumbar Spine, 2nd edn. W B Saunders, Philadelphia, pp 524–537

Kambin P, Gellmann H 1983 Percutaneous lateral discectomy of the lumbar spine. Clin Orthop 174: 127–132

Keller T 1996 Historical perspective: Victor Horsley's surgery for cervical caries and fracture. Spine 21: 398–401

Keller T, Holland M C 1997 Some notable American spine surgeons of the 19th century. Spine 22: 1413–1417

King D 1944 Internal fixation for lumbosacral fusion. Am J Surg Arch Surg 66: 357

Knuttson F 1942 Volum und Formulariationen des Wirbelkanals bei Lordosierung und Kyposierung und ihre Bedeutung für die Myelographische. Acta Rad Diag 23: 431–443

Lange F 1910 Support of the spondylolytic spine by means of buried steel bars attached to the vertebrae. Am J Orthop Surg 8: 344

Leyden E von 1874 Klinik der Rückenmark-Krankheiten. August Hirschwald, Berlin

Lister J 1867 On the antiseptic principles in the practice of surgery. Lancet ii: 353–356, 688–689

Love J G 1939 Removal of intervertebral discs without laminectomy. Proc Staff Meet Mayo Clin 14: 800

Luque E R 1974 Anatomy of scoliosis and its correction. Clini Orthop 105: 298

Luque E R 1984 Segmental Spinal Instrumentation: The State of the Art. New York, Slack, pp 1–11

MacClennan A 1922 Scoliosis. Br Med J 2: 864–866

Macnab I 1977 Backache. Williams & Wilkins, Baltimore

Magerl F 1981 Clinical application of the thoracolumbar junction and the lumbar spine with a fixateur interne. In: Mears D C (ed) External Skeletal Fixation. Williams & Wilkins, Baltimore, pp 353–366

Main C J et al 1992 the distress and risk assessment indices. A simple classification identify distress and evaluate the risk of poor outcome. Spine 17: 42–52

Mansfield P, Maudsley A 1977 Medical imaging by NMR. Br J Rad 50: 188–194

Marks D, Thompson A, Piggott H 1995 The long term results of combined anterior and posterior convex fusion for congenital scoliosis due to hemivertebra. J bone Joint Surg 77B (suppl. II): 156

Marsolais B E, Kobetic R 1988 Development of practical electrical stimulation for restoring gait in the paralysed patient. Clin Orthop 233: 64–74

Mathews H H et al 1995 Laparoscopic discectomy with anterior lumbar interbody fusion. Spine 20: 1797–1802

Mehlman C T, Crawford A H, Wolf R K 1997 Video-assisted thoracic surgery. Spine 22: 2178–2182

Ménard V 1895 Traitement de la paraplégie du mal de Pott par le drainage lateral: costotransversectomie. Revue d'Ortopédie 6: 134–146

Mixter W J, Barr J S 1934 Rupture of the intervertebral disc with involvement of the spinal canal. N Engl J Med 211: 210–215

Moe J H 1987 Historical aspects of scoliosis. In: Bradford D S et al (eds) Moe's Textbook of Scoliosis and Other Spinal Deformities, 2nd edn. W B Saunders, Philadelphia, pp 1–6

Moe J H 1958 A critical analysis of methods of fusion for scoliosis. J Bone Joint Surg 40A: 529

Nash C L, Schatzinger L, Lorig R 1974 Intraoperative monitoring of spinal cord function during scoliosis surgery. J Bone Joint Surg 56A: 765

Nolte L-P et al 1995 Computer assisted fixation of spinal implant. Image Guid Surg 1: 88–93

Quigley M R, Maroon J C 1994 Laser discectomy: a review. Spine 19: 53–56

Resina J 1963 Redressment et stabilisation immédiate des scolioses par un tuteur métallique. Association Européenne contre la poliomyélite. Masson, Paris, pp 421–429

Resina J, Ferreira Alves A 1977 A technique of correction and internal fixation for scoliosis. J Bone Joint Surg 59B: 159–165

Roaf R 1966 Scoliosis. Churchill Livingstone, Edinburgh

Röentgen W C 1895 Über eine neue Art von Strahlen. Sitzungsberichte der Physische-Medizinische Gesellschaft Würzburg 137: 132–141.

Roy-Camille R et al 1970 Pedicle screws for spinal fixation. Press Med 78: 1447–1448

Royle N D 1928 The operative removal of an accessory vertebra. Med J Australia 1: 467

Smith A G 1829 Account of a case in which portions of three dorsal vertebrae were removed for the relief of paralysis from fracture with partial success. N Am Med Surg J 8: 94–97

Steindler A 1929 Diseases and Deformities of the Spine and Thorax. C V Mosby, St Louis

Taneichi H et al 1997 Risk factors and probability of vertebral body collapse in metastases of the thoracic and lumbar spines. Spine 22: 239–245

Vauzelle C. Stagnara P, Jouvinroux P 1973 Functional monitoring of spinal cord during spinal surgery. Clin Orthop 93: 173

Virchow R 1857 Untersuchung über die Entwickelung des Schadelgrund. G Reimer, Berlin

Waddell G et al 1980 Nonorganic physical signs in low back pain. Spine 5: 117–125

Wilkins B F 1888 Separation of the vertebrae with protrusion of hernia between the same: operation, cure. St Louis Med Surg J 54: 340–341

Williams R W 1977 Microlumbar Discectomy in Surgical Techniques. Codman, pp 1–10

Wiltse L 1968 The paraspinal sacrospinalis splitting approach to the lumbar spine. J Bone Joint Surg 50A: 919

Wiltse L L 1992 History of pedicle screw fixation of the spine. In: Arnold D M, Lonstein J E (eds) Spine: State of the Art Reviews Hanley & Belfus, Philadelphia, 6, pp 1–10

Zdeblick T 1993 A prospective randomised study of lumbar fusion. Spine 18: 983

Zielke K, Pellin B 1976 Neue Instrumente und Implante zur Erganzung des Harrington Systems. Z Orthop Chir 114: 534–537

12

Development of foot and ankle surgery

Leslie Klenerman

Much of early orthopaedic surgery was on the foot and ankle. Indeed the principles of most of the common procedures were established by 1900. This is in contrast to hand surgery that only started to develop after the First World War (see Chapter 9). However, paradoxically subspecialisation in foot and ankle surgery started only about twenty years ago.

One of the earliest books about the foot and ankle was *Ober den bestern Shoen* (1781) by Pieter Camper (1722–89), Professor of Medicine, Surgery and Anatomy in Amsterdam. (It was translated into English as *The Best Form of Shoe* by James Dowie in 1861.) Camper had clear views on the height of heels. He considered that the centre of gravity of the whole body was displaced by unreasonably high heels and that anyone wearing high heels would walk less securely and were at risk of falling and spraining their ankles. He stated 'that the arrangements of the bones and muscles of the feet prove that we might move them in many ways, were those members not entirely neglected and rendered useless by shoes and boots constructed as it were on purpose to destroy their mechanism'.

Delpech, George Frederick Louis Stromeyer and William John Little had used subcutaneous tenotomy for correction of club foot deformities, but open corrective surgery was only possible after the introduction of anaesthesia and antisepsis in the mid- and latter half of the nineteenth century.

An early textbook *Operative Surgery of the Foot and Ankle* by Henry Hancock was published in London in 1873. The contents were quite different from what one would expect to find in a modern textbook. Besides a section on anatomy, there were chapters on Tubercular Disease of the Foot, Syme's Amputation, Subastragaloid Amputation, Excision of the Astragalus, Excision of the Ankle Joint, Chopart's Amputation and Resection of Os calcis, which give an indication of the common clinical problems at that time.

The operation and word 'arthrodesis' were introduced in 1882 by Edward Albert (1841–1900). However, Henry Park in Liverpool in 1781 had already carried out the first bone and joint excision of a tuberculous joint with a fixed flexion deformity instead of an above-knee amputation as was the practice at the time. The joint fortuitously ankylosed (Kirkup 1991). Albert was at first Professor of Surgery in Innsbruck in 1883 and he later moved to Vienna (Le Vay 1990). He conceived the idea of stabilisation of the ankle in a paralysed foot. He excised the articular cartilage from the body of the talus and the ankle mortise and then immobilised the lower leg in plaster. Subsequently he proceeded to stiffen other joints such as the talonavicular and calcaneocuboid. Albert also originated the temporary excision and subsequent replacement of the talus to ensure thorough excision of the articular surfaces of the ankle and subtalar joints, a procedure which has fortunately long since been abandoned. Deliberate fusion of a tarsal joint was performed before 1884 by Alexander Ogston of Aberdeen (Kirkup 1992) when he fused the talonavicular joint for painful flat feet. After the removal of articular cartilage the joint was fixed with two pegs derived from ivory knitting needles. He reported seventeen cases and sixteen were said to be cured. A variety of combinations of arthrodeses in the foot were developed, which included the triple arthrodesis, i.e. subtalar and midtarsal joints. This operation allowed the patient to give up wearing costly and cumbersome braces. Naughton Dunn of Birmingham recommended combined fusion of the subtalar and midtarsal joints in 1919 for paralytic calcaneocavus. In *The Robert Jones Birthday Volume* (Dunn 1928) he analysed the results of 535 cases of tarsal arthrodesis. There were only eight subtalar fusions. Lambrinudi (1927) designed a triple arthrodesis for the drop-foot so as to stabilise the ankle by use of the posterior tubercle of the talus. The posterior part of the talus is in contact with the tibia as a physiological bone block and the remainder of the foot is brought up to the talus. Dunn advocated removal of the whole or part of the navicular to allow the foot to be displaced backwards under the bones of the leg. Triple arthrodesis is still used today for rheumatoid disease, after trauma or after the late diagnosis of a ruptured tibialis posterior tendon. The basic technique is unchanged, but the use of internal fixation has improved the quality of the results.

Another operation for flail joints following poliomyelitis was tendon transfer. Nicoladoni of Innsbruck introduced this in 1882 when he attached peroneus brevis and longus tendons to the tendo achillis for a paralytic calcaneocavus deformity. This important contribution subsequently lay dormant for many years. Vulpius and Lange revised the principle in Germany at the beginning of the twentieth century. Vulpius sutured tendon to tendon and Lange tendon to bone. Biesalski and Leo Mayer further refined the technique.

Astragelectomy (talectomy) for tuberculosis and resistant club foot was practised in the second half of the nineteenth century (Evans 1928).

In 1901, Royal Whitman of the then Hospital for Ruptured and the Crippled in New York (now the Hospital for Special Surgery) performed the first astragalectomy for paralysis and a calcaneal deformity (Whitman 1901). Talectomy is still done today, but infrequently, and is reserved for the rigid deformity that occurs with arthrogryposis multiplex congenita.

Ankle arthroplasty was first attempted by Themistocles Gluck (1853–1942) (see Chapter 3), who was an innovative surgeon, ahead of his time, but who lacked the appropriate supporting technology effectively to put his ideas into practice (Fig. 12.1). His ankle prosthesis was anchored by prongs into the metatarsals and made of ivory and metal. His joint replacements eventually suppurated or developed tuberculous sinuses and by 1891 he admitted his failures (Le Vay 1990). Many varieties of ankle arthroplasty such as the Mayo, Imperial College and London Hospital, and Bath ankle have been produced since the 1970s, but the success rate was low. More recently Kofoed and his team in Copenhagen have been successful with an arthroplasty that takes account of the importance of restoring the normal tension of the collateral ligaments to ensure both gliding and rolling movements. He used a three-component device. There are metal coverings for the tibia and talus with a polythene meniscus that is congruent with both metal components. He has reported on one hundred consecutive patients treated for osteoarthritis or rheumatoid arthritis with a median six-year follow-up (Kofoed 1999). The results for patients with traumatic osteoarthritis were equally good in patients younger or those more than fifty years of age and those for rheumatoid arthritis were similar.

Osteotomy of the calcaneus, nowadays a common operation on the hindfoot for correction of valgus or varus deformities, was first performed by Gleich (1893) in Germany who sawed the calcaneus in an oblique direction and shifted the posterior fragment forward and downward for a patient with a marked valgus deformity. This increased the angle between the calcaneal axis and the floor. He used a stirrup incision under the foot and reported on three operations (Silver et al 1967).

THE FOREFOOT: BUNIONS AND HALLUX VALGUS

According to Lewis Durlacher, Surgeon Chiropodist to the Royal Household during the times of George IV, William IV and Queen Victoria, in his *Corns and Bunions* of 1845, the use of the word 'bunion' should be

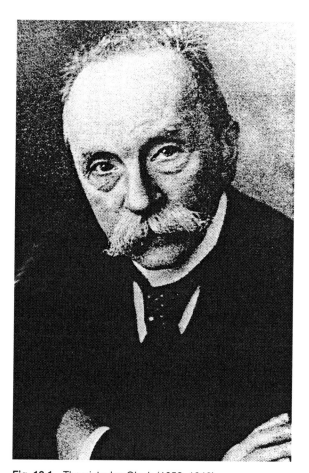

Fig. 12.1 Themistocles Gluck (1853–1942)

restricted to designate an enlargement of the great or little toe at the articulation with the metatarsal bone, produced by pressure or some other cause effecting a change in the position of the adjacent phalanx (Durlacher 1845). The word 'bunion' is probably a modification of *oignion* (onion), which was used in France to describe the disease. He goes on to state that although not a scientific term, 'that enlargement does in a measure resemble a skinned onion in smoothness and roundness'. Karl Hueter (1838–82) first introduced the term 'hallux valgus' in 1871. He described the deformity as an 'abduction' contracture in which the toe deviated from the median plane of the body. It is anomalous that valgus, i.e. abduction, is due to or at least aggravated by adductor hallucis! With reference to each foot alone, the valgus of the hallux is a varus deformity that uses the second metatarsal as the reference line.

As early as April 1884 an operation for hallux valgus was described in *The Lancet* by A. E. Barker of University College. A medially based wedge osteotomy of the first metatarsal was performed 'according to the strictest antiseptic precautions'.

In 1894, H. H. Clutton in the *St Thomas' Hospital Reports* gave a detailed description of the technique of arthrodesis of the metatarsophalangeal joint of the great toe. He used an ivory peg to maintain the position and stressed the importance of the position of the proximal phalanx. He stated that 'the phalanx and the metatarsal bone should be absolutely in a straight line, as regards the inner border of the foot, but a very slight inclination to dorsal flexion is an advantage for easy progression'.

In April 1887 John Neville Davies-Colley described the condition of hallux flexus, which would today be called hallux rigidus. He had operated on five patients. In two cases he had excised the proximal half of the proximal phalanx and left the head of the metatarsal intact. In October 1904, Colonel W. L. Keller of the US Army described a procedure that has remained popular for many years. He removed the medial exostosis and base of the proximal phalanx with a Gigli saw while carefully preserving the tendon of flexor halluxis longus. He mentioned that simple removal of the exostosis would be followed by a recurrence of the deformity. Keller was not especially interested in the development of his procedure and went on to achieve fame in general surgery.

An alternative operation done by Charles Mayo in 1908 was an arthroplasty of the metatarsophalangeal joint, with resection of the cartilage-bearing surface of the head of the first metatarsal. Hueter had first recommended this procedure in 1871. The remnant is remodelled and a 'U'-shaped flap of bursal tissue was turned into the joint. In 1936 E. J. Lloyd compared the results of Keller's and Mayo's operations in patients with

bilateral hallux valgus in which Keller's operation was done on one foot and the Mayo operation on the other. There were twenty patients in the series with a followup of one to three years. The results showed little difference between the two procedures.

McBride described a soft tissue correction in 1935. He moved the tendons of adductor hallucis from its insertion into the base of the proximal phalanx to the head of the metatarsal and removed the exostosis. In 1945 Hawkins, Mitchell and Hedrick described the double osteotomy of the neck of the first metatarsal now commonly referred to as Mitchell's osteotomy. The operation was a development of procedures described by Hohman and Peabody and corrected the metatarsus primus varus (intermetatarsal angle). They noted that excessive shortening of the first metatarsal predisposed to metatarsalgia by shifting weight from the first metatarsal to the head of the second and third. Narrowing of the intermetatarsal angle is the basis of all the many present-day metatarsal osteotomies. This is supported by the work of Hardy and Clapham (1951), who were the first to show a statistical relationship between the intermetatarsal and hallux valgus angles. However, it was not until 1990 that the first randomised comparison of two procedures, Keller's arthroplasty and first metatarsophalangeal arthrodesis for symptomatic hallux valgus or hallux rigidus, in patients over forty-five yeas of age was published by O'Doherty et al (1990). In eighty-one patients (110 feet) with a minimum followup of two years, both procedures gave a similar degree of satisfaction to the patient and relief of symptoms. The incidence of metatarsalgia was also similar. As six patients with an arthrodesis required a revision operation, the authors suggested that Keller's operation was preferable for these patients.

Alfred Swanson introduced a silicone elastomer replacement of the proximal third of the proximal phalanx in 1968 in patients with rheumatoid arthritis, hallux valgus and hallux rigidus. Later he developed a flexible double hinge implant to allow more correction of the deformity with removal of bone from both articular surfaces of the first metatarsophalangeal joint (Swanson et al 1979). There have been reports of the development of foreign body reactions to particles of silicon elastomer abraded from prostheses in the toes. Bone lesions (Gordon & Bullough 1982) and lymphadenopathy (Christie et al 1977) have also been reported. Histologically, particles indistinguishable from silicone elastomer have been found in synovium. As correction of the common deformities of the great toe can be achieved by operations that do not involve the insertion of foreign material, it does not seem necessary to use these silastic spacers routinely.

MORTON'S NEUROMA

The pain of a Morton's Neuroma was first described by the chiropodist Lewis Durlacher in *Corns and Bunions* in 1845. 'It is a kind of neuralgia seated between the toes, but which fortunately is not very common. It constitutes a most troublesome and severe complaint and one very difficult of removal.'

The patient complains of a severe pain between two of the toes, along the inside of one or the other, generally the second and third, he can seldom tell which. The pain extends up the leg and is increased when the toes are pressed together more particularly after walking.

In 1876 Thomas G. Morton, Surgeon to the Philadelphia Orthopaedic Hospital, described 'A peculiar and painful affliction of the fourth metatarsophalangeal articulation', the symptoms of which have now become well known as Morton's Metatarsalgia. His treatment was complete excision of the irritable metatarsophalangeal joint with the surrounding soft parts. A. E. Hoadley of Chicago described six patients in 1893. He operated on only one and cut down on the sole of the foot and 'without any difficulty' found the digital branches of the lateral plantar nerve. He found a small neuroma on the nerve, seven-eights of an inch long and nearly one-eighth of an inch in diameter. Resection of the nerve produced a prompt and perfect cure. His other patients improved by shoe modification, which consisted of reinforcement of the sole of wide shoes. Robert Jones considered excision of the metatarsal head, excision of the joint or amputation of the toe as possible surgical solutions to the problem.

Hoadley's observations do not seem to have aroused great interest amongst his contemporaries until nearly forty years later in 1935 when Sir Harold Stiles was operated on for long-standing metatarsalgia (Hoadley 1893). The nerve between the third and fourth toes was resected by Norman Dott (Nissen 1948), a neurosurgeon. In 1940 L. O. Betts of Adelaide reported ten patients on whom he had resected the fourth plantar digital nerve through a plantar incision. McElvenny (1943) reported twelve neuromas in eleven patients and advocated a dorsal web-splitting incision. In 1951 J. D. Mulder of Amsterdam described a clinical test for Morton's Neuroma in which a click is elicited from the affected foot by exerting pressure around the forefoot with the left hand and at the same time using the right thumb to put pressure on the sole at the site of the suspected neuroma. One may reproduce the characteristic pain with a palpable click. More recently Morton's Metatarsalgia has been shown to be a typical entrapment syndrome (Guiloff et al 1984) similar to median nerve compression at the wrist and ulnar neuritis at the elbow.

FLAT FOOT

Although flat feet, i.e. feet with flattening of the longitudinal arch, were recognised for many years, a clear understanding of the problem only really began with the work of Harris and Beath who in 1947 published a study of foot problems in 3600 recruits in the Royal Canadian Army. They subdivided flat feet into three groups: flexible flat foot, flexible flat foot with short tendo achillis and peroneal spastic or rigid flat foot (2%). They found that the first group (6%) rarely caused symptoms. They showed that in the young male, the hypermobile flat foot, with a tight tendo achillis, produced a marked reduction in locomotor efficiency in 0.7% of those admitted to the army and a mild reduction in 5.5% (Rose 1991).

With the advance of basic scientific studies, notably by Hicks (1951, 1954), a much better understanding of the arch mechanism of the foot has gradually emerged. The role of muscles has been found to be necessary for function and balance, but not for structural integrity. The plantar plates of the metatarsophalangeal joints and the intervening deep transverse metatarsal ligaments form a tranverse tie bar capable of controlling splay of the metatarsal heads (Stainsby 1997). The deeper layer of the plantar aponeurosis with Hicks' windlass mechanism provides a dynamic longitudinal tie bar system supporting the five metatarsal rays of the longitudinal arch structure of the foot. Work by McNeil Alexander and his team have explained the spring-like nature of the long arch (Ker et al 1987). The flexible flat foot has generally been accepted as normal, one has only to look at black athletes.

RIGID FLAT FOOT

Recognition of the clinical significance of a tarsal coalition was first noted by Holl in 1880. In spite of Sir Robert Jones's clinical description of a peroneal spastic flat foot in 1897 it was not until the work of Slomann (1921), Badgeley (1927), and Harris and Beath (1948) that tarsal coalitions were conclusively linked with the peroneal spastic flat foot. Subsequently triple arthrodesis and much more recently treatment by excision of calcaneonavicular and talocalcaneal bars has been advocated.

It is interesting to read Jones's description (1897). He noted many flat feet were accompanied by spasm, but one variety exhibited characteristic symptoms and the spasm proved to be the sole cause of the deformity. He had operated on forty patients and found nothing short of resection of portions of the peroneal tendons (brevis and longus) relieved symptoms. The foot was then placed in a varus position for a fortnight and the patient allowed to walk with an altered boot in three weeks. This is an interesting example of a surgical solution for symptoms, but without the knowledge of the underlying pathology.

Acquired flat foot in adults due to dysfunction of the tibialis posterior tendon has been gradually recognised as a cause for pain and discomfort and is nowadays recognised as a common problem. It arises in adults who have low longitudinal arches. Kulowski in 1936 (Pomeroy et al 1999) is given the credit for the first description of tenosynovitis of the posterior tibial tendon. Almost twenty years later Fowler (1955) discussed the tibialis posterior syndrome and described a series of patients who had had operative treatment for the condition. Williams (1963) described the operative treatment for tenovaginitis of the posterior tibial tendon. Kettelkamp and Alexander (1969) reported on the repair of spontaneous rupture of the tendon. Gradually an awareness of this problem has developed and a variety of treatments has been developed starting with decompression of the tendon of tibialis posterior in the early stages and use of a side-to-side transfer of flexor digitorum longus, or half the width of the tibialis anterior tendon for the ruptured tendon. Tendon transfer may be combined with a medial displacement osteotomy of the calcaneus. For more advanced disease subtalar or triple arthrodesis may be necessary.

CAVUS FOOT

The first description of pes cavus is credited to Nicholas Andry. Guillaume Benjamin Armand Duchenne of Boulogne (1806–75) systematically tested every susceptible muscle and learned what the function was in the normal state and the abnormal situation in disease or paralysis. Duchenne studied the functional and anatomical collapse of the foot and identified the lesions. He identified three patterns of cavus foot, i.e. due to contracture of peroneus longus, calcaneocavus due to weak triceps surae and a cavus foot due to intrinsic muscle atrophy (Fig. 12.2). There is a variety of possible deformities. Pes cavus refers to a fixed equinus deformity of the forefoot in relation to the hindfoot which results in an abnormally high arch. The forefoot equinus is often accompanied by clawing of the toes. The heel may be neutral, varus, valgus, calcaneus or equinus. Duchenne showed how weakness of the interossei allows the proximal phalanx to be held in a doriflexed position, thereby depressing the metatarsal heads. A weak tibialis anterior in the presence of a normal peroneus longus can cause depression of the first metatarsal head. A weak peroneus brevis results in hypertrophy of the peroneus longus which depresses the first metatarsal head and

causes the forefoot to swing into a pronated position. This latter observation has been confirmed by Tynan using MRI and histology (Tynan et al 1992).

Approximately half the patients with cavus feet present with an obvious neurological disease such as Hereditary Motor-Sensory Neuropathy Type 1 (Charcot–Marie–Tooth disease) spina bifida, cerebral palsy and poliomyelitis. Corrective procedures used for cavus feet have

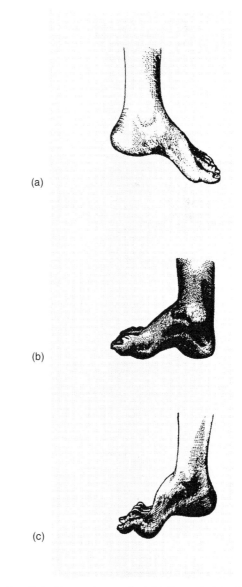

(a)

(b)

(c)

Fig. 12.2 Types of cavus foot. (a) Cavus foot due to contracture of the peroneus longus. (b) Calcaneocavus foot due to weak triceps surae. (c) Cavus foot due to intrinsic muscle atrophy; all from Duchenne

been varied and even today there is no clear consensus as to the optimal approach. As recently as 1949, McMurray in his *A Practice of Orthopaedic Surgery* suggested a tenotomy of the plantar fascia, or more extensive stripping of the undersurface of the calcaneus as described by Steindler, followed by 'a thorough and systematic stretching of the sole by means of the Thomas wrench, and immobilisation in plaster for eight weeks'.

Jones's tendon transfer of extensor hallucis longus to the neck of the first metatarsal first described in 1916 has stood the test of time. This is valuable for correction of the depression of the first metatarsal head and is combined with arthrodesis of the proximal interphalangeal joint of the great toe. Girdlestone's transfer of the flexor to the extensor of the lesser toes is a valuable adjunct to synchronous correction of the great toe (Taylor 1951). Other well-tried procedures that may be used are calcaneal osteotomy, as originally advocated by Dwyer (1959), and triple arthrodesis.

RHEUMATOID FOOT

Rheumatoid arthritis affects both the forefoot and hindfoot. When conservative treatment has failed surgery may be necessary. The commonest hindfoot problem is valgus deformity due to involvement of the subtalar joint. Sometimes the ankle joint is also involved. The standard procedures for hindfoot disorders are used such as triple arthrodesis, ankle arthroplasty or arthrodesis. For the forefoot when the lesser toes become clawed and dorsally dislocated at the metatarsophalangeal joints with rigidus or valgus a variety of operations have been devised from 1912 when Hoffman excised all the metatarsal heads through a plantar incision (Hoffman 1912). Other popular procedures have been Fowler's operation (Fowler 1959), which involved a proximal hemiphalangectomy of all five toes and trimming of the metatarsal heads. A dorsal incision was used with division of all the extensor tendons and removal of a plantar ellipse of skin to bring the toes into a plantarflexed position. In 1960 Flint and Sweetnam advocated amputation of all toes with a long plantar flap and trimming of the metatarsal heads (Flint & Sweetnam 1960). In 1967 Kates, Kessel and Kay described an operation very similar to that of Hoffman with the addition of the excision of a wedge of skin from the sole. Recently there has been an attempt to preserve the metatarsal heads and correct the deformities of the toes by proximal hemiphalangectomy and stabilisation of the toe by suture of the extensor tendon to the flexor at the level of the metatarsophalangeal joint and by replacing the plantar plates underneath the metatarsal heads (Stainsby 1997).

INGROWN TOENAIL (OR NAIL GROWING INTO THE FLESH)

According to Fowler (1958) a logical, simple and effective operation was described by Quénu in 1887. The procedure is the typical wedge excision of the nail and nail bed which is popular today and if the nail is affected on both sides the whole nail matrix can be excised. Colles in an article in 1843 mentioned the use of caustics and Quénu's operation has been reintroduced as Zadik's operation. F. J. W. Porter, a Captain in the Royal Army Medical Corp, in 1900 reported in the *British Medical Journal* his use of phenol on the exposed matrix of the resected wedge of nail removed for an ingrowing nail (Porter 1981). He was at the time stationed in Bloemfontein during the Boer War. Phenolisation of the nail bed is still very commonly used today.

BIOMECHANICS

The work carried out by Verne Inman (1905–80) and his team on the fundamental aspects of human walking at the University of California, San Francisco has extended knowledge of the biomechanics of the lower limb. A number of techniques were used including motion pictures, force plates, interrupted lights, inserted pins, glass walkways and electromyography. The dynamics of human walking was studied and measurements of normal gait were used as a basis for comparison with that of handicapped people. In addition, the development of precise measurements of the pressures beneath the bare foot and insole measurements has been made possible by pedobarography. A variety of techniques have been produced of which the EMEDF apparatus with 1344 capacitance transducers (Hughes et al 1993) is probably the most sophisticated. Four main types of foot pressure measurements exist: optical systems, force plates and load cells, insoles, and pressure pads. More than forty different systems have been documented.

ARTHROSCOPY

This invaluable technique has over the years been adapted for use in the ankle joint, the subtalar joint and, most recently, in the metatarsophalangeal joint of the great toe. New developments in video technology, power tools and holders for the foot and ankle have allowed the arthroscopist to assess and treat a variety of disorders. Although most procedures are excisional in nature, techniques for arthrodesis have been developed which have raised the incidence of successful fusion to 95%. Hinterman et al (2000) reported a prospective series of ankle fractures which were all initially inspected by arthroscopy and provided accurate information of damage to the articular surfaces which may affect the final outcome. Arthroscopy will gradually allow foot and ankle surgeons to develop their knowledge of ankle pathology and raise standards of treatment.

MANAGEMENT OF THE FOOT IN DIABETES

The work of Paul Brand has clearly indicated the role of the orthopaedic surgeon in the management of the foot in diabetes. He applied his experience of management of the insensitive foot in leprosy with the help of his colleagues at Gillis W. Long Hansen's Disease Centre in Carville, Louisiana (Brand 1991). The results of treatment of forefoot ulceration were poor until the introduction of plaster immobilisation by Khan (1939). As the padding in casts becomes compressed, Brand introduced the concept of the total contact cast with minimal padding and a rocker on the sole. He considered that as the calf is conical it will take weight and that there will be a reduction of both shear and vertical force at the sites of high pressure in the sole (Bauman et al 1963). These casts can also be used to prevent deformity and collapse of the hind and midfoot. This type of control can be supplemented by surgery, triple arthrodesis or ankle arthrodesis, but the penalty for failure due to infection or non-union is amputation. The orthopaedic surgeon familiar with the biomechanics of the foot and normal gait is well suited to deal with the neuropathic feet in diabetes uncomplicated by major vascular disease.

THE FUTURE

Foot and ankle surgery has gradually progressed since it started in the first half of the nineteenth century with subcutaneous tenotomy. This has been due to increased knowledge of the physiology and pathology as a result of biomechanical studies, improvements in imaging, accurate gait analysis and pressure measurements. Operative surgery has improved with new techniques of internal and external fixation and become less invasive with arthroscopy. There has been much greater interest in the foot and ankle as shown by the number of national societies and an international society, the International Federation of Foot and Ankle Societies, with new textbooks in two and three volumes and journals devoted to the subject. Indeed the International Federation of Foot and Ankle Societies was founded in 1999 and now unites the societies of foot and ankle surgery in Europe, North America and the Far East. With this intense activity further progress is certain. Foot and ankle surgery is now an accepted subspecialty and has taken its place alongside hand, hip and knee surgery.

Club foot and amputations of the foot and ankle have been omitted from this chapter as these topics are covered in Chapters 10 and 13.

REFERENCES

Badgeley C E Coalition of calconeus and novicular. Arch. Surg. 15: 75–88, 1927

Barker A E 1884 On operation for hallux valgus. Lancet i: 2

Bauman J H, Girling J P, Brand P W 1963 Plantar pressures and trophic ulceration. J Bone Joint Surg 45B: 652–673

Betts L O 1940 Morton's metatarsalgia, neuritis of fourth digital nerve. Med J Australia 1: 514–515

Brand P W 1991 The insensitive foot including leprosy. In: Jahss M H (ed) Disorders of the Foot, vol. 3. W B Saunders, Philadelphia, pp 2170–2186

Camper P 1781 Ober den bestern Shoen. Amsterdam; trans. as The Best Form of Shoe by Dowie J 1861. Handwick, London

Christie A J, Weinberger K A, Dietrich M 1977 Silicone lymphadenopathy and synovitis. J Am Med Assoc 237: 1463–1464

Clutton H H 1894 The treatment of hallux valgus. St Thomas' Hospital Reports 22: 1–12

Davies-Colley J N C 1887 Contraction of the metatarsophalangeal joint of the great toe. Br Med J 1: 728

Duchenne G B Physiology of motion-translated and edited by Emmanuel B Kaplan. Philadelphia. J B Lippinott Conpeny 1949. Original Book 1862

Dunn N 1928 In: Suggestions based on ten years' experience of arthrodes of the tarsus in the treatment of deformities of the foot. Fairbank H A T (ed) The Robert Jones Birthday Volume. Oxford University Press, Oxford, p 395

Durlacher L 1845 A treatment on corns and bunions, the disease of nails and the general management of the feet. Simpkins, Marshall & Co, London

Dwyer F C 1959 Osteotomy of the calcaneum for pes cavus. J Bone Joint Surg 41B: 80–86

Evans E 1928 Laming astragelectomy. In: Fairbank H A T (ed) The Robert Jones Birthday Volume. Oxford University Press, Oxford, p 375

Flint M, Sweetnam D R 1960 Amputation of all toes. J Bone Joint Surg 42B: 90–96

Fowler A W 1955 Tibialis posterior syndrome. J Bone Joint Surg 37B: 520

Fowler A W 1959 A method of forefoot reconstruction. J Bone Joint Surg 41B: 507–513

Fowler A W 1958 Excision of the germinal matrix: a unified treatment for embedded toe-nail and onychogryphosis. Br J Surg 45: 382–387

Gordon M, Bullough P G 1982 Synovial and ossous inflammation of failed silicone prostheses. J Bone Joint Surg 64: 514–580

Guiloff R J, Scadding J W, Klenerman L 1984 Morton's metatarsalgia. J Bone Joint Surg 66B: 586–591

Hancock H 1873 On the operative surgery of the foot and ankle joints. J & A Churchill, London

Hardy R H, Clapham J C R 1951 Observations on hallux valbus. J Bone Joint Surg 36B: 272–293

Harris R I, Beath T 1948 Etiology of peroneal spastic flat foot. J Bone Joint Surg 30B: 624–634

Harris R J, Beath T 1947 Army Foot Survey. An investigation of foot ailments in Canadian soldiers. National Research Council of Canada, Ottawa

Hawkins F B, Mitchell L, Hedrick D W 1945 Correction of hallux valgus by osteotomy. J Bone Joint Surg 27: 387–394

Hicks H 1954 Mechanics of the foot. Plantar aponeurosis and arch. J Anat 88: 25

Hicks J H 1951 The function of the plantar aponeurosis. J Anat 85: 414

Hinterman B, Reggazoni P, Lampert C, Statz G, Gechter A 2000 Arthroscopic findings in acute fractures of the ankle. J Bone Joint Surg 82B: 345–351

Hoadley A E 1893 Six cases of metatarsalgia. Chicago Med Recorder 5: 32–37

Hoffman P 1912 An operation for severe grades of contracted or clawed toes. Am J Ortho Surg 9: 441

Hughes J, Clark P, Lings K, Klenerman L 1993 A comparison of two studies of the pressure distribution under the feet of normal subjects using different equipment. Foot and Ankle International 14: 514–519

Jones R 1916 Claw foot. Br Med J 1: 749

Jones Sir R 1897 Peroneal spasm and its treatment. Liverpool Medico-Chirurgical J 17: 442

Kates A, Kessel L, Kay A 1967 Arthroplasty of the forefoot. J Bone Joint Surg 49B: 552–557

Keller W L 1904 Surgical treatment of bunions and hallux valgus. NY Med J Philadelphia Med J 80: 141–142

Ker R F, Bennett M B, Bibby S R, Kester R C, Alexander R McN 1987 The spring in the arch of the human foot. Nature 325: 147–149

Kettelkamp D B, Alexander H H 1969 Spontaneous rupture of the posterior tibial tendon. J Bone Joint Surg 51A: 759–764

Khan J S 1939 Treatment of leprous trophic ulcers. Leprosy in India: 11–19

Kirkup J 1991 Bone and joint excisions of the foot. Foot 1: 165–166

Kirkup J 1992 Arthrodeses of the hindfoot. Foot 2: 55–56

Kofoed H 1999 Ankle arthroplasty in patients younger and older than 50 years. Foot and Ankle Intl 20: 501–506

Lambrinudi C 1927 New operation on drop foot. Br J Surg 15: 193–200

Le Vay D 1990 The History of Orthopaedics. Parthenon, Carnforth

Lloyd E J 1936 Hallux valgus – a comparison of the results of two operations. Br J Surg 24: 341–345

Mayo C 1908 Surgical treatment of bunions. Ann Surg 48: 300–302

McBride E D 1935 Conservative operation for bunions. J Am Med Asson 105: 1164–1168

McElvenny R T 1943 The aetiology and surgery of intractable pain about the fourth metatarsophalangeal joint (Morton's toe). J Bone Joint Surg 25: 675

McMurray T P 1949 A Practice of Orthopaedic Surgery, 3rd edn. Edward Arnold, London

Morton T G 1876 A peculiar and painful affliction of the fourth metatarsophalangeal articulation. Am J Med Sci 71: 37–45

Mulder J D 1951 The causative mechanism in Morton's metatarsalgia. J Bone Joint Surg 33B: 94–95

Nissen K I 1948 Plantar digital neuritis. J Bone Joint Surg 30B: 84–94

O'Doherty D P, Lowrie I G, Magnussen P A, Gregg P J 1990 The management of the painful first metatarsophalangeal joint in older patients. Arthrodesis or Keller's arthroplasty. J Bone Joint Surg 72B: 839–842

Pomeroy G C, Pike R H, Beals T C, Manoli A 1999 Acquired flatfoot in adult due to dysfunction of the tibialis posterior tendon. J Bone Joint Surg 81A: 1173–1182

Porter F J W 1981 The treatment of affections common in military practice. Br Med J ii: 476

Rose G K 1991 Pes Planus. Chapter 37. In: Jahes M (ed) Disorders of the Foot and Ankle. W B Sanders, Philadelphia Pg 892–920

Silver C M, Simon S D, Spindell E, Litchman H M, Scale M 1967 Calcaneal osteotomy for valgus and varus deformities of the foot in cerebral palsy. J Bone Joint Surg 49A: 232–246

Slomann H C 1921 on Coalitie Calcaneo-navicularis J. Orthop. Surg. 3: 586–601. 1921

Stainsby D 1997 Pathological anatomy and dynamic effect of the displaced plantar plate – deep transverse ligament tie bar. Ann Roy Coll Surg Engl 79: 58–68

Swanson A B, Lumsden R M, Swanson G de G 1979 Silastic implant arthroplasty of the great toe. Clin Ortho 142: 3–43

Taylor R G 1951 The treatment of claw toes by multiple transfers of flexor into extensor tendons. J Bone Joint Surg 33B: 539–542

Tynan M C, Klenerman L, Helliwell T R, Edwards R H T, Hayward M 1992 Investigations of muscle imbalance in the leg in symptomatic forefoot cavus. Foot and Ankle International 13: 489–501

Whitman R 1901 The operative treatment of paralytic talipes of the calcaneous type. Am J Med Sci 122: 593–601

Williams R 1963 Chronic non specific tendovaginitis of the tibialis posterior. J Bone Joint Surg 45B: 542–545

13

Amputation surgery from 1800 to the present

Kingsley P. Robinson

By 1800 many of the basic principles of the management of amputees were already established. Jean Ullrick Bilguer the Prussian Military Surgeon and advocate of debridement (1764) for many of the battlefield injuries that had previously been treated by amputation defined the indications for major limb amputation as follows:

- Gangrene spread to reach bone.
- Severe fracture or disruption.
- Violent contusion of soft parts.
- Wounds of larger vessels.
- The incurable infection of bone.
- Part attacked by cancer.

He shared this conservative approach to major limb amputation with John Hunter (1728–93) who although he had a very limited experience of military surgery in Portugal is widely recognised for his contribution to general surgical principles. The high mortality rate associated with amputation was due to the inability to treat the initial consequences of trauma, haemorrhage and what was at one time referred to as shock, followed by inevitable infection and its feared consequence of septicaemia, infective gangrene and secondary haemorrhage.

At that time there was a dispute between the military surgeons about the best management of severe limb trauma and gunshot wounds. There was considerable animosity between the proponents of conservatism, debridement and early active intervention with immediate amputation.

Dominique Jean Larrey (1766–1842), with the French army of Napoleon, had a phenomenal record for the speed and number of amputations, but more important was his organisation of a stretcher-bearing contingent 'ambulance volante' organised to pick up the injured from the battlefield in a manner that was followed with success in recent modern conflicts (Larrey 1817).

He also organised the administration of fluids and broth made from the slaughtered horses for the injured who would otherwise have died from progressive neglect and dehydration. Nevertheless in company with G. J. Guthrie (1785–1842) of the British Forces he insisted that the sooner an amputation was performed the more likely the outcome would be favourable (Guthrie 1815) (Fig. 13.1).

It was well recognised at that time that any surgery carried out in a crowded military or civilian hospital was attended with a high incidence of hospital fever, suppuration and mortality. The Liverpool surgeon Edward Alanson (1747–1823) made the cogent observation 'many hospitals so tainted by unwholesome effluvia, that they are rather a pest than a relief to the object they contain' and he made the following recommendations abbreviated here 'that each ward should be cleared and cleaned at least once in four months and that bedsteads should be ironed to allow easy cleaning, bedding should be frequently changed, bedding should be aired in the open and that patients on admission should be bathed and attired in fresh clean clothing while their own clothing was cleaned to be returned to them at discharge' (Alanson 1782). He emphasised the importance of ventilation and suggested chronically infected patients with leg ulcers should not be admitted to treatment wards but segregated and that surgical patients should be in well-ventilated, frequently cleaned special wards. The hospital should not be overcrowded, the nurses should ensure that every patient's hands and face are washed every morning and their feet once a week. Some convalescent facility should be provided remote from the main hospital.

In addition to these common-sense recommendations for hygiene Alanson also made a major contribution to the practice of amputation surgery. He reviewed the practice of his colleagues and felt that too little skin was

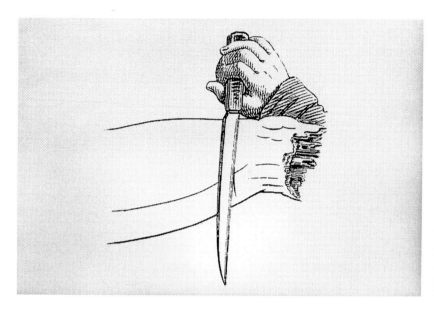

Fig. 13.1 Illustration from James Guthrie from his treatise of gunshot wounds, published in 1815 which shows the backhanded technique of making a circular amputation

saved in most amputations and as the muscles were divided perpendicularly, union by first intention was not attempted. He was concerned that when securing the arteries by transfixion, the ligature frequently included nerves, veins and adjacent parts which he felt contributed to muscle spasms, fever, haemorrhage, purulent discharge and retraction of the muscles. He therefore proposed that a skin flap of sufficient length should be produced while the muscles were divided circularly. The incision was inclined to leave the cut end of the bone at the apex of a conical scar. He was particularly careful to dissect the arteries clean and clear, ligating the artery with a forceps rather than by transfixion. He cleansed the wound thoroughly before closure and advised accurate skin apposition with sutures and adhesive strips.

At this time amputations were carried out as speedily as possible, with the patients premedicated with alcohol and laudanum available as an opiate. Ischaemia with a tourniquet was attempted and sometimes digital pressure on a major nerve prior to the operation was used. Control of primary haemorrhage was obtained by the application of a tourniquet before the surgery commenced. Mechanically efficient tourniquets were pioneered by Bouchet (1966) and a wide variety of winch, windlass and screw devices were applied. The rubber tourniquet of Esmarch (1873) was not introduced until 1857.

Controversy and uncertainty persisted about the best surgical technique. The use of flaps had been described and illustrated since the first account by Lowdham and by Verduyn in 1657.

Every possible variant of circular incision was practised before sophisticated flaps were used. A guillotine

technique literally with a weighted blade was used by one surgeon and a single blow with a heavy cutting instrument had also been used for distal lower and upper limb amputations. The circular amputation cutting from outside inward appears to have been the most commonplace and sickle-shaped knives were designed and used to facilitate this procedure as illustrated in the famous – but now lost – painting in the Royal College of Surgeons (Fig. 13.2).

A modification in which the skin was circumscribed distally, retracted so that the fat and fascia were divided, then the muscles and most proximally the bone, as described by Hey (1803) and Bell (1888) became a favoured technique, particularly with the military surgeons, despite the obvious disadvantage of a terminal scar.

The transfixion method to obtain a flap originally described by Garengot in 1720 became increasingly adopted in which a double-edged knife was thrust as close to the centre of the limb as possible so that cutting outwards from the bone could produce either a vertical incision and a guillotine type of amputation or the incision could be inclined distally to produce an obliquity and the formation of a myocutaneous flap. There appeared to be difficulties in handling the amount of soft tissue that resulted so that defined skin flaps were developed to cover the muscle and bone end. A single skin and fascia flap was described by Carden in 1854. A rectangular long and short myocutaneous flap was recommended by Teale in 1855, which produced a posterior scar and musculocutaneous cover for the bone end. He performed this successfully many years prior to

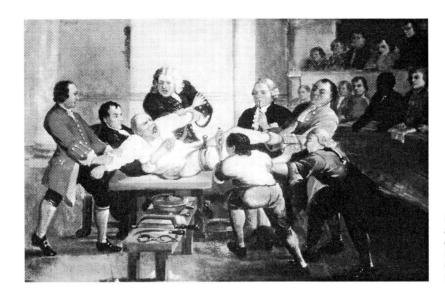

Fig. 13.2   Amputation without anaesthesia at St Thomas's operating theatre, Guy's Hospital. By kind permission of the Royal College of Surgeons of England, London

the introduction of anaesthesia and claimed considerable advantage in the use of a prosthesis, which could have an appreciable degree of end bearing.

Disarticulation appears to have been unpopular at this time. It was felt that synovial tissue was susceptible to infection and synovial fluid had an inhibitory effect on wound healing. Disarticulations were essentially avoided but through-knee amputation had been described by Velpeau (1830) who did not support this view and renewed interest in knee disarticulation. In 1843, James Syme's ankle disarticulation operation was carried out for the first time for tuberculosis of the tarsus and became the established technique for amputation at the ankle. In 1845 he described a modification of knee disarticulation.

Robert Liston in 1837 was established as the fastest surgeon for major limb amputation closely rivalled by Sir William Ferguson, Charles Bell, Syme and Sir Astley Cooper, all prestigious surgeons of their day. An amputation taking more than a few minutes was considered to be unnecessarily prolonged.

A first-hand record of the recent changes was made by Sir Henry Carden in a lecture read at Birmingham in 1864:

under these impressions I commenced hospital practice in 1838; when chloroform the handmaid of conservative surgery, was unknown and when the celerity of execution was the order of the day; when we were taught to stab the limb with Lisfrancs long knife and having made two cuts outward with the rapidity of lightning, and sawn the bone with breathless haste, to consign the severed limb to the sawdust in less than sixty seconds. I adopted these somewhat theatrical performances at that time, operating by the watch as others did; and, I believe with about the same amount of satisfaction and success.

In 1798 Mr Cheselden had reported the case of a miller – Samuel Wood, whose arm was caught in revolving machinery and who avulsed the whole arm and survived the injury requiring only dressings to achieve a full recovery (LeDran et al 1749) (Fig. 13.3). This case contrasted with the severe mortality rate still encountered in major limb amputs, particularly of the lower limb where amputation at above or below knee level might be expected to have a one-third mortality rate in civilian trauma or disease, while on the battlefield the same amputations would result in a 50% mortality rate, a situation that had not improved with the introduction of general anaesthesia and which was largely due to the high incidence of surgical sepsis. Despite the observations of Alanson (1782) it took the circumstances of the conflict in the Crimean War (1854–56) and the American Civil War (1861–65), in which large numbers of amputations were carried out under very poor conditions, to emphasise the importance of cleanliness and the humanitarian management of patients with major injuries.

A most important development was the introduction of antisepsis into surgical practice by Lord Lister in 1867. Despite his convincing evidence of the efficacy of the antiseptic management of wounds, injuries and infections, his methods were only reluctantly adopted into general surgical practice. The concept of asepsis rather than antisepsis was progressively accepted and shown to have as good results. Before the routine use of antiseptic measures and later aseptic principles, vessels were ligated with silk or cotton thread which was left long, protruding through the wound, so that once the vessel thrombosed and sloughed the ligature material

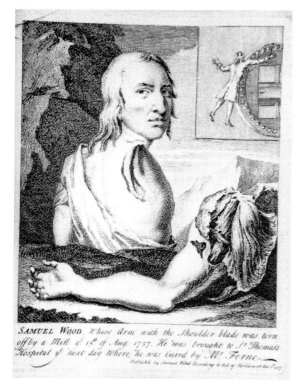

Fig. 13.3 Samuel Wood, the patient quoted by Mr Cheselden in whom a traumatic amputation of the forequarter was healed with simple dressings and without serious sepsis

could be pulled out. It was only the later introduction of catgut as an absorbable ligature material that caused this practice to be abandoned.

With the advances in antisepsis, anaesthesia and haemostasis many variations in amputation techniques were proposed in order to improve healing and produce a more satisfactory residual limb (Fig. 13.4). The introduction of Esmarch's rubber bandage tourniquet (1857) enabled a bloodless field to be obtained, which allowed accurate application of haemostats and saved blood loss as the limbs were emptied of blood (Esmarch 1873). Although a spring-closing front application, forceps of the 'bec de corbin' (crows beak) type had been available from the time of Ambroise Pare the advent of the tip-applied scissors-type of locking forceps devised by Pean and Spencer Wells (Kirkup 1999), became available and brought new precision to ligation of vessels. Despite this in 1916 a tourniquet forceps was described in which a long-bladed forceps with one probe-pointed blade was introduced blindly through a stab incision to run behind a pulsating artery and on closure to compress the artery against the outer blade which remained on the skin surface. This was the tourniquet forceps of Lynn Thomas (1916).

Carden (1864) reported his observation that where skin cover of the amputation was obtained a scar remote from the bone end produced a much more satisfactory stump and he described a technique with the reflection of a skin and fatty flap amounting to half the circumference at the site of amputation with which to cover what was virtually a conventional circular amputation

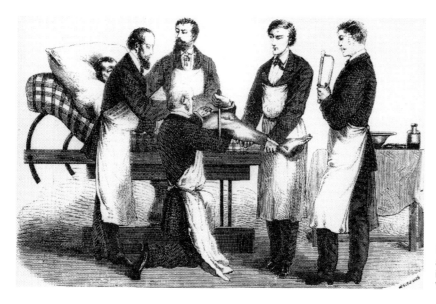

Fig. 13.4 Malgaigne performing an amputation under anaesthesia in 1874. By kind permission of the Welcome Library, London

performed by transfixion. He reported thirty-one patients treated by this technique with five postoperative deaths. Alanson (1782) had previously described the modification of the circular amputation in which the bone was sectioned proximal to the soft tissue.

The circular operation was progressively modified to take on a sleeve configuration. Hey (1803) had described a method in which the skin cut longer than the muscles, the muscles cut longer than the bone so that soft tissue could turn in over the bone end to leave a terminal scar. Teale (1855) of Leeds proposed that a back cut from the circular incision should be utilised to make an anterior and posterior myocutaneous flap where the anterior flap was long and the posterior flap short, except at the transtibial level when the longer flap was posterior. The long single myocutaneous flap described originally by Pierre Verduyn in 1669 was a well-known procedure. The essential principle of the Teale operation was that the longer flap would fold over the bone end and be sutured to the shorter flap. This was the first attempt at a myoplasty to provide adequate soft tissue cover over the bone end. It is recorded that the lower limb stumps produced in this way were favourably viewed by artificial limb-makers of the day who were able to allow a degree of end-bearing on these stumps.

As the basic techniques of amputation developed, the methods of performing the less frequently performed amputations became more sophisticated and new methods were described. A number of ankle and foot procedures in addition to that of Syme had already been described such as the Chopart operation (1814) with disarticulation at the talonavicular and calcaneocuboid joints and the Lisfranc (1815) amputation, disarticulation of the metatarsals along the cuboid and cuneiform articulations. Pirogoff (1991) introduced his osteoplastic amputation at the ankle retaining the posterior half of the calcaneus in the heel flap to obtain bony union with the transected tibia. This became the first of many attempts to improve on the Syme procedure which has been largely adopted as the standard technique for ankle disarticulation. The Gordon Watson (1917) and the Boyd (1939) procedures remove the talus and require a tibiocalcaneal fusion and a similar effect is produced by the Marquardt (1950) procedure. Contemporaries of Pirigoff, Baudens, Rue, Morrel, Chopart, Supa, Sabatier and Velpeau all contributed variations on the method of achieving amputation and disarticulation at this level. Of all these the classic Syme procedure has remained supreme with the ability to stand and walk on the residual limb without a prosthesis. This has been the most important benefit, particularly as most of the amputations at this level were performed for trauma or tuberculosis. Wagner (1977) described a two-stage procedure for use in diabetic patients.

The transtibial level of amputation produced almost as much controversy. There was wide variation in the proposed length of the below knee stump, it being felt for a long time that the longer the stump, the better the function and certainly the smaller the chance of the knee flexors being destroyed. A long anterior flap was recommended by Ferguson (1846) but the long posterior flap has been described by Verduyn and illustrated in Heisters textbook of surgery 1712 and revived in 1956 by Kendrick. Sagittal flaps were described by Sedillot (1835). Every surgeon claimed advantages in healing and function. Even after the introduction of antiseptic surgery and anaesthesia, the place of open amputation was still recognised. Military surgeons recommended that a penetrating wound involving a joint, open contaminated fractures, with nerve or arterial damage should be treated by an unsutured open procedure.

AMPUTATIONS AT THE KNEE

Amputation at the knee is a technically easy operation and its proponents in Hoin, Brasedor, Velpeau (1830) and Symes (1843) all recognised the problem of tenuous soft tissue cover of the large bony condyles, but felt this was offset by the ability of the stump to support the weight of the patient (Fig. 13.5). However the technique was and remains controversial and many attempts have been made to modify it by Mazet (Mazet & Hennessy 1966), Burgess (1977), Baumgartner (1989), Bowker (Bowker & Poonekar 1998) with only marginal improvements to avoid the problem of covering the large condular area. A higher level of amputation at the supracondylar site was proposed by Dr Ricardo Gritti (1857) and subsequently by Dr William Stokes in Dublin (1870) with the modification of retaining the patella in the quadriceps expansion. The articular surface was removed from the patella and attached to the exposed cancellous bone of the cut end of the femur. The knee flexor muscles were attached to the residue of the patellar tendon. The patella was attached using ligatures through drill holes. Subsequently it was shown that if the patella is inclined slightly upwards posteriorly, the tension of the extensors and flexors would hold it securely in place and minimise the chance of malunion. The operation utilised a long anterior flap of knee skin and was intended to be suitable for weight bearing, with a slender shape that allowed more elegant prosthetic fitting. However, pain from non-union made use of a prosthesis uncertain. The supracondylar Gritti–Stokes amputation was not used for gunshot and battlefield injuries which required primary closure. Despite good

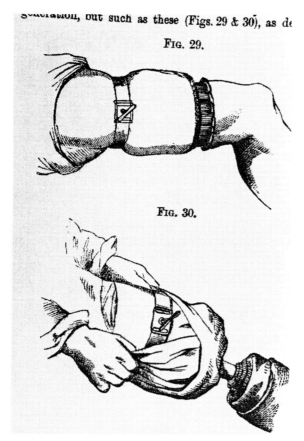

Fig. 13.5 Illustration from the June 1865 lecture on amputation by William Ferguson demonstrating the standard technique for circular amputation below a tourniquet at above knee level

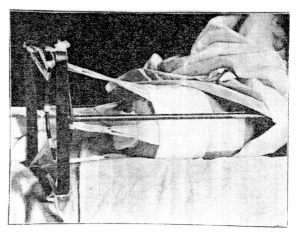

Fig. 13.6 A patient who has had a guillotine amputation at the transfemoral level with the system of skin traction used in 1916 to improve the soft tissue cover of the stump

Dederich (1961) with a more recent study of the function of thigh adductors by Gottschalk and Stills (1992).

In the 1914–18 War under conditions of heavy contamination from trench warfare, the guillotine amputation was reintroduced and performed close to the point of injury and where possible skinflaps were formed and turned back with a view to secondary suture. Later skin traction through adhesive plaster strapping applied to the skin was utilised to prevent undue soft tissue retraction. To avoid the formation of bony spurs, any muscle attached in the vicinity of the bone end was dissected away from the bone and the periosteum was left intact.

AMPUTATION AT THE HIP

Amputation at the hip was the most adventurous and hazardous amputation first performed by Baron Jean Larrey (1817) and James Guthrie (1815) (Fig. 13.7) in the Napoleonic Wars and not long after by John Warren in the USA. The initial operation was a disarticulation leaving the open acetabulum covered with equal flaps of skin which turn in to provide a terminal cicatrix. This amputation proved particularly difficult to fit with a socket prosthesis and subsequently a trend emerged to transect the residual femur at trochanteric level or above with the intention that the residual bone would provide a flatter and wider contour for the application of the socket. Control of haemorrhage from the femoral vessels was dependent on manual pressure; although compressive forceps could be applied they carried the high risk of damage to the external iliac vein and a

initial results the supracondylar amputation without the patella, Weale (1969) has been limited on account of the better function of the transfemoral amputation which allows 12 cm distance beyond the stump to accommodate a knee mechanism in the prosthesis.

The transfemoral amputation was the most widely used with considerable variation in the recommended ideal length termed 'Site of Election' which was specified particularly during the War years (Fig. 13.6). Five inches of femur from the greater trochanter was the minimum length for a satisfactory artificial limb. The distance measured downwards in inches from the greater trochanter varied. Initially the amputation level was close to supracondylar and as distal as possible to allow for the easy placement of the tourniquet, the smallest amount of soft tissue incision and at the same time the greater accessibility of the femoral vessels and sciatic nerve.

Myodesis, the attachment of functioning muscle to bone, was described by Bier (1895), Ertle (1981) and

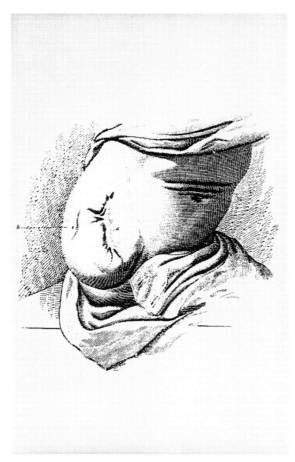

Fig. 13.7 The first patient with hip disarticulation treated in 1820 by James Guthrie

mechanical pressure device that pressed on the aorta was both uncomfortable and complicated by the possibility of damage to the small bowel within the abdomen if adhesions were present.

The prosthesis of the day consisted of a bucket socket with a hinge below at approximately the point corresponding to the acetabulum and controlled with a variety of cords, springs and rubber stops – an arrangement that produced such uncertain function that the majority of amputees with hip disarticulation preferred to mobilise without a prosthesis and use axillary crutches. The hip disarticulation and hip amputation was a feared operation until the advent of blood transfusion although with meticulous technique it was possible to perform the operation without an acceptable mortality rate. The prosthesis was greatly improved with the introduction of the Canadian Tilting Table artificial leg McLaurin (1957).

Hemipelvectomy, or as it was initially known, hind quarter amputation, developed as an elective procedure for tumours of the pelvis, principally chondromata and chondrosarcoma, which was hardly feasible prior to the availability of transfused blood. It should also be remembered that in the 1920s and 1930s the skills of arterial and venous reconstruction and repair by direct suture were uncertain and difficult due to the unsuitable needles and suture materials available at the time and therefore beyond the capability of the general and orthopaedic surgeons of the day. The whole system of surgery was devised to avoid life-threatening blood losses and damage or loss of control of major vessels and nowhere was this more appropriate than in the hind quarter operation. The hind quarter amputation was first carried out by Bilroth in 1891 for a soft tissue sarcoma without survival of the patient. The first survival from the operation was in 1895 and the operation was performed by Giraud (1895). Sir Gordon-Taylor (Gordon-Taylor & Monro 1952) took a special interest in the operation, and his work was continued by Gerald Westbury of the Westminster Hospital, London. Both drew attention to the necessity of early control of the tributaries of the common iliac vein, which are otherwise responsible for considerable venous haemorrhage. The resulting residual tissue makes a soft and rather unsatisfactory basis for a prosthetic socket particularly where a large proportion of the pelvic bony structure ring has had to be resected. The socket is essentially unstable and requires a wide restraining band with a shoulder strap resulting in a heavy and rather cumbersome arrangement, which the patient may choose to discard. For these reasons the operation in which the pelvic resection is carried out with radical principles but with the blood supply and nerve preservation to allow a flail limb to be retained is preferable where it can be achieved (the Tickhoff–Lindberg procedure).

Aust (Aust & Absolon 1960) and Miller (Miller et al 1966) pioneered the translumbar amputation for uncontrolled localised malignancy of the whole pelvis or pelvic osteomyelitis in paraplegia. With a urinostomy and colostomy L2/3 or 3/4 transection can be achieved, with rehabilitation in a trunk socket and wheelchair. This is fortunately a rarely performed procedure in carefully selected patients.

UPPER LIMB AMPUTEES

Upper limb digital amputations have been performed since the earliest days for ritual and other reasons. The bone divided through the base of a phalanx, where possible, to retain the attachment of long tendons and short muscles. The transverse scar is orientated to the dorsal aspect of the digit, taking extreme care to avoid incorporation of Pacinian corpuscles or nerve endings which can produce troublesome pain and neuromata. Disarticulations are less satisfactory but the principal consideration is to retain all functional tissue possible. From the earliest times amputation of a whole digit has raised the problem of whether the associated metacarpal should also be partially resected, a decision related to the patient's needs and occupation. The same principles are applied to the thumb and residue of the hand in severe injury.

Anterior and posterior flaps have evolved as the most satisfactory for major amputations to the upper limb at wrist level. Soft tissue cover is dictated by the residual soft tissue, as is the case in forearm amputations where the principles of myoplasty are applied. The carefully shaped bone ends are an important feature. Elbow disarticulation and transhumeral amputation have changed little. The problems of nerve entrapment were well illustrated by the case of Admiral Lord Nelson in 1794, when postoperative pain was only relieved after the brachial artery ligature sloughed away five months later (Power 1931).

The principles used for upper arm prostheses were established in 1844. The body-powered prosthesis has become progressively more sophisticated by the use of double-action mechanisms, return springs and the incorporation of passive movements operated by the opposite arm. The more severe operation of forequarter amputation, claviculoscapular resection, carried an initial high mortality rate from the difficulty in controlling the vessels as it was impossible to use any sort of tourniquet or mechanical device. It was Guthrie who showed how the subclavian artery could be digitally compressed against the first rib to allow control until the amputation gave access for a ligature. The possibilities of the operation were demonstrated by the successful case of Cheselden (1737) (LeDran et al 1749) in which the forequarter was avulsed by machinery and the patient survived the initial haemorrhage and required only dressings to achieve a full recovery. The need for scapuloclavicular amputation of the arm has been considerably reduced in oncological surgery by the use of massive bone replacements and the occasional acceptance of a flail limb rather than a radical amputation.

The cineplastic procedure devised by Vanghetti (1912) and performed by Ceci (1906) exteriorised tendons in a skin bridge to transmit their function to an arm prosthesis. While effective it is little used. The simpler Krukenberg procedure (1917) to separate and cover with skin the residual radius and ulna to form opposable jaws provides excellent function. Unfortunately this procedure finds little aesthetic acceptance and is therefore limited to bilateral forearm amputees with visual loss. In underdeveloped countries it is an extremely effective method of restoring function without the need for any prosthesis (Mathur et al 1981).

Progress in general principles was made in successive conflicts. The need for an open amputation as an emergency procedure for the mangled or shattered limb, heavily contaminated or with major nerve or blood vessel damage, has been relearned from the Napoleonic conflicts. The surgical practice is well recorded in the American Civil War, the Crimean War and the Boer War, followed by the First and Second World Wars. There was increasing efficiency of casualty retrieval and the organisation of field hospital or casualty-clearing facilities with improved evacuation to both forward and base hospitals. The essential management has been an early debridement. But where there is a clear indication a place remains for a distal simple or even guillotine amputation with an open technique, followed by a secondary closure or re-operation when the patients had reached adequate treatment facilities. Chloroform anaesthesia was first widely used in the latter part of the American Civil War and was uniformly available in the First World War, but despite established principles, contamination left the problem of gas gangrene, clostridial myositis and other infections as a major cause of loss of life and the need for amputation.

Prior to the introduction of antibiotics a considerable advance was made in 1937 when Winnett Orr (1929) and Trueta (Trueta & Barnes 1940) described the technique of debridement followed by plaster immobilisation for complex limb injuries with open fractures and soft tissue loss. This method was applied with success in the Spanish Civil War and later adopted as a first line of treatment for British Forces. It was improved further for the lower limb immobilisation with a Thomas' splint which was incorporated in a plaster of Paris. As a result of its success in the Western Desert Campaign, it was known as the Tobruk splint.

The adoption of this more conservative regimen resulted in a considerable reduction in the number of battle amputations. By 1940 sulphonamides were available and by 1942 penicillin became widely available to the Armed Forces. Evacuation procedures became increasingly sophisticated. The increased use of air transport resulted in earlier access to base hospitals for major surgical management. The introduction of helicopters for frontline casualty evacuation was not established until the Korean conflict and the Vietnam War when their extensive use for casualty retrieval produced a significant reduction of time to primary treatment and a diminution in amputation rates.

During the Second World War (1939–45) amputation technique in general was improved with education of service medical officers and surgical staff due to increased cooperation with centres which dealt with primarily the amputees. Queen Mary's Hospital, Roehampton was the largest and dealt with 26,262 amputees from the First World War and twenty thousand more disabled and two thousand civilian casualties in the Second World War. This centre initiated the close cooperation between the limb-makers, the limb-fitting facilities and the casualties producing an association that generated a sound basis for education and practice.

An important development in Germany was the introduction of the osteomyoplasty to the transtibial amputation to improve the muscle function in young amputees. The procedure designed by Ertl (1981) in which part of the fibula was utilised as a bony bridge across which the gastrocnemius/soleus mass could act efficiently as a strong knee-flexor, constituted an osteomyoplasty. Although not frequently carried out now, the principle added to the observations of Bier (1895) and Teale (1855) that functioning muscle in an amputation stump was an advantage for better function.

Major amputations continue to be caused by transport accidents, particularly road and rail traffic, but are also due to terrorist activities and land mine injuries are emerging as a major problem, during and after regional conflict. The latter are responsible for a high incidence of transtibial amputations. While there are reports of primary suture with antibiotic adminis-tration, the principles of thorough debridement, with delayed primary suture at three to five days, are restated by Coupland (1991).

PROSTHESES

Prior to the commencement of the nineteenth century an articulated prosthesis for below knee amputees had been designed by Verduyn in 1696. In 1775 an ankle spring had been devised and in 1796 a flexible foot had been produced. In 1800 James Pott had produced pros-theses for above knee amputees with articulations at knee and ankle in which flexion of the knee produced plantar flexion of the foot. The basic construction was carved from wood. This leg became known as the Anglesey leg as it was used by the Earl of Anglesey following his amputation at the Battle of Waterloo (1815). This leg became the pattern for prostheses in America and was further developed in 1839 by William Selpo, Benjamin Palmer and J.E. Hanger. A rubber foot was introduced in 1860 and in 1863 D.D. Parmalee introduced an above knee prosthesis with a suction socket, polycentric knee joint and a multiarticulated foot. Dr Heather Bigg (1885) in London, who is best described as a limb-fitting surgeon dealing with servicemen from the Crimean War, was able to prescribe

a simple carved socket peg leg for the amputee veterans while the officers were prescribed articulated limbs. He emphasised the importance of the shape of the bone in an amputation stump and devised a conical reamer to obtain the optimum shape. The principle of ischial weight bearing had been developed in 1831. Until the introduction of the sheet metal aluminium socket by Desouttar in 1922, the majority of sockets were block leather with lacing or carved wood. This led to a vogue for an all metal limb which was essentially exsoskeletal in design. As an initial or temporary limb the pylon was widely used. It was essentially a leather socket with side irons, a simple hinge knee, a sliding lock and a rocker foot piece. This was superseded by the pneumatic walking aid. The advent of new materials had a dramatic effect on prosthetic development, with the use of resin polymers, composites and polypropylene. These enabled accurate production of the socket from casts. More recently computerised design and manufacture has given additional precision. Production of a suction socket was greatly facilitated and the principle of the patellar tendon-bearing socket for transtibial amputees could be readily applied without any thigh corset. The Patellar Tendon-bearing prosthesis designed in California by Radcliffe and Foorte (1961) became sophisticated and gave the below knee amputee the ability to run, climb and take part in sporting activities with little difficulty. Development of the prosthetic foot with energy-storing springs has increased athletic capa-bility. Carbon fibre and composite materials have reduced the weight and increased the strength of components of the above knee prosthesis. The socket has become total contact with either ischial contain-ment or ischial weight bearing. The prosthesis has become endoskeletal frequently using modular compo-nents. There have been continuing developments of the knee joint mechanism incorporating inertia locks, swing phase controls, hydraulic damping and, most recently, computerised adjustment of the swing characteristics to match the patient's mode of walking. In a knee joint util-ising parallelogram geometry, the four-bar linkage provides stability when extended and free movement when flexed. It has the particular advantage that the geometric centre of flexion can be above the unit making it invaluable for the through knee prosthesis where the alternative would be hinges below or on either side of the already wide knee.

PROGRESS

Great progress has been made in the retention of lower limb prostheses. The rigid pelvic band with external hip hinge is less frequently required, as is the Silesian belt with its strap across the shoulder. The suction socket has become highly sophisticated for the transfemoral amputee and some close-fitting total-contact sockets are self-retaining. For the transtibial amputee the suspension has progressed from a suprapatellar strap to the condylar grip of the patellar tendon suspension type of socket to suspension by means of a silicone sleeve, an elastic stocking and, most recently, by a silicone sock in the Iceross and Icex system where a ratchet-locking device is incorporated in the silastic to engage the socket and provide secure fixation Kristinsson (1993). This principle can also be applied to the transfemoral amputee. When other techniques cannot be tolerated by the patient, the prosthesis fixed to bone using the osseo-integration principle is a possibility.

In the upper limb the prostheses have developed from carved, wooden-jointed extremities passively operated by the opposite hand to highly sophisticated controlled and motorised prostheses. In 1818, a dentist, Peter Baillif, suggested the use of cords running from the trunk and shoulders to operate mechanical fingers moving against the rigid thumb, which was improved by Eichler. The principle has been applied to above elbow prostheses to obtain flexion and extension of the elbow, as well as finger movement, also powered from the shoulders, with pronation and supination of the wrist and forearm being passive, operated by the opposite hand. In 1886 Claeseu devised a more powerful hand, but the later Carnes arm (1904) was more successful, although heavy. Gears drove a powerful grip, while elbow flexion was combined with supination. In the bilateral amputee, body power can be utilised with a satisfactory cosmetic appearance in the fully dressed patient. The simplicity and effectiveness of body power has limited the usefulness of the cineplastic procedures necessary to obtain finger function.

There is much enthusiasm for the mechanical hand and arm prosthesis, with sophisticated control mechanisms and internal power sources. Great efforts and resources were devoted to producing such prostheses for the victims of the thalidomide disaster and a whole range of upper limb prostheses powered by compressed gas or electric battery power were devised. Sophisticated control mechanisms were operated mechanically by contraction of a proximal muscle or, in the case of thalidomide patients, with the residual fingers of the vestigial hand at shoulder level. The myoelectric control has proved extremely satisfactory and dramatic improvement in rechargeable nickel cadmium batteries has made electric power the best option with micro-actuators that can produce sophisticated finger and thumb function. There are now many patients using myoelectric arm prostheses to great advantage, particularly those with

bilateral arm amputations. However there are many patients who following a trial of the myoelectric prosthesis elect for the lightweight and simplicity of the body-powered prosthesis preferring the split hook to a prosthetic hand except on occasions when appearance is all important. A non-functioning silicone hand can deceive all but the closest inspection. There remain a considerable number of unilateral arm amputees who rapidly become proficient for all life requirements using the remaining arm and accept their disability without any prosthesis at all.

The rapid increase in the number of amputations for arterial ischaemic disease in the 1950s affecting an ageing population demanded some means of early walking. At that time most were transfemoral amputations, and M. B. Devas (1971) pioneered the use of an improvised socket and second-hand parts from discarded prostheses to make temporary walking appliances for the patients to use as soon as their amputation stumps were healed. He demonstrated the considerable benefit to the patients by the early activity.

In a similar situation the Femurett walking aid was devised, a manufactured, preshaped, transfemoral amputation socket with a simple leg extension for use before a definitive prosthesis was prescribed. The alternative where a limb-fitting facility was available was at that time to supply a simple pylon with a rocker foot, simple knee lock and leather or metal socket, which could be replaced with a definitive prosthesis when the stump was mature and the patient showed that they were able to make effective use of a prosthesis.

The Jobst Company in the USA had introduced a pneumatic inflatable cylinder as a first aid method for immobilising limb fractures. It was suggested that this might be used as an early walking aid. The most successful adaptation was the pneumatic walking aid adapted and designed by Professor Little (1971) in Sydney, who advised its use in the way that the immediate plaster socket for the prostheses was used, applied on the operating table and then used to allow the patient to stand and later walk in the postoperative period. This was achieved by making the pneumatic cylinder the centre of a frame bearing a rocker foot. At Roehampton this device was tried and enthusiastically accepted (Fig. 13.8). Some redesign by Redhead et al (1978) resulted in increased stability and a range of sizes was produced commercially so that the per-operative amputation mobility device was retained for use in the walking training school and applied to the patients attending for rehabilitation and also to the patients being managed in the specialist rehabilitation centre and the surgical unit for amputees at the hospital. The pneumatic aid provided all the advantages of early walking, retention of muscle function, and

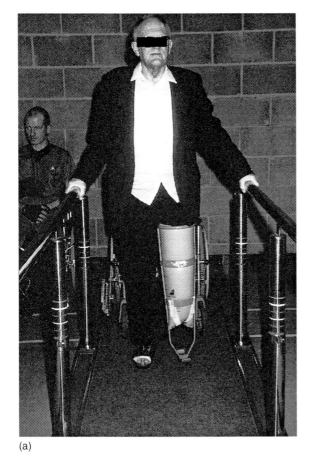
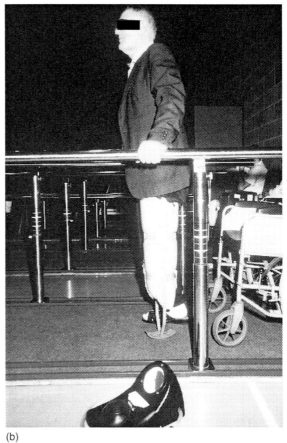

(a)   (b)

Fig. 13.8a,b   A patient demonstrating the use of the pneumatic walking aid as an effective device for early walking within forty-eight hours of amputation surgery (1997)

balance, control of oedema and psychological encouragement without the hazard of a plaster socket.

The experience provided by the immediately fitted plaster socket and prosthesis (Vitali & Redhead, 1967) and subsequently by the pneumatic walking aid resulted in the evolution of an integrated multidisciplinary team and later to the establishment of a specialist unit for amputation surgery and management at Roehampton. The success of this multidisciplinary approach was widely accepted and has been maintained worldwide since that time.

IMMEDIATE FITTING OF A PROSTHESIS

The idea of a plaster socket to be applied to the stump on the operating table was an attractive one, so that function could start as soon as possible after the amputation (Figs. 13.9 and 13.10). Berlemont (1961) in France described a method of immediate per-operative fitting of a prosthesis (IPOFP) also applied by Weiss in Poland (1969). Large-scale evaluation and development was carried out by Burgess and Romano (1968) in Seattle, USA, with the support of the Veteran's administration.

Burgess and Romano realised that the conventional transtibial amputation was unsuitable for use in the plaster socket and they adopted the long posterior flap procedure and found as an incidental finding that they achieved a higher percentage of patients with healing of their transtibial amputations than most of the published results at that time. It was also apparent that they achieved a much higher rate of below knee amputations than the experience of other centres suggested in patients with vascular disease (Fig. 13.11).

The method was widely used in the USA and some European centres, but a voice of caution was introduced when a few centres reported less than favourable results,

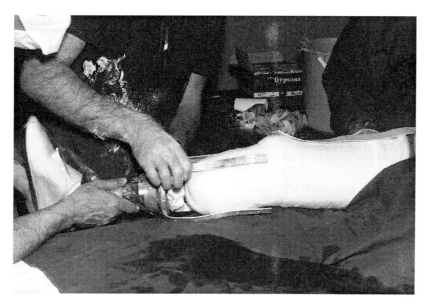

Fig. 13.9 A patient who has had a plaster socket and leg extension applied on the operating table, shown at the conclusion of the operation (1969)

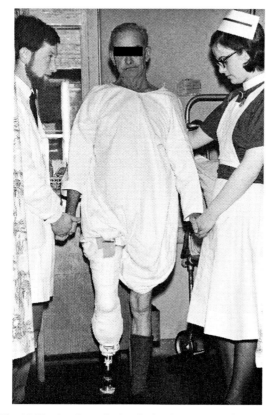

Fig. 13.10 A patient who has had a plastercast socket applied on the operating table (see Fig. 13.9) with the leg extension piece, shown on the third postoperative day with assistance to make ground contact with the prosthesis (1967)

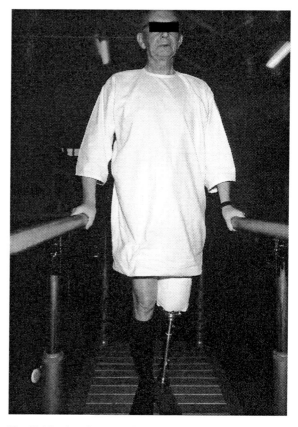

Fig. 13.11 A patient standing with partial weight bearing one week after immediate per-operative fitting of plaster socket to transfemoral amputation. Burgess technique (1969)

but possibly where the facilities for rapid plaster change were not available, or the protocol of the Seattle team not accurately observed. The method was used in London but increasing anxiety about the risk of a recent amputation concealed in a close-fitting plaster and the occurrence of one patient out of the series of twelve in our series who required a re-amputation for gas gangrene led to a search for an alternative. However in the upper limb, a different situation was encountered.

The early development of one-handiness and the failure to accept a prosthesis can be effectively eliminated by the provision of a temporary prosthesis, with a plaster socket on the operating table at the time of surgery (Fig. 13.12). A small series was carried out at Roehampton and the advantages demonstrated. The low incidence of primary arm amputations and the practical difficulties of providing the temporary prosthesis has prevented the technique being widely accepted.

RECENT ADVANCES

The bony attachment of a limb prosthesis has been a distinct prospect for amputees who have been unable to tolerate a conventional prosthetic socket. The first use of metal penetrating a living bone was by Malgaigne in 1843. Experimental work on a bone-fixed prosthesis had been small-scale and sporadic, often poorly recorded in the literature. A project to develop this in 1942 in the USA was rejected. In 1946 Dr Dummer in Germany commenced a study of metal-implanted limb extensions in sheep, extending into a study on human patients, four of whom had metal-implanted prostheses. When one became infected, the implants were removed from all four

patients and the study discontinued. In the USA Mooney fitted a prosthesis to the humerus in a triple amputee but, following increased leakage, the implant was removed after a few months. A study of penetrating implants to a fixed prosthesis was carried out by Esslinger (1965), Hall and Rospoter (1980) who had a considerable degree of success with implants into the hind limbs of Spanish goats; out of twenty only two failed over fourteen months.

While engaged in research in Oxford the now Professor Branemark studied microcirculation in bone and adapted the Clarke Sanderson observation chamber for microscopy of living tissue for the study of blood flow in bone and bone marrow. He made a tubular funnel into the bone marrow, and the material chosen for this was titanium. When each individual study was completed it was necessary to remove the chamber and this was found to be technically extremely difficult as the metal surface appeared to be integrated with the bone structure.

As a result a commercially pure titanium implant was developed that could be secured in the medullary cavity of the long bones. A sophisticated design and attachment system has been evolved at the Branemark Institute in Sweden (Gunterburg et al 1998). The implant consists of an internal tubular component with an internal screw thread to accept the retention bolt which secures the abutment extension, which is inserted into the distal end of the implant (Fig. 13.13). This type of implant is most satisfactory in a tubular section of bone and is therefore the best applications for the humerus, radius, ulna and femur. While a much smaller version is for use in the metacarpals and phalanges for reconstruction of digital, thumb and part hand losses.

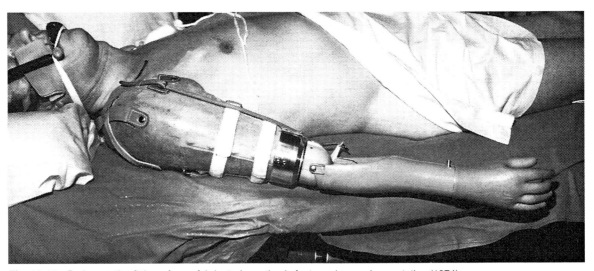

Fig. 13.12   Peri-operative fitting of a prefabricated prosthesis for trans-humeral amputation (1974)

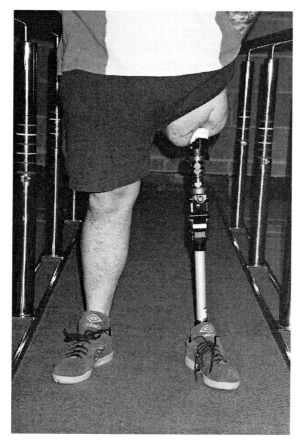

Fig. 13.13 A patient with a bony fixed prosthesis using the Branemark technique (1998)

The external component, the abutment, at its distal end is shaped into a square-section rectangular portion for the fixation of the prosthesis which is secured to this by a screw clamp, operated by an Allen key, which can be inserted through the side of a cosmetic cover of the artificial limb.

This technique has been applied to fifty patients in Sweden and five in the UK. The implant is inserted at a preliminary operation and the stump closed for at least six months in the lower limb for healing and 'osseo-integration' to take place. A second operation is required to insert the abutment, which penetrates the skin at the distal part of the stump to which the prosthesis is attached. A further period is required before mechanical load can be applied. All the patients are those in whom conventional prosthetic use has proved impossible. Infection and loosening had occurred, but only in a very small number of patients, most achieving good prosthetic function.

Reference has been made to the use of internal prosthetic replacement for excised bone in limb surgery.

Silastic implants have been used experimentally to improve the characteristics of the bone end in amputations but have not proved their worth for routine practice.

PAIN

Pain in amputation stumps has been a long-term problem. Ambroise Pare is credited with the first description of 'Phantom Pain', and the pain experienced by Admiral Lord Nelson is well documented due to the inclusion of a nerve trunk in the brachial artery ligature.

Neuromata have been recognised and pain attributed to their formation. To avoid these, it was recommended that the nerve should be crushed and ligated in the area just proximal to the nerve division. This was standard practice in the 1914–18 War. Now division of the major nerves under traction is advised, so that the nerve section is above the healing tissue. Many attempts have been made to implant the nerve in a muscle or a drill hole in the bone. Adhesives have been applied and various caps have been used to encase the cut end of the nerve. The most elegant technique is to split the nerve and anastomose the cut ends to inhibit neurofibril formation.

In the Boer War painful stumps were treated by percussion, now superseded by the TENS (transcutaneous nerve stimulation), which has had some limited success. Proximal nerve and central nervous system surgery has met with little success, while spinal cord stimulation is still under evaluation.

SECONDARY SURGERY

Secondary surgery to correct faults in the residual limb has become increasingly accepted, with scar revision, where necessary meshed skin grafting, soft tissue microvascular transfer, bone lengthening by the Ilizarov technique (Latimer 1990), remodelling of unsatisfactory bone ends with the incorporation of myodesis or myoplasty to restore the best possible function. Where a painful stump has a trigger point that may represent entrapment of a nerve in scar tissue or a neuroma surgical exploration is frequently successful.

Advances in the field of plastic and reconstructive surgery have brought the involvement of these disciplines to amputation. The use of microvascular vessel and nerve anastomosis techniques for tissue transfer can avoid some amputations in severe trauma where soft tissue loss, for example from the sole of the foot or the soft tissue over a joint or complex compound fracture, would otherwise require an amputation. Alternatively they secure an additional length of residual limb by making up the defect in soft tissue at the end of the stump. A feature of some importance is the use of skin and vascularised tissue from the amputated extremity to be used to gain length in the residual limb and where re-implantation of the extremity severed in a traumatic amputation may be considered.

The decision for re-implantation remains one of the most difficult. In the lower limb re-implantation has proved disappointing, with an end result inferior to that of an amputation and a satisfactory prosthesis, but in a child a lower limb re-implantation is extremely worthwhile and re-implantation of the upper limb at all ages is advantageous when it can be satisfactorily achieved and the more distal the loss the better the result is likely to be. The nerve regeneration and reconnection and the time involved to achieve this has emerged as the main limiting factor for success or failure. Overall re-implantation must represent the pinnacle of achievement of amputation management while the use of the same technology for limb transplantation has been demonstrated in the upper limb and depends on the long-term safety of the necessary immunosupression to determine its practical value for the future. Advances in this field may yet bring the miracle of Sts Cosmos and Damien, described in the fifteenth century, to reality (see Chapter 14).

REFERENCES

Alanson E 1782 Practical Observations on Amputations and the After Treatment, 2nd edn. Johnson, London

Aust J B, Absolon K B 1962 A successful lumbo-sacral amputation, hemicorporectomy. Surgery 52: 756–759

Baumgartner R 1989 Knee exarticulation: technique for amputation of ischaemic extremities. Langenbecks Arch Chir (suppl.)

Bell J 1888 A Manual of the Operations of Surgery. Oliver Boyd, Edinburgh, pp 47–111

Berlemont M 1961 Notre experience de l'appariellage precoce des amputes de membre inferieur aux establisments Helio–Marins de Berck. Ann De Medicine physique 4: 4

Bier A 1895 Weitere Mittheilungen uber tragfaluge Amputationsstumpfe in Bereiche der Diaphysen. Archiv Klin Chir 50: 356, 127: 1

Bigg H R 1885 Artificial Limbs and the Amputations which Afford the Most Appropriate Stumps in Civil and Military Surgery. Heather Bigg, London

Bilguer J U, 1764 De membrorum amputatione rarisime administrada, aut quasi abroganda. Magdeberg: 1761 trans. as A Dissertation on the utility of the Amputation of Limbs. Baldwin, London

Bouchet A 1966 De l'amputation des membres et des instrument que lui sont necessaires. Rev Lyon Med 15: 927–936

Bowker J H, Poonekar P D 1998 Knee disarticulation, an anatomic study. In: Proceedings of the 7th World Congress, ISPO

Boyd H B 1939 Amputation of the foot, with calcaneotibial arthrodesis. J Bone Joint Surg 21: 997–1000

Burgess E M 1977 Disarticulation at the knee, a modified technique. Arch Surg 112: 1250–1255

Burgess E M, Romano R L 1968 The management of lower extremity amputees using immediate post surgical protheses. Clin Orth Rel Res 57: 137–146

Carden H D 1864 On amputation by single flap. Br Med J i: 416

Ceci A 1906 Presse Medical 14: 745

Coupland R M 1991 Amputation for anti-personnel mine injuries of the leg; preservation of the tibial stump using a medial Gastronemius myoplasty. Ann Roy Coll Surg Engl 71: 405–408

Dederich R 1963 Plastic treatment of muscles and bone in amputation surgery. J Bone Joint Surg 45B: 60–66

Devas M B 1971 Early walking of geriatric amputees. Br Med J 1: 394–396

Ertl JW von 1981 Die versorgung von amputationsstumpfen durch osteo-myplastic nach V. Ertl. Z Plast Chir 5: 184–189

Esmarch F 1873 Ueber Kunstliche Blutleere bei Operateonen. Samml Klin Volr no. 58 (Chir 19): 373–384

Esslinger J O 1965 Highlights of V.A. contractual research programme—prosthetics. Bull Prothat Res 10: 197

Fergusson W 1846 System of Practical Surgery, 2nd edn. Churchill, London

Fergusson W 1865 On amputation. Lancet ii: 29–34

Gordon-Taylor Sir G, Monro R 1952 The technique and management of the 'hind-quarter' amputation. Br J Surg 39: 536

Gordon Watson C 1917 A method of amputation at the ankle joint which leaves the heel intact. Tibio-calcaneal resection with amputation of the remainder of the foot. Br J Surg 5: 390–397

Gottschalk F A, Stills M 1994 Biomechanics of transfemoral amputation. Prosthet Orthot Int 18: 12–17

Gritti R 1857 Dell'amputazione del femore al terzo inferiore e della disarticulazione del genoulies. Annals University Milano 161: 5–32

Gunterburg B, Branemark P I, Branemark R, Bergh P 1998 Osseo-integration prostheses in lower limb amputation. XIth World Congress, ISPO, Amsterdam, pp 137–139

Guthrie G J A 1815 A Feature on Gunshot Wounds of the Extremities Requiring Amputation. Burgess & Hill, London

Hall C W, Rostoker W 1980 Permanently attached artificial limbs. Bull Prosthetic Res 17: 98–100

Hey W 1803 Practical Observations in Surgery, illustrated with cases. Cadell & Davies, London

Kendrick R R 1956 Below knee amputation in arterio-sclerotic gangrene. Br J Surg 44: 13–17

Kirkup J R 1999 The history and evolution of surgical instruments. X. Clamps, haemostats and related pivot controlled forceps. Ann R Coll Surg Engl 81: 420–428

Kristinsson O 1993 The ICEROSS concept: a discussion of a philosophy. Prosthet Orthot Int 17: 49–55

Krukenberg H 1917 Ueber plastische Umwertung von Amputationsstumpfen. Enke, Stuttgart

Larrey D 1817 Memoires de Chirugie Militaire et Campagnes. Paris, pp 176–177

Latimer H A (1990) Lengthening of below the knee amputation stumps using the Ilizarov technique. J Orthop Trauma 4: 411–414

LeDran H F, Gataker T, Chelselden W 1749 The Operations in Surgery of Mon. Le Dran with Remarks by William Cheselden. Hitch, London

Lisfranc J 1815 Nouvelle methode operatoire pour l'amputation hastrelle due pied daus sousarticulation tariometatatsienne method precides des noumbrance modification qui a subies celle de Chopart. Gabon, Paris

Lister J 1867 On the antiseptic principle in the practice of surgery. Lancet ii: 353–356, 668–669

Liston R 1837 Practical Surgery. Churchill, London

Little J M 1971 A pneumatic weight bearing temporary prosthesis for below knee amputees. Lancet i: 271–273

Marquard W 1950 Gliedmassenamputationen und Gliederersatz. Wissenshaftliche, Stuttgart

Mathur B P, Narang I C, Piplani C L, Majid M A 1981 Rehabilitation of the bilateral below-elbow amputee by the Kruckenberg procedure. Prothet Orthot Int 5: 135–140

Mazet R Jr, Hennessy C A 1966 Knee disarticulation: a new technique and a new knee mechanism. J Bone Joint Surg 48A: 126

McLaurin C A 1957 The evolution of the Canadian type hip disarticulation prosthesis. Artificial Limbs 44: 22–29

Miller T R, Mackenzie A R, Randall H T, Tigner S P 1966 Hemicorporectomy. Surgery 69: 988–993

Pirogoff N I 1854 Resection of bones and joints and amputations and disarticulation of joints. Trans 1991. Clin Orthop 266: 3–11

Power Sir D'A 1931 Some bygone operations in surgery, VI. Amputation the operation on Nelson in 1797. Br J Surg 19: 171–175, 351–355

Radcliffe C W, Foorte E 1961 The Patellar Tendon Bearing Below Knee Prosthesis. Biomechanics Laboratory, University of California, Berkeley

Redhead R G, Davies B C, Robinson K P 1978 Post amputation pneumatic walking aid. Br J Surg 65: 611–612

Sedillot W 1835 Traite complete l'anatormie de l'homme comprennent la Medicine operatoire, 6 vols. Bourgery & N H Jacob

Stokes W Jr 1870 On supracondylar amputation of the thigh. Med Clin Trans 53: 176–186

Syme J 1843 Amputation at the ankle joint. Edinburgh Monthly Journal of Medical Science no. XXVI, no. 11: 93–96

Syme J 1845 Amputation at the Knee. Lond Edinb Mon J Med Sci 5: 337–341

Teale T P 1855 On Amputation by a Long and a Short Rectangular Flap. J Churchill, London

Thomas L 1916 Emergency amputation in military surgery. Br Med J ii: 482

Trueta J, Barnes JM 1940 Immobilisation in the treatment of infected wounds. Br Med J 2: 46

Vanghetti G 1912 Plastica e prostesi cinematiche. Transversari, Empoli

Velpeau A 1830 Memoire sur l'amputation de la jambre dans L'articulation de genou et description d'un nouveau procede pour pratiquer cette operation. Arch Gen Med 24: 44–60

Verduyn P H F 1657/1969 Dissertatio epistolares de nova artenum decurtandorum ratione. Wolters, Amsterdam

Vitali M, Redhead R G 1967 The modern concept of the general management of amputee rehabilitation, including immediate post-operative fitting. Ann Roy Coll Surg Engl 40: 261–263

Wagner F W Jr 1977 Amputation on the foot and ankle. Current status. Clin Orthop 122: 62–69

Weale F E 1969 The supra-condylar amputation with patellectomy. Br J Surg 56: 589–593

Weiss M 1969 Physiologic amputation, immediate prosthesis and early ambulation. Prosthet Int 8: 38–44

Winnett Orr H 1929 Osteomyelitis and Compound Fractures. Henry Kimpton, London

14

History of the treatment of musculoskeletal tumours

Henry J. Mankin

ANCIENT HISTORY

There is little doubt that cancerous limbs were well recognised by ancient societies and their physicians although little was known about the nature of the lesions, particularly in the early years of our civilisation. The Egyptians reported cancerous growths on various parts of the body in the Ebers papyrus believed to have been written *c.*1500 BC (Bryan 1930, Ebbell 1937). The manuscript recommended cauterisation of benign lesions but warned of the 'cruel nature' of fungating or ulcerating tumours. It was pointed out that those tumours that involved peripheral parts of the body sometimes required amputations or resections and it is likely that some of these procedures were done for cancerous limbs (Olson 1989). In fact, studies of the bones of Egyptian mummies have shown lesions consistent with benign and malignant tumours of bone and cartilage, myeloma and metastatic carcinoma (Struhal 1976, Allison 1980).

The early concepts of the causes of cancer were dominated by the views of two individuals, Hippocrates and Clarissimus Galen. Hippocrates recognised various forms of cancer and attributed them to the pervasiveness of 'black bile', one of four humoral elements he postulated to be responsible for all disease (Hippocrates/Jones 1953–57, Barrow 1972). It was his view that cancer was a systemic disease related to this humoral abnormality rather than a localised process. He coined the word 'karkinos' for the hard lump seen in places such as the breast, likening cancer to a crab because of its way of growth. Galen wrote a treatise on abnormal swellings in 192 AD (Lytton & Resuhr 1978, Kardinal & Tarbro 1979). He advanced the humoral theory and listed an array of abnormal swellings including *karkinoi* and *karkinoma* in many sites, further enlarging the description of the hard nodules originally defined as

cancer by Hippocrates (Lytton & Resuhr 1978). He is also believed to have introduced the word 'sarcoma' for lesions clearly arising in the soft tissues.

These writings provided the world before and shortly after the birth of Christ with views as to the nature of cancerous growth and, equally importantly, the need for concern about the outcome and effective treatment for these lesions. It was not until the sixteenth and seventeenth centuries, however, that the black bile humoral theory was rejected, mainly on the basis of the observations of morbid anatomists such as Vesalius (1543) and others (Olson 1989) who postulated that cancer grew at one site and then spread via the lymphatics or blood stream to other areas of the body. These views were supported in part by John Hunter who felt that coagulated lymph or blood was in large measure responsible for the genesis of tumours and metastases that occurred via these vascular and lymphatic pathways (Dobson 1959).

Two early references to cancer affecting the extremities are included in the canonical literature. The first was most extraordinary and consisted of a 'miracle' performed by Saints Cosmas and Damian in the sixth century AD (Gerlitt 1939, Rinaldi 1987, Julien et al 1993). The saints were twin physicians born in the third century AD in the town of Egea in Cilicia in Asia Minor (modern Turkey). They travelled widely in Greece and Asia Minor and went to Rome, treating ailments of all sorts and refusing payment for their services. They somehow angered the Emperor Diocletian (284–305) and after a variety of attempts to kill them, they and their three brothers were beheaded and buried in a grave in Egea in 287 (Curie & Curie 1898, Ewing 1919b). They returned however in the fifth century to a basilica in the Roman Forum, which now bears their name, where Deacon Justinian, a faithful church retainer with a cancerous limb was so exhausted by his pain that he fell asleep during his prayers. There came to him in a dream the twin physicians who after amputating the limb of a Moor who had died that morning replaced the diseased part with the obtained allograft implant. The procedure, known as the Miracle of the Black Leg, was reportedly successful and because of that the twins were subsequently canonised, receiving their sainthood c.550. Of note is the fact that the occasion and drama associated with the procedure was so extraordinary that it captured the imagination of first the Florentine painter Fra Angelico and then many other artists (Cosmas and Damian were also the patron saints of the ruling Florentine Medici family); and literally hundreds of some of the most extraordinary paintings depicting the procedure can now be found in many of the world museums (Rinaldi 1987) (Fig. 14.1).

A second miracle occurred in the case of St Peregrine Laziosi who lived in the fourteenth century (Jackson 1971). After an initial rebellious and anti-religious youth, the Virgin Mary came to Peregrine in a vision asking him to mend his ways. He responded instantly by becoming a devout Catholic and subsequently a priest in Siena and then Forli. In his latter years he developed a cancer of the foot and leg, which caused him great pain. The surgeons advised him to have an amputation but on the night before the procedure after praying to God he fell asleep and awoke without a trace of the tumorous process. For this miracle, as well as for his life of great giving, he was canonised in 1726 (Fig. 14.2).

EARLIEST IDENTIFICATIONS OF BONE TUMOURS

The earliest views of bone tumours in historical data were that they were simply cancers of the limbs rather than neoplasms arising from connective tissue. Thus when early authors spoke of bone cancer they were of the opinion that they were simply neoplasms associated with other lesions rather than tumours arising from bone or soft tissue and this concept is clearly supported by the much higher incidence of carcinomas than sarcomas and indeed the frequency with which breast, lung and prostate primary carcinomatous metastases afflict the skeleton. It should be noted that histological evaluation of tumours depended on the microscope which was not

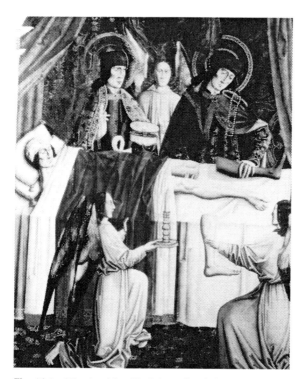

Fig. 14.1 *Miracle of the Black Leg*, oil painting by an anonymous fifteenth-century Netherlands artist. Cosmas and Damian are applying the allograft component after the resection of the cancerous limb

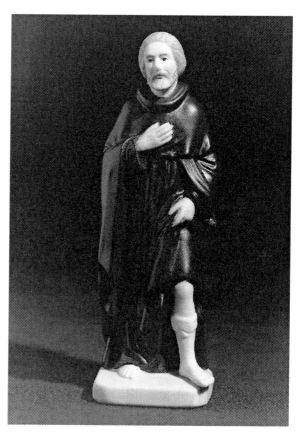

Fig. 14.2 St Peregrine. Note the bandaged limb. Prayer cured the tumour before the amputation could take place

in common use for that purpose until the mid-nineteenth century and of perhaps greater importance was the fact that Wilhelm Conrad Röntgen did not introduce X-ray imaging until 1895 (Röntgen, 1895). Recognition of tumours of bone and soft tissue and their histological definition and origin were at best rudimentary early in the nineteenth century. It was therefore not until the latter part of that century that imaging allowed sophisticated recognition of tumorous processes in the bones and histology allowed speculation as to cellular origin of the tumour. These limitations made non-surgical or conservative treatment programmes less reliable than amputation above the level of the lesion. Clearly there were also limitations on amputation, which were fraught with the hazards of infectious and other types of complications.

The first description of a tumour arising within connective tissue probably was that of Abernethy (1764–1831) who in 1803 described a neoplasm of the limb of probably soft tissue origin (Abernethy 1804). He is alleged to have reintroduced the term 'sarcoma' from the Greek term for tumours of soft tissue, suggesting that tumours of connective tissue may have substantially different cellular origins. It was shortly thereafter in 1805 that Baron Guillaume Dupuytren further defined the entity of osteosarcoma (describing it as an aggressive lesion arising from bony elements) and alluded to its malignancy and ability to metastasise (Dupuytren, 1805). However, it was not until 1845 that histological evidence of a lesion arising in bone was presented and documented as containing cells that seemed bony in origin. In that year Hermann Lebert described a case of giant-cell tumour of bone, the cells of which resembled bone cells, particularly the osteoclasts seen in normal tissues. Subsequently, Rudolf Ludwig Karl Virchow (1863–67) and Sir James Paget (1853) showed convincing histological evidence that the giant-cell tumour had some of the same cellular elements that existed in bone and was almost surely bony in origin. The investigators further showed that the giant-cell tumour could and did locally destroy the bone of origin (Lebert 1845, Virchow 1863–67). In his exceptional three-volume work published from 1863 to 1867, Virchow, considered by many to be the father of modern pathology and certainly one of the famous pathologists of the nineteenth century, expressed the opinion that although there were examples such as the giant-cell tumour and others such as fibrosarcoma, myxosarcoma, osteosarcoma and chondrosarcoma, tumours arising primary in bone were much rarer than other tumours that metastasised to bone. These concepts are considered to be the foundation of modern understanding of cancer (Wilson 1947).

Of critical importance to this system was the use of the microscope in the definition of tumours. Despite the earlier discovery of optics and the lens and the microscope, the technology was not applied to the body tissues and more specifically tumours until the mid-nineteenth century (Olson 1989). The first positive identification of tumorous tissues was attributed to Hermann Lebert who published an illustrated atlas entitled *Physiologie Pathologique* in 1845, which not only contained pictures of the histological structures of tumours, but also some of these were in colour. In the same year, the Scottish clinician and anatomist John Hughes Bennett described microscopic differences between benign and malignant cells. In 1853, Donaldson reported on the microscopic characteristics of cancer, and in the following year Lionel Beale a Professor at King's College wrote *The Microscope in its Application to Practical Medicine* (1858), a treatise in which he proposed some histological markers which distinguished normal from cancerous tissue (Beale, 1858). All these techniques were very useful to the surgeon who was resecting a tumorous growth, but were only available on examination of the histological section of a specimen submitted to the pathology department. Specifically, none were available during the operative procedure, which was considered a serious problem. It was not until 1891 that surgeons and pathologists collaborated in providing a diagnosis of malignant disease on a rapidly performed frozen section, thus allowing the surgeon to alter his surgical procedure by such measures as increasing the size of the resection margins or moving to another portion of the anatomy (Bloodgood 1927, Wright 1985).

Perhaps the first real identification of the nature of bone tumours was the report of Samuel Gross, a Professor of Surgery in Philadelphia who in 1879 published 'Sarcoma of the long bones, based on a study of one hundred and sixty five cases' in the *American Journal of Medical Science*. His paper stated that of the 165 tumours, seventy could be histologically identified as giant-cell tumours, forty-five were what might be currently termed parosteal osteosarcomas and twenty-eight were central sarcomas. Of that last group of twenty-eight, sixteen were considered to be forming a matrix (probably osteosarcoma or chondrosarcoma) and twelve consisted of small round cells (probably Ewing's sarcoma). He also noted that these tumours frequently metastasised to the lung and much less commonly to lymph nodes. Because of the nature of these lesions and their aggressive character, he recommended amputation as the treatment of choice.

At about the same time, a number of studies defined the tumour population which is considered haematopoetic in origin. In 1848 Dalrymple in a paper in the *Dublin Quarterly* described the entity of myeloma (Clemp 1967,

Bergsagel & Rider 1985) and in the same year Henry Bence-Jones described the characteristics of the urinary protein in these patients that bears his name and is believed to be diagnostic for that disease (Bergsagel & Rider 1985). Similarly several authors described bone lesions with a greenish colour that became known as chloromas and which were established as having a relationship and indeed being diagnostic of leukaemia.

TUMOUR RECOGNITION AND BIOLOGICAL BEHAVIOUR

The next thirty-five years was a time of development of an understanding of connective tissue tumours, based not only on the discoveries of the nature and characteristics of an array of these lesions, but also by establishing some concept of their biological behaviour. It was the period when the great pathologists of the twentieth century contributed to our knowledge and established an order to the prior chaos. The contributors of this era included Paget, von Recklinghausen, Erdheim, Bloodgood, Jaffe, Ewing, Coley, Geschickter, Copeland, Phemister, Schmorl, Codman, Fischer, Albright, Lichtenstein, Schajowicz, Enzinger, Dahlin and many more. It should be noted that these individuals not only defined and graded the tumour populations, but also described the histological and in some cases the radiological characteristics of a variety of other non-neoplastic diseases, including hyperparathyroidism (von Recklinghausen), fibrous dysplasia (Albright, Jaffe, Lichtenstein, von Recklinghausen), Paget's disease (Paget, Schmorl), eosinophilic granuloma (Jaffe), haemangiomas of bone (Erdheim), neurofibromatosis (von Recklinghausen), rickets (Albright) and a large number of other disorders of the skeleton.

Several of these contributors stand out. Earnest A. Codman (1896–1940) was a general surgeon at the Massachusetts General Hospital who was interested and quite knowledgeable about bone disease and, more specifically, tumours. In 1920 in an effort to define the field of orthopaedic oncology further, he wrote letters to surgeons to obtain information about their patients with malignant tumours of bone and collected over four hundred replies. These replies were the basis and beginning of a Bone Tumor Registry that he, in collaboration with James Ewing and Joseph Bloodgood, established in 1927 (Codman 1922, 1925). He became fascinated with the shoulder and published a book on that subject in 1934 in which he not only described the anatomical structure and particularly the rotator cuff, but also described and defined the entity of chondroblastoma (known since as Codman's tumour) (Codman 1931, 1934). Codman is also responsible for describing the periosteal lifting seen

on a radiograph at the margin of high-grade tumours such as osteosarcoma, which is now known as Codman's triangle (1925).

James Ewing (1866–1943) was a pathologist born in Pittsburgh. He developed an osteomyelitis of the femur from which he was never cured (Stewart 1954). He became fascinated with the microscope and with bone disease based in part on his illness and became a pathologist in New York City around the turn of the century. He was the first Chief of Pathology at Cornell University and as well as being the Chief of Pathology at Cancer Memorial Hospital, he served as Director of that Hospital for a number of years. He was interested in radiation effects on bones and was one of the first to describe deleterious effects (Ewing 1922); he also established a classification system for tumours (Ewing 1919a, b). He, Codman and Bloodgood collaborated in starting the first Bone Tumor Registry in the early 1920s (Codman 1922) and he was a founder of the American Cancer Society. Ewing described the tumour that bears his name in 1921 calling it diffuse endothelioma of bone, indicating the highly malignant nature of the lesion.

Henry L. Jaffe (1896–1979) (Fig. 14.3) and his colleague Louis Lichtenstein (1906–77) were perhaps the most prolific contributors to our knowledge of bone tumours. Jaffe was born in New York City and at the early age of thirty-two became Chief of Pathology at the Hospital for Joint Diseases, a position he held from 1928 to 1965. He was an excellent educator, an astute clinical scientist and an ardent collector. Based in large measure on his well-catalogued and massive collection of tumour material, he beautifully enhanced the description of some already known entities and described some new ones. He and in some cases his colleague Lichtenstein added substantially to our knowledge of the pathology of giant-cell tumour (Jaffe et al 1940) and chondroblastoma (Jaffe & Lichtenstein 1942), and he also initially described the entities of osteoid osteoma (Jaffe 1934), pigmented villonodular synovitis (Jaffe et al 1941), osteoblastoma (Jaffe 1956, Lichtenstein 1956), aneurysmal bone cyst (Jaffe 1950), chondromyxoid fibroma (Jaffe & Lichtenstein 1946) and solitary eosinophilic granuloma (Jaffe & Lichtenstein 1944). Jaffe wrote two monumental texts, the first in 1958 (Jaffe 1972) and the second in 1970 (Jaffe 1972) and Lichtenstein another (1959), and all are still in use today. There is little doubt that Jaffe did more than most of the pathologists of the day in terms of not only detailing the histological nature of the lesions, but also by keeping track of the patient's outcome, developing some concept of the malignant nature of the tumour. He and Lichtenstein clearly indicated the state of the science in their time with two cardinal statements from their texts regarding the major lesions. They declared that osteosarcoma has a bad prognosis (a survival rate of only 10%) and that Ewing's sarcoma is a lesion from which patients only rarely survived.

Joseph Bloodgood (1867–1935) was a student of Halsted and gained renown as a tumour surgeon at The Johns Hopkins Hospital where he subsequently became Director of Surgical Pathology. In 1912 he became fascinated with the entity of giant-cell tumour, partly because most patients survived, despite the malignant appearance of the lesion. In a seminal paper he concluded that conservative management for this entity was much more logical than amputation (Bloodgood 1923), and he was the first to suggest that the cavity of the tumour be washed with phenol after curettage, and then implanted with autograft to support the bony structure (Bloodgood 1924). Bloodgood helped develop the Bone Tumor Registry in 1921 and was a major contributor (Codman 1922). The Registry prospered during the first part of the twentieth century but after the Second World War became a part of the Armed Forces Institute of Pathology. He also proposed the name myxoma for what was probably a myxoid chondrosarcoma (Bloodgood 1924).

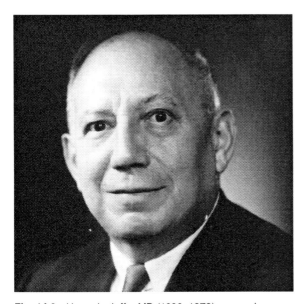

Fig. 14.3 Henry L. Jaffe, MD (1896–1979) was perhaps the greatest contributor to the knowledge of bone tumours. He was also a great teacher and collector and was the person who stimulated the author to enter the field of bone and soft tissue tumours

William B. Coley (1862–1936) was one of the early treating physicians at the Memorial Hospital in New York and defined the natural history of osteosarcoma (Coley 1924) and the effect of radiation on high-grade cancers of bone (Coley 1905). He was impressed with the amazing remission of a patient with widespread malignant disease which appeared to coincide with the development of erysipelas. He introduced 'Coley's toxins', a sterilised bacterial solution that appeared to act on the patient's immune system to help ameliorate neoplastic disease (Coley 1893). This is considered by some to be the first example of adjuvant therapy for cancer.

Charles Geschickter and Murray Copeland published *Tumors of Bone (Including the Jaws and Joints)* (1936) that established the state of the science and specifically the pathology at the time for bone tumours and subsequently identified the entity known as parosteal osteosarcoma and indicated its less malignant nature than the centrally placed lesions (Geschickter & Copeland 1951). Several years later George Pack and Irving Ariel did the same for soft tissue tumours but with special emphasis on surgical management (Pack & Ariel, 1958). Several authors defined the development of a peculiarly virulent bone sarcoma in patients with Paget's disease (Brailsford 1938, Schajowicz 1942, Poretta et al 1957). In 1913, Bernhard Fischer described adamantinoma of bone which was almost always peculiarly located principally in the tibia (Fischer 1913). Friedrich von Recklinghausen defined neurofibromatosis of soft tissue (von Recklinghausen 1882). He also is for the most part responsible for describing the histological changes in hyperparathyroidism (osteitis fibrosa cystica generalisata) (von Recklinghausen 1891).

A word or two must be added about famous collectors who maintained vast numbers of specimens along with, in many cases, pictures of the gross tumours and X-ray imaging. For some the specimens were the basis of a book about tumours, their clinical and histological characteristics and their prognosis and in some cases proposed treatment and outcome. These great collectors include Jakob Erdheim, Henry Jaffe (1972), Louis Lichtenstein (1959), Bradley Coley (1949), Fritz Schajowicz (1981), David Dahlin (1975, 1967, Dahlin & Henderson 1962, Dahlin & Coventry 1967), David Bloodgood (1924), Albert Kolodny (1927), Fuller Albright (Albright et al 1937, Albright & Reifenstein 1948), Dallas B. Phemister (1930), Charles Geschickter and Murray Copeland (1936), Mario Campanacci (1999), Arthur Purdy Stout (1953), William F. Enneking (1983), Franz Enzinger and Sharon Weiss (1983), Howard Dorfman (1998) and many others. These studies have been enormously advantageous. Using these reports as background data, and with the advent of new techniques of imaging, i.e. bone scan (Malmud & Charkes 1975), tomography, angiography, computed tomography (Hounsfield 1973a, b) and magnetic resonance imaging (Damadian 1971, Damadian et al 1973) it was now possible more effectively to define the extent and nature of the tumour and plan effective treatment.

A special comment must be added about teachers. There have been a number of individuals starting historically with Hippocrates who by their interest and enthusiasm for the subject of bone tumours have stimulated others to enter the field and add to our knowledge. Many of the people listed above stand out in this regard but there are some special individuals. Jakob Erdheim was a teacher in Vienna who stimulated Schajowicz, Jaffe, Phemister and many others to study pathology of bone lesions. With the German Anschluss, he bequeathed his collection to Jaffe and it still exists today at the Massachusetts General Hospital (as is a large component of the Jaffe collection).

Dallas B. Phemister was born in 1882, trained in Vienna and then served at the University of Chicago as a surgical chief for many years (Bick 1957). He is responsible for aspects of our understanding of chondrosarcoma, osteonecrosis, bone grafting as well as the nature of osteomyelitis and other disorders (Phemister 1930, 1940, 1945). One of his claims to fame however was the development of a teaching programme in oncology at the University of Chicago which was carried on by C. Howard Hatcher after Phemister's death and resulted in stimulating the interest of many of the latter day orthopaedic oncologists, including Crawford Campbell, Mary Sherman, Michael Bonfiglio, Eugene Mindell, Thomas Brower and William F. Enneking. These people in turn have done the same and many of the current oncological programmes are based on the educational stimulation of the directors by one or several of these great teachers.

MANAGEMENT OF BONE AND SOFT TISSUE TUMOURS

The management of malignant bone and soft tissue tumours was until the mid-twentieth century and somewhat beyond a very discouraging area. Benign tumours were managed well with little major problem aside from a high local recurrence rate for such tumours as giant-cell tumour or osteoblastoma (Johnson & Dahlin 1959, Goldenberg et al 1970, Campanacci 1999). The malignant tumours such as Ewing's tumour or osteosarcoma or high-grade soft tissue tumours had very high local recurrence, metastasis and death rates. High-grade chondrosarcoma had a lower rate of metastasis but those lesions about the pelvis did poorly (Phemister 1930, Enneking 1983). The great changes that occurred

in the last thirty years arose principally because of the use of chemotherapeutic agents, radiation oncological treatments and improved imaging technology.

Shortly after Röntgen discovered the X-ray as an imaging technique in 1895, radiation was considered as a potential treating agent for cancer (Lyon 1896, Lederman 1981, Bernier 1995). The Curies provided a radioactive source of considerable strength in 1898. In 1900 Kienbock reported some experiments with rats that were radiated and underwent an unmistakable series of effects; and it was then agreed that radiation might well be of value in the management of patients (Kienbock 1900). Armed with this information, the treating radiologists became concerned about sources of radiation (Miller 1950, Lederman 1953, Bernier 1995), the amount of radiant energy delivered to the patient (Bordier 1907, Quimby 1941, Berry & Andrews 1964) and the dosage required to treat disease (Johns et al 1952, Hall 1972). It should be noted however that in 1933 Emil Grubbe of Chicago reported that he had treated a patient with breast cancer in 1896 and also noted the occurrence of dermatitis (in his own hands). He also was allegedly the first to use lead shields to reduce the amount of radiation to unaffected anatomical parts (Grubbe 1933). Radium or Crooke's tubes and subsequently radon seeds were initially the sources of the radiation but devices to shield and focus the beam became an essential part of the system (Lysholm 1923, Lederman & Greatorex 1953, Lederman 1981). The first treatment of a sarcoma with radiation was reported by Coley in 1905 and soon thereafter with better equipment the radiation technology became an essential part of oncological management of patients with bone and soft tissue tumours (Coutard 1934).

It became apparent early on that the radiation was of value in the management of patients with cancer but it also was strongly suspected that overuse or abuse of the system might cause cancer (Steiner 1965). Such a case was suggested by Martland et al (1925) and supported strongly by a classic paper written by Howard Hatcher in 1945. Of considerable importance however was the systematic application of high-energy, well-defined dosages of radiation to a specific anatomical part in an effort to eliminate the neoplasm, or at least to serve as either neo- or adjuvant therapy. Foremost amongst the pioneers in connective tissue disease was Herman Suit of the Massachusetts General Hospital and Harvard Medical School. Suit and his co-workers devised both adjuvant and neo-adjuvant systems for the management of patients with lymphoma (Dorfman & Czerniak 1998), osteosarcoma (Suit 1975) and soft tissue sarcomas (Suit & Russell 1975, Suit et al 1973, 1975, 1981, 1988) which have greatly increased the rate of survival for the patients and improved the functional status of patients after limb-sparing surgery.

In terms of chemotherapy, the earliest approaches were those of Coley (1893) (Coley's toxins) and Sullivan with L-phenylalanine mustard (Sullivan et al 1963) but neither was considered successful. It was not until 1954 that Sidney Farber reported successful treatment of several children with Wilm's tumours with actinomycin D (Foley 1974), which began the period of discovery for chemotherapeutic agents. In 1973, Norman Jaffe, Sidney Farber and co-workers introduced high-dose methotrexate with leukovorin rescue for the treatment of osteosarcoma (Jaffe et al 1973, 1974). At almost the same time, Cortes and Holland and others reported the effect of adriamycin on osteosarcoma and found that they could bring the survival rate to greater than 40% (Cortes et al 1972, 1974, Sinks & Mindell 1975). *Cis*-platinum was introduced in 1979 by Baum and shortly thereafter Marti introduced ifosfamide, thus establishing the four principal drugs in the chemotherapeutic regimen for this and other malignant connective tissue neoplasms (Sutow et al 1976, Olson 1989). In the 1970s Rosen introduced the concept of neo-adjuvant therapy, which allowed the treating physicians to assess the impact of the drugs chosen on the tumour prior to resective surgery and thus allow possible changes in protocol (Rosen et al 1974, 1982, Rosen 1987). This brought the curve up further and also made limb-sparing resective surgery considerably safer. These drugs and the neo-adjuvant approach have shifted the curve for all the high-grade tumours such that the average long-term survival rate for osteosarcoma is as much as 70% and an equal or even greater rate for Ewing's sarcoma (Jaffe & Watts 1976, Goorin et al 1985, Rosen 1987). Lymphoma and most of the soft tissue sarcomas have been reported to respond to both adjuvant therapy and especially radiation (Dosoretz et al 1983). We owe a debt to the intrepid pioneers in this important field who have provided us with these adjuvants that offer the patients a much greater chance at local control and prolonged disease free survival.

ORTHOPAEDIC MANAGEMENT OF PATIENTS WITH SARCOMAS

Until the 1940s, tumour management was difficult at best and at least for high-grade tumours the patients usually had amputations performed (mostly for osteosarcoma or chondrosarcoma) or received radiation (principally for Ewing's sarcoma, lymphoma, myeloma or metastatic carcinoma). Reconstructive surgery had little place in their care and limb-sparing surgery was a very rare event. Local resection could be performed but often failed because the surgeon had limited ability to know the extent of the lesion or to provide a wide

enough margin to prevent recurrence. The success of local resection depended on the site of the tumour, the proximity of adjacent neural or vascular structures and whether sufficient skin or soft tissue could be maintained to avoid problems with wound closure. Such surgery was made more difficult by the fact that without modern imaging techniques, planning was difficult and without frozen sections at the time of definitive surgery the assessment of the proximity of the tumour to the surgical margin was often inaccurate.

It should be clearly evident that amputation was the method of choice for malignant bone or soft tissue tumours unless the lesions were small or remarkably accessible (Sweetnam 1973). Mott in 1828 reported on having performed a resection of the clavicle for osteosarcoma and Langenbeck reported on a complete scapular resection for a cartilage tumour in 1850. Morris partially resected a forearm for a giant-cell tumour successfully and reported the procedure in 1876 and Hinds introduced 'scraping' for palliative treatment of myeloma in 1895 (Hinds 1898). Amputations could be modified such as with the 'turn-about' procedure as designed by Van Nes (1950) and applied to the management of sarcomas by Kotz and Salzer (1982) (Fig. 14.4). With this procedure the distal femur was removed en bloc, the leg below it turned around 180° and the vessels anastamosed and the bones connected with a plate and screws. The turned about foot (now pointing posteriorly) served as a knee joint in a special prosthesis. Another similar approach for tumours of the upper end of the femur was the 'turn up-plasty' advocated by Sauerbruch in 1922. In this procedure the entire femur is resected and the tibia brought up and the medial malleous articulates with either the proximal femur or the acetabulum (Fig. 14.5). Partial ablations of the shoulder for tumours that spare the arm to maintain function were reported initially by Linberg (1928) and subsequently by Marcove et al (1977). Despite problems with surgical complications, Pringle reported on two interpelvic abdominal resections in 1916.

In an effort to maintain a functional limb surgeons of the time turned to autograft transplants to replace resected tumour-containing bone. One of the earliest such reports was that of Bloodgood in 1912 for giant-cell tumour. Additional approaches were defined in the remarkable reports by Albee (1936), Bloodgood (1923), Coley and Higgenbotham (1948), D'Aubigne and Dejournay (1958), Johnson and Dahlin (1959), Wilson and Lance (1965), Marcove et al (1970), Campanacci (1979) and Enneking et al (1980a). One of the more creative approaches was that suggested by Enneking and Shirley (1977) who used autograft to

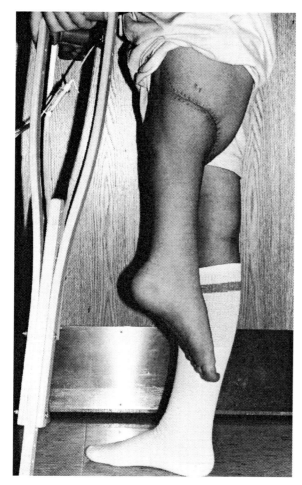

Fig. 14.4 A fifteen-year-old patient treated for an osteosarcoma of the distal femur with a Van Nes turnabout. The ankle will serve as the knee joint in a special prosthesis

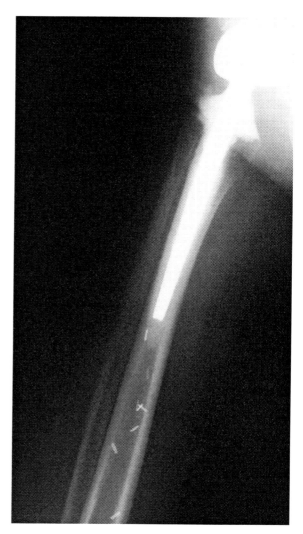

Fig. 14.5 A 'turn up-plasty' in a thirty-year-old woman with a high-grade sarcoma of the proximal femur. The entire femur was resected and the tibia and fibula 'turned up'. A total hip replacement prosthesis driven into the medial malleolus is articulating with the acetabulum

arthrodese the knee joint after resection of tumours and in separate reports by Enneking (1966), Enneking and Dunham (1978) and Johnson (1978) novel approaches were described for the reconstruction of the pelvis after tumour resection.

It should be apparent however that none of these specialised surgical procedures could have been done earlier. Orthopaedic management of patients with bone and soft tissue tumours has advanced considerably since the early part of the twentieth century and have established new and exciting variations in treatment of these difficult and unpredictable lesions. There are several reasons for these advances:

1. For both benign and malignant lesions, the knowledge of the nature of the lesion has made behaviour more predictable and allowed the surgeons and physicians greater leeway in planning the patient's therapy (Dahlin 1967).

2. Vastly improved imaging technology using radiographs (Brailsford 1948, Deeley 1983), bone scans (Subramanian & McAfee 1971), computed tomography (Damadian 1971, Damadian et al 1973, Weis et al 1978) and magnetic resonance imaging (Hounsfield 1973a, b) have allowed the surgeons to define with greater certainty the anatomical position of the tumour and what would be necessary to remove it (Hudson et al 1983) (Fig. 14.6).

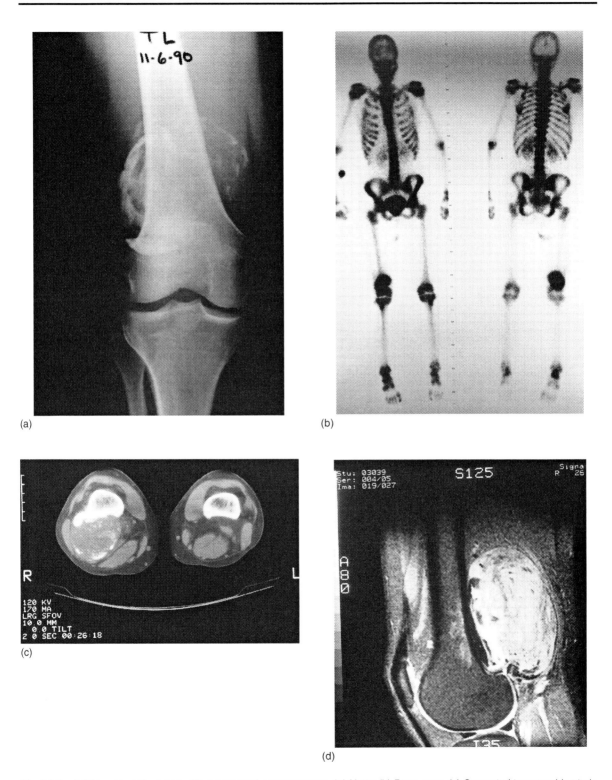

(a)

(b)

(c)

(d)

Fig. 14.6 A thirty-year-old woman with a parosteal osteosarcoma. (a) X-ray. (b) Bone scan. (c) Computed tomographic study. (d) Magnetic resonance image. The tumour was successfully resected and replaced with an allograft

3. A staging technique for bone and soft tissue tumours has advanced our ability to predict outcome and define the goals of treatment (Enneking 1980b) (Table 14.1); and another system has been introduced to evaluate end results (Enneking 1987).

4. Clearer assessment of biopsy technology has made it possible to know in advance what the tumour's behaviour is likely to be (Ottolenghi 1955, Wilson 1971, Mankin et al 1982).

5. The use of neo-adjuvant chemotherapy and radiation has made marginal or wide surgery safer than in the past and allows better and far less disabling limb-sparing surgery (Sweetnam 1975, Simon et al 1986, Suit et al 1988).

6. The ability effectively to treat lung metastases with chemotherapy and resection thus enhancing the patient's chance at survival (Muhm 1977, Marcove et al 1975, Spanos et al 1976, Campanacci 1999).

7. Modern technology for construction of custom or modular prostheses has made it possible to replace joints and adjacent bony parts (Scales et al 1984, Chao & Sim 1985, Johnston 1987, Salzer et al 1987).

8. Allograft banks have allowed a supply of good bony segments with attachment sites for ligaments and tendons, and improved selection and harvest technology has made grafts biologically safer and more successful (Tomford et al 1989, Contreras et al 1998, Tomford & Mankin 1999).

The goal in the management of patients with benign or low-grade tumours of bone or soft tissue is one of achieving the highest rate of pain relief and functional competence possible. Osteoid osteoma can be treated with partial or complete resection or now with heat ablation with little difficulty for the patient (Rosenthal et al 1998). Giant-cell tumours until recently have had a high rate of recurrence and the treatment proposed in the past is now considered excessive for such lesions (Goldenberg et al 1970), even when they threaten the joint or recur after incomplete surgery (McCarthy 1980). Similarly low-grade cartilage tumours have only a limited likelihood of significant effect on the survival and functional competence of patients with the disease, which suggests that the simpler, less destructive methods of treatment are logical. Techniques such as curettage and treatment with phenol, liquid nitrogen (Malawer et al 1987, Otis & Lane 1987) or burring of the adjacent bone (Campanacci 1999) and packing with plaster of Paris (Peltier 1961) cement or with auto- or with allograft chips or occasionally resection and allograft replacement can be logically applied to such lesions as aneurysmal bone cyst, parosteal osteosarcoma, osteoblastoma, giant-cell tumour, enchondroma, some central chondrosarcomas, peripheral chondrosarcomas, etc. without great threat of recurrence or metastasis. Some of these as well as desmoblastic fibroma, osteoblastomas, chondromyxoid fibromas, etc. and other benign tumours with a high recurrence rate can be effectively treated with marginal resection and allograft replacement (Mankin et al 1996). Similarly, lipomas, myxomas, neurofibromas and even desmoid tumours can be successfully removed with little threat of local recurrence or damage to

Table 14.1 Staging system for bone and soft tissue tumours adopted by Enneking with the help of the Musculoskeletal Tumor Society in 1980. Note that tumours are classified according to grade (G, high or low), anatomical site (T, intra- or extracompartmental), and the presence or absence of metastases (M) and then the stage is defined as 1A to 3. This system is highly successful and provides an excellent assessment of the potential of the tumour to metastasise or recur locally

Stage	Grade (G)	Anatomical site (T)	Metastases (M)
IA (G_1, T_1, M_0)	low (G_1)	intracompartmental (T_1)	none (M_0)
IB (G_1, T_2, M_0)	low (G_1)	extracompartmental (T_2)	none (M_0)
IIA (G_2, T_2, M_0)	high (G_2)	intracompartmental (T_1)	none (M_0)
IIB (G_2, T_2, M_0)	high (G_2)	extracompartmental (T_2)	none (M_0)
III ($-$, $-$, M_1)	any	any	present (M_1)

adjacent anatomical structures (Campanacci 1999) while the high-grade soft tissue sarcomas are often effectively treated by surgical resection preceded or followed by radiation (Pack & Ariel 1958, Suit et al 1973, 1981, 1988, Simon & Enneking 1976).

The current objectives of treating such patients with high-grade sarcomas of bone must be to provide them with the best chance for survival and only then should one consider the relief of pain and the maintenance of function as important goals to be achieved. All of these are major issues. As indicated above adjuvant and especially neo-adjuvant therapy chemotherapy and radiation have made the surgery more successful in terms of survival and avoidance of local recurrence and this has been a major factor in orthopaedic oncological patient management.

Metallic implants

Just as the hip and knee and shoulder surgeons developed metallic implants for relief of arthritis of these joints, the tumour surgeons proposed devices that would provide artificial joints, usually hinged and with attachment sites for ligaments and tendons. Earliest among these systems was Austin Moore who was amongst the first to use vitallium devices (Moore & Bohlman 1943). In 1965, Joseph Buchman reported the results of the use of a custom total femoral endoprosthesis and in 1971 J. N. Wilson of the Royal National Hospital in London reported on two such cases and subsequently, in 1975, he, Jackson Burrows and John Scales presented a larger series and defined the use of the custom prosthesis designed by Scales in a presentation in 1987 (Bradish et al 1987). Additional programmes that used the devices included the group at Birmingham under the direction of Rodney Sneath and the team at the Middlesex Hospital led by Rodney Sweetnam. Similarly the materials produced by Albert Burstein for the staff at the Hospital for Special Surgery in New York City were utilised by Ralph Marcove (Marcove et al 1977), Joseph Lane (Otis & Lane 1987) and the group at Memorial Hospital in New York. The Mayo Clinic oncology group including Frank Sim and Douglas Pritchard introduced proximal humeral replacements (Bos et al 1987). Mario Campanacci and his group at Bologna performed similar surgery (Campanacci & Costa 1979), but all of these custom systems required a waiting period on the part of the patient and always held the threat of poor fit despite measurement. Kotz and co-workers in Austria produced a system that was initially custom (Ramach et al 1987) but subsequently was in part modular and in some cases was cementless (Ritschl et al 1987, Salzer et

al 1987) and has reportedly been successful in a larger number of cases. Modular systems for the proximal humerus and shaft of the bone were produced by the Mayo Clinic and showed some success, although bony ingrowth into the device was less than optimal (Chao & Sim 1985). The current modular systems are often more successful and patients in whom the devices are placed have good function and a low complication rate. There are a number of reports of prolonged use of these systems which appear to be best in the proximal femur and a little less successful but still of considerable value in the distal femur (Sim & Chao 1979, Sim et al 1987). Proximal tibial systems are difficult because of the difficulty of connecting the patellar tendon to the metallic implant but some techniques have been advanced which make it functional (Malawer & McHale 1989, Eckardt et al 1991) (Fig. 14.7).

In recent years the use of expandable devices for young children has been advocated by Lewis et al (1987) and by the group at Stanmore, and although as yet not universally successful they have added considerably to our armimentarium in the management of osteosarcoma or Ewing's tumours in the child with open physes.

Modular systems in metal are the leading technology for limb-sparing surgery, particularly for proximal and distal femoral and proximal humeral resective surgery. The relatively low number of infections, the ease of implantation and the rapid recuperative rate make this system more attractive than autograft arthrodesis or allograft implantation. The length of time such devices have been observed is still shorter than some of the other systems and there is some early evidence to suggest that late failures will occur and possibly require a more complicated repair system than some of the other systems (Clarke et al 1998, Stauffer et al 1991).

Allograft replacements

In his exhaustive report on the history of allografting, Burwell (1993) records several attempts by individuals over the many years that followed, but the world recognises the first report of a successful allograft to be that of Macewen in 1881. In that procedure, Macewen transplanted segments of bone from a rachitic patient to the humerus of a three-year-old child who had lost a portion of the shaft as a result of osteomyelitis. The major effort however in the early part of the twentieth century was that of Lexer, who in 1908 reported on four such procedures about the knee and in 1925 described a reasonable success rate on eleven half joint and twenty-three whole joints using fresh cadaveric tissue. Sporadic case reports and short series were presented over the next twenty or so years, but it was a Russian group

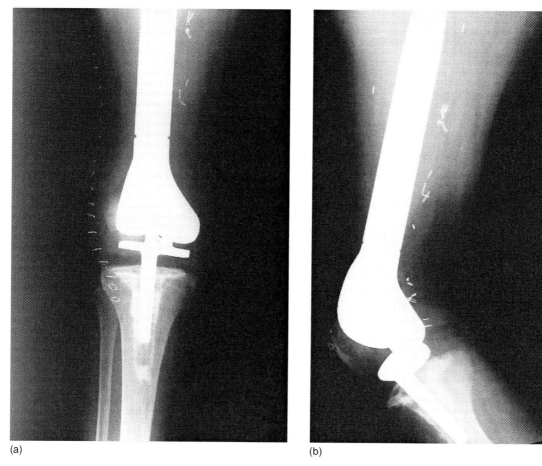

(a)   (b)

Fig. 14.7 Anteroposterior (a) and lateral (b) radiographs of a modular prosthesis implanted after resection of large tumour of the distal femur. The knee joint is a rotating hinged device that provides the patient with a relatively normal gait pattern

under the direction of Volkov (1970) that reported a large series of successful procedures using processed but not frozen cadaveric bone. On the basis of a sophisticated group of experimental studies, Curtiss, Chase and Herndon (Herndon & Chase 1954, Curtiss et al 1959) proposed the concept that freezing the cadaveric bony parts would reduce immunological activity and thus reduce the rejection rate. This also made it possible to develop bone banks in which the bony parts obtained at surgery or autopsy (or subsequently at harvest) were stored in a freezer at −20 to −70°C and thawed prior to implantation (Friedlaender et al 1976, Tomford et al 1989, Tomford & Mankin 1999).

Following the Second World War, the US Navy became interested in preservation of allograft tissue and in 1950 founded the Navy Tissue Bank under the direction of George Hyatt (Contreras et al 1998). Subsequently, when Kenneth Sell became head he recruited a number of

Fellows to rotate through the system and perform research on graft technology. The list of graduates of Kenneth Sell's programme included some very distinguished investigators such as Andrew Bassett, Gary Friedlaender, Theodore Malinin, William Tomford and Michael Strong, all of whom started their own banks and also along with others performed very competent research (Friedlaender et al 1976, Tomford 1983, Schachar & McGann 1991, Schachar et al 1994). Their work not only advanced the field in terms of improved success of the implant, but also added greatly to the safety of the host in relation to infectious bacterial and especially virus transmission (Lord et al 1988, Buck et al 1989, Conway et al 1990, Loty et al 1990, Tomford et al 1990, Hernigou et al 1991, Strong et al 1991).

On the basis of these pioneer efforts, two major sets of experimentation started. The first was clinical. Frank Parrish in Houston, Texas, acting in part on the reported success of Volkov, performed a series of surgical procedures in which frozen allografts were implanted after removal of a bone tumour (Parrish 1966, 1973). He carefully followed the patients and reported the complications of the procedure. Carlos Ottolenghi in Buenos Aires started a similar series and reported in 1966 on successes and most importantly on the causes of failures. Stimulated by these efforts, several other groups including especially the active programme at the Massachusetts General Hospital began to look at allografting as a possibly better solution than metallic implants (Mankin et al 1982, 1987, 1996, Hejna et al 1997, McGoveran et al 1984, Mankin 1983, Matley et al, Jofe et al 1988, Delloye et al 1988, Gouin et al 1996, Ortiz-Cruz et al 1997, Tan & Masnkin 1997, Friedlaender et al 1999, Hornicek et al 1999) (Figs 14.8 and 14.9).

During this same period, several investigators recognised that the complications including infection, fracture and non-union severely compromised the results in the clinical series and were probably based on the immune response (Lord et al 1988, Berrey et al 1990, Muscolo et al 1996, Alho et al 1998). A group in Canada headed by Langer demonstrated that the response to allografting in animals was markedly reduced by freezing the graft, thus suggesting that a blocking antibody was produced by the temperature reduction (Langer et al 1978). Most recently the studies of Alho et al (1998) strongly implicated the immune response as being responsible for the complications of infection, fracture and non-union. Friedlaender, Strong and Mankin showed that the clinical result was significantly improved in patients who achieved a match with MHC Class II antigens than with MHC Class I or with mismatch (Friedlaender et al 1976, 1999, Strong et al 1996).

Simultaneously the rules regarding bone banking were being established in a number of centres. The

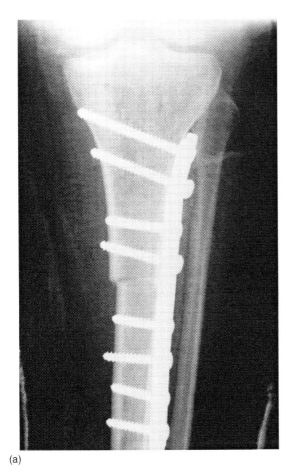

(a)

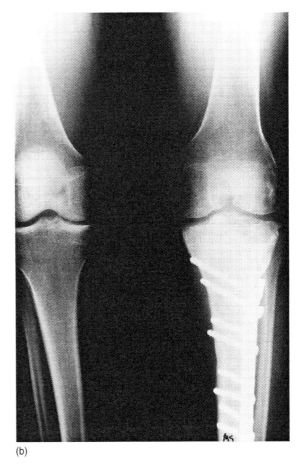

(b)

Fig. 14.8 (a) Anteroposterior radiograph of a proximal femoral allograft shortly after implantation for a recurrent giant-cell tumour in 1980. (b) Radiograph of the same patient taken in 1999. Function remains good

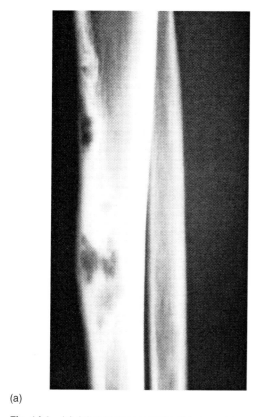

(a)

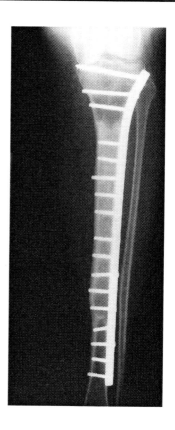

(b)

Fig. 14.9 (a) Adamantinoma of the tibia in a sixteen-year-old female treated with resection and an allograft in 1988. (b) Radiograph showing that in 1999 the patient had normal function

methods of testing the donor for bacterial or viral diseases were established as well as the approaches to the optimal rules for freezing and thawing (most believe slow freeze and rapid thaw) and the value and the drawbacks of radiation to the graft (Loty et al 1990). It seemed sensible to maintain cartilage at least partially alive during the freezing and thawing process and the use of glycerol or dimethylsulphoxide was proposed to achieve this important goal (Tomford 1983, Schachar & McGann 1991, Schachar et al 1994). Establishing the Bone section of the American Association of Tissue Banks and promulgating guidelines was a major step forward and allowed safe bone banks to spring up throughout the USA and Europe (Tomford et al 1989, Tomford 1999).

DEVELOPMENT OF CENTRES OF EXCELLENCE

As has been clearly demonstrated in a number of countries, bone and soft tissue neoplasms do not represent a major health hazard, particularly when compared with breast, prostate and lung cancers. Nevertheless they are the subject of enormous interest in orthopaedic surgery partly because so much can now be done to save a life and also to spare a limb. Children with osteosarcoma or Ewing's tumour can survive and live reasonably normal lives and most of those great accomplishments are based on the talents and achievements of the clinicians and scientists of the past as listed above. Bone and soft tissue tumours are no longer a mystery but continue to remain a challenge and indeed a very special one.

It should be apparent from the sparse numbers of such tumours, the complexity of their diagnosis and treatment protocols, and the number of disciplines involved that 'centres of excellence' are necessary for the management of these lesions. Each such centre must by definition include a knowledgeable pathologist, an interested and experienced bone and soft tissue radiologist, a capable and innovative radiation oncologist, skilled and knowledgeable medical and paediatric oncologists and, of course, orthopaedic oncological surgeons who can deal with problems throughout the axial and appendicular skeleton and perform the necessary limb-sparing surgery without compromising the life and function of the patient. Additionally, skilled anaesthetists, psychiatrists, social workers, nurses and other support personnel make such programmes possible with a minimum of anxiety and suffering for the patients and their families. Of considerable importance is the need for the centre to be a 'collection depot' for patient data, histological and biochemical material and careful tracking for outcome studies.

Some of these centres are well known, some are new and just beginning to develop and acquire talent and a referral base, but all have the same demands and principles. All must be prepared to care for the patient no matter what the disorder is; all must teach students, residents, fellows and staff; all must be dedicated to clinical and if possible basic research in tumour management. Each country has such centres and they through the mechanism of such organisation as the musculoskeletal societies in Europe, the USA and the Far East and especially through the medium of the International Society for Limb Sparing all must communicate with each other with candour and not fear trying new approaches for the benefit of patients.

SUMMARY

Perhaps there is no area within the specialty of orthopaedic surgery where there has been such a spectacular achievement in dealing with potentially life-threatening disease. In the early days, virtually everyone with high-grade sarcomas succumbed and if there was a surgical solution to their problem it was an amputation. Over the decades that followed those dreadful early days, the pathologists contributed knowledge about the tumours and identified their features and the radiologists their cardinal findings on radiological imaging. The medical oncologists provided drugs in adjuvant and neo-adjuvant protocols and the radiation oncologists offered better means of safely radiating the lesional area, both of which vastly enhanced the patient's survival rate. The orthopaedic surgeon provided a means of staging the patient and developing a protocol for assessing the patient's degree of disease and stage and at least in part predicting the outcome. In addition based on the modern technology of surgery and the information gained as a result of the staging studies, the treating team has developed protocols for the resection of the bone and soft tissue tumours which are safe and cause the least damage to adjacent muscular, vascular and neurological structures. Finally the orthopaedic surgeons and their engineering and tissue-banking

colleagues have developed methods of replacing safely and functionally a part of the skeleton after resection of the tumours. No greater success or achievement has been recorded in tumour treatment.

REFERENCES

Abernethy J 1804 Surgical Observations on Tumors. Longman & Rees, London

Albee F H 1936 The treatment of primary malignant changes of the bone by radical resection with bone graft replacement. J Am Med Assoc 107: 1693–1698

Albright F, Butler A M, Hampton A O, Smith P 1937 Syndrome characterized by osteitis fibrosa disseminata, areas of pigmentation and endocrine dysfunction with precocious puberty in females. Report of 5 cases. N Engl J Med 216: 727–746

Albright F, Reifenstein E C 1948 The Parathyroid Glands and Metabolic Bone Disease. Williams & Wilkins, Baltimore

Alho A J, Eskola J, Ekfors T, Manner I, Kouri T, Hollmen T 1998 Immune responses and clinical outcome of massive human osteoarticular allografts. Clin Orthop 346: 196–206

Allison M J 1980 Metastatic tumor of bone in Tiahuanaco female. Bull NY Acad Med 56: 581–587

Barrow M V 1972 Portraits of Hippocrates. Med Hist 16: 85–88

Beale L 1858 The Microscope in its Application to Practical Medicine. John Churchill, London

Bennett J H 1845 Introductory address to a course of lectures on histology and the use of the microscope. Lancet i: 517–522

Bergsagel D E, Rider W 1985 Plasma cell neoplasms. History. In: DeVita V T, Hellman S, Rosenberg S (eds) Philadelphia, Lippencott. Cancer: Principles and Practices of Oncology, pp 1753–1754

Bernier J 1995 Radiation Oncology: A Century of Progress and Achievement. European Society of Therapeutic Radiology and Oncology, Brussels

Berrey W H Jr, Lord C F, Gebhardt M C, Mankin H J 1990 Fractures of allografts. Frequency, treatment and end-results. J Bone Joint Surg 72A: 822–833

Berry R J, Andrews J R 1964 The response of mammalian tumor cells *in vivo* to radiation of differing ionization densities (LET). Ann NY Acad Sci 114: 48–59

Bick E M 1957 Phemister of Chicago (1882–1951). Clin Orthop 10: 1–5

Bloodgood J C 1912 The conservative treatment of giant cell sarcoma with the study of bone transplantation. Ann Surg 56: 210–239

Bloodgood J C 1923 Benign giant cell tumor of bone. Its diagnosis and conservative treatment. Am J Surg 37: 105–116

Bloodgood J C 1924 Bone tumors. Myxoma. Ann Surg 80: 817–833

Bloodgood J C 1927 When cancer becomes a microscopic disease, there must be tissue diagnosis in the operating room. J Am Med Assoc 88: 1022–1023

Bordier H 1907 Determination of the quantity of X-rays absorbed by various tissues of the body. Arch Rontgen Ray 12: 199–202

Bos G, Sim F, Pritchard D, Shires T, Rock M, Askin L, Chao E 1987 Prosthetic replacement of the proximal humerus. Clin Orthop 224: 178–191

Bradish C F, Kemp H B, Scales J T, Wilson J N 1987 Distal femoral replacement by custom-made prosthesis. Clinical follow-up and survivorship analysis. J Bone Joint Surg 69B: 276–284

Brailsford J F 1938 Paget's disease of bone. Its frequency, diagnosis and complications. Br J Radiol 11: 507–532

Brailsford J F 1948 The Radiology of Bones and Joints, 4th edn. J & A Churchill, London

Bryan C P 1974 The Papyrus Ebers. Ares, Chicago

Buchman J 1965 Total femur and knee joint replacement with a vitallium endoprosthesis. Bull Hosp Joint Dis 26: 21–34

Buck R E, Malinin T I, Brown M D 1989 Bone transplantation and human immunodeficiency virus. An estimate of risk of acquired immunodeficiency syndrome (AIDS). Clin Orthop 240: 129–136

Burrows H J, Wilson J N, Scales J T 1975 Excision of tumours of humerus and femur with restoration by internal prostheses. J Bone Joint Surg 57B: 148–159

Burwell R G 1993 History of bone grafting and bone substitutes with special reference to osteogenic induction. In: Urist M R, O'Connor B T, Burwell R G (eds) Bone Grafts, Derivatives and Substitutes. Butterworth-Heinemann, Oxford, pp 3–102

Campanacci M 1999 Bone and Soft Tissue Tumors. New York, Springer

Campanacci M, Costa P 1979 Total resection of distal femur or proximal tibia for bone tumors. J Bone Joint Surg 61B: 454–463

Chao E Y, Sim F H 1985 Modular prosthetic system for segmental bone and joint replacement after tumor resection. Orthopedics 8: 641–651

Clarke H D, Berry D J, Sim F H 1998 Salvage of failed femoral megaprostheses with allograft prosthesis composite. Clin Orthop 356: 222–229

Clemp J R 1967 Some aspects of the first recorded case multiple myeloma. Lancet 7530: 1354–1356

Codman E A 1922 The registry of cases of bone sarcoma. Surg Gyne Obstet 34: 335–343

Codman E A 1925 Bone Sarcoma. Paul B. Hoeber, New York

Codman E A 1931 Epiphyseal chondromatous giant cell tumors of the upper end of the humerus. Surg Gyne Obstet 52: 543–548

Codman E A 1934 The Shoulder. Thomas Todd Co., Boston

Coley B L 1949 Neoplasms of Bone and Related Conditions, 2nd edn. Paul B. Hoeber, New York

Coley B L, Higgenbotham N L 1948 Conservative surgery in tumors of bone. With special reference to segmental resection. Ann Surg 127: 231–242

Coley W B 1893 The treatment of malignant tumors by repeated innoculations of erysipelas: with a report of ten original cases. Am J Med Sci 105: 487–511

Coley W B 1905 Final results in the X-ray treatment of cancer including sarcoma. Ann Surg 42: 161–184

Coley W B 1924 Prognosis in giant-cell sarcoma of the long bones. Based upon the end-results in a series of 50 cases. Ann Surg 79: 321–357

Contreras T J, Blair P J, Harlan D M 1998 Brief history of the United States Navy Tissue Bank and Transplantation Programme. Captain Kenneth Sell's living legacy. In: Phillips G O, Strong D O, von Versen R, Nather A (eds) Advances in Tissue Banking, vol. 2. World Scientific, River Edge, pp 21–28

Conway B, Tomford W W, Hirsch M S, Schooley R T, Mankin H J 1990 Effects of gamma irradiation on HIV-1 in a bone allograft model. Trans Orthop Res Soc 15: 225

Cortes E P, Holland J F, Wang J J, Sinks L F 1972 Doxorubicin in disseminated osteosarcoma. J Am Med Assoc 221: 1132–1138

Cortes E P, Holland J F, Wang J J, Sinks L F, Blom J, Senn H, Bank A, Glidewell O 1974 Amputation and adriamycin in primary osteosarcoma. N Engl J Med 291: 998–1000

Coutard H 1934 Principles of X-ray therapy of malignant disease. Lancet ii: 1–12

Coventry M B, Dahlin D C 1957 Osteosarcoma. A critical analysis of 430 cases. J Bone Joint Surg 39A: 741–757

Curie P, Curie M 1898 Sur une substance nouvelle radioactive, contenue dans la pechblende. Compt Rendus Acad des Sci Paris 127: 175

Curtiss P H, Powell A E, Herndon C H 1959 Immunological factors in homogeneous bone transplantation. III. The inability of homogeneous rabbit bone to induce circulating antibodies in rabbits. J Bone Joint Surg 41A: 1482–1488

D'Aubigne M, Dejournay J P 1958 Diaphyseo-epiphysial resection for bone tumors about the knee. J Bone Joint Surg 40B: 385–395

Dahlin D C 1967 Bone Tumors: General Aspects and Data on 3987 Cases, 2nd edn. Charles C. Thomas, Springfield

Dahlin D C 1975 Pathology of osteosarcoma. Clin Orthop 111: 23–32

Dahlin D C, Coventry M B 1967 Osteogenic sarcoma: a study of six hundred cases. J Bone Joint Surg 49A: 101–110

Dahlin D C, Henderson E D 1962 Mesenchymal chondrosarcoma. Further observations on a new entity. S Cancer 15: 410–417

Damadian R 1971 Tumor detection by nuclear magnetic resonance. Science 171: 1151–1153

Damadian R, Zaner K, Hor D, Dimaio T 1973 Human tumors by NMR. Physio Chem Phys 5: 381–402

Deeley T J 1983 A brief history of cancer. Clin Radiol 34: 597–608

Delloye C, DeNayer P, Allington N, Munting E, Coutelier L, Vincent A 1988 Massive bone allografts in large skeletal defects after tumor surgery: a clinical and microradiographic evaluation. Arch Orthop Trauma Surg 107: 31–41

Dick H M, Malinin T I, Mnaymneh W A 1985 Massive allograft implantation following radical resection of high-grade tumors requiring adjuvant chemotherapy treatment. Clin Orthop 197: 88–95

Dobson J 1959 John Hunter's views on cancer. Ann Roy Coll Surg Engl 25: 167–181

Donaldson F 1853 The practical application of the microscope to the diagnosis of cancer. Am J Med Sci 25: 43–70

Dorfman H D, Czerniak B 1998 Bone Tumors. Mosby, St Louis

Dosoretz D E, Murphy G F, Raymond A K, Doppke K P, Schiller A L, Wang C C, Suit H D 1983 Radiation therapy for primary lymphoma of bone. Cancer 51: 44–46

Dupuytren G 1805 Tumors of bone. Bull Ecole Med de Paris 2: 13–24

Ebbell B 1937 The Ebers Papyrus: The Greatest Egyptian Medical Document, Copenhagen

Eckardt J J, Matthews J G, Eilber F R 1991 Endoprosthetic reconstruction after bone tumor resections of the proximal tibia. Orthop Clin N Am 22: 149–160

Enneking W F 1966 Local resection of malignant lesions of the hip and pelvis. J Bone Joint Surg 48A: 991–1007

Enneking W F 1983 Musculoskeletal Tumor Surgery. Churchill Livingstone, New York

Enneking W F 1987 A system for evaluation of the surgical management of musculoskeletal tumors. In: Enneking W F (ed) Limb Salvage in Musculoskeletal Oncology. Churchill Livingstone, New York, pp 145–150

Enneking W F, Dunham W K 1978 Resection and reconstruction for primary neoplasms involving the innominate bone. J Bone Joint Surg 60A: 731–746

Enneking W F, Eady J L, Burchardt H 1980a Autogenous cortical bone grafts in the reconstruction of segmental skeletal defects. J Bone Joint Surg 62A: 1039–1058

Enneking W F, Shirley P D 1977 Resection-arthrodesis for malignant and potentially malignant lesions about the knee using an intramedullary rod and local bone grafts. J Bone Joint Surg 59A: 223–236

Enneking W F, Spanier S S, Goodman M A 1980b Current concepts review: the surgical staging of musculoskeletal sarcoma. J Bone Joint Surg 62A: 1027–1030

Enzinger F M, Weiss S W 1983 Soft Tissue Tumors. C V Mosby, St Louis

Ewing J 1919a A review and classification of bone sarcomas. Arch Surg 4: 485–533

Ewing J 1919b Neoplastic Diseases: A Textbook of Tumors. W B Saunders, Philadelphia

Ewing J 1921 Diffuse endothelioma of bone. Proc NY Path Soc 21: 17–24

Ewing J 1922 An analysis of radiation therapy in cancer. Trans Coll Phys Phila 44: 190–235

Fischer B 1913 Ueber ein primares adamantinoma der tibia. Frankfurt Z Path 12: 422–441

Foley G E 1974 Sidney Farber (1903–1973). CA Cancer J Clin 24: 294–296

Friedlaender G E, Strong D M, Sell K W 1976 Studies on the antigenicity of bone. I. Freeze-dried and deep-frozen bone allografts in rabbits. J Bone Joint Surg 58A: 854–858

Friedlaender G E, Strong D M, Tomford W W, Mankin H J 1999 Long term follow up of patients with osteochondral allografts. A correlation between immunologic responses and clinical outcome. Orthopedic Clin N Am 30: 583–590

Galen C 192 De Tumoribus Praeter Naturam

Gerlitt J 1939 Cosmas and Damian, the patron saints of physicians. Ciba Found Symp 1: 118–121

Geschickter C F, Copeland M M 1936 Tumors of Bone (Including the Jaws and Joints). American Journal of Cancer, New York

Geschickter C F, Copeland M M 1951 Parosteal osteoma of bone: a new entity. Ann Surg 103: 790–807

Goldenberg R R, Campbell C J, Bonfiglio M 1970 Giant cell tumor of bone. An analysis of two hundred and eighteen cases. J Bone Joint Surg 52A: 619–662

Goorin A M, Abelson H T, Frei E 1985 Osteosarcoma fifteen years later. N Engl J Med 313: 1637–1643

Gouin F, Passuti N, Verriele V, Delecrin J, Bainvel J V 1996 Histological features of large bone allografts. J Bone Joint Surg 78B: 38–41

Gross S W 1879 Sarcoma of the long bones: Based on the study of one hundred and sixty-five cases. Am J Med Sci 78: 2–57, 338–377

Grubbe E H 1933 Priority in the therapeutic use of X-rays. Radiol 21: 156–162

Hall E J 1972 Radiation dose rate: a factor of importance in radiobiology and radiotherapy. Br J Radiol 45: 81–97

Hatcher C H 1945 The development of sarcoma in bone subjected to rontgen or radium irradiation. J Bone Joint Surg 27: 179–195

Hejna M J, Gitelis S 1997 Allograft prosthetic composite replacements for bone tumors. Sem Surg Oncol 13: 18–24

Herndon C H, Chase S W 1954 The fate of massive autogenous and homogenous bone grafts including articular surfaces. Surg Gynec Obstet 98: 273–290

Hernigou P, Delepine G, Goutallier D 1991 Infections after massive bone allografts in surgery of bone tumors of the limbs. Incidence, contributing factors, therapeutic problems. Rev Chir Orthop 77: 6–13

Hinds F 1898 Case of myeloid sarcoma of the femur treated by scraping. Br Med J 1: 555

Hippocrates, trans. W H S Jones, 4 vols. Heinemann, London, 1953–57

Hornicek F J, Gebhardt M C, Sorger J I, Mankin H J 1999 Tumor reconstructions. Orthopedic Clin N Am 30: 673–684

Hornicek F J, Mnymneh W, Lackman R D, Exner G U, Malinin T I 1998 Limb salvage with osteoarticular allografts after resection of proximal tibia bone tumors. Clin Orthop 352: 179–186

Hounsfield G N 1973a Computerized transverse axial scanning (tomography): Part 1: Description of system. Br J Radiol 46: 148–149

Hounsfield G N 1973b Computerized transverse axial scanning (tomography): Part 2: Description of system. Br J Radiol 46: 1016–1022

Hudson T M, Scheibler M, Sprigfield D S, Hawkins I F, Enneking W F, Spanier S S 1983 Radiologic imaging of osteosarcoma: role in planning surgical treatment. Skel Radiol 10: 137–146

Jackson R 1971 St. Peregine, OSM – Patron saint of cancer patients. Canad Med Assoc J 111: 824–827

Jaffe H L 1934 Osteoid osteoma: a benign osteoblastic tumor composed of osteoid and atypical bone. Arch Surg 31: 709–728

Jaffe H L 1950 Aneurysmal bone cyst. Bull Hosp Joint Dis 11: 3–13

Jaffe H L 1956 Benign osteoblastoma. Bull Hosp Joint Dis 17: 141–151

Jaffe H L 1958 Tumors and Tumorous Conditions of Bones and Joints. Lea & Fèbiger, Philadelphia

Jaffe H L 1972 Metabolic, Degenerative and Inflammatory Diseases of Bones and Joints. Lea & Fèbiger, Philadelphia

Jaffe H L, Lichtenstein L 1942 Benign chondroblastoma of bone. A reinterpretation of the so called calcifying or chondromatous giant cell tumor. Am J Pathol 28: 969–983

Jaffe H L, Lichtenstein L 1944 Eosinophilic granuloma of bone. Arch Pathol 37: 99–118

Jaffe H L, Lichtenstein L 1946 Chondromyxoid fibroma of bone. A distinctive benign tumor likely to be mistaken for chondrosarcoma. Arch Pathol 45: 541–551

Jaffe H L, Lichtenstein L, Portis R B 1940 Giant cell tumor of bone. Its pathologic appearance, grading, supposed variants and treatment. Arch Pathol 30: 993–1031

Jaffe H L, Lichtenstein L, Sutro C J 1941 Pigmented villonodular synovitis, bursitis and tenosynovitis. Arch Pathol 31: 731–765

Jaffe N, Farber S, Traggis D, Geiser C, Kim B S, Das L, Frauenberger G, Dierassi I, Cassady J R 1973 Favorable response of osteogenic sarcoma to high dose methotrexate with citrovorum rescue and radiation therapy. Cancer 31: 1367–1373

Jaffe N, Frei III E, Traggis D, Bishop Y 1974 Adjuvant methotrexate and citrovorum factor treatment of osteogenic sarcoma. N Engl J Med 291: 994–997

Jaffe N, Watts H 1976 Multidrug chemotherapy in the treatment of osteosarcoma. J Bone Joint Surg 58A: 634–635

Jofe M H, Gebhardt M C, Tomford W W, Mankin H J 1988 Osteoarticular allografts and allografts plus prosthesis in the management of malignant tumors of the proximal femur. J Bone Joint Surg 70A: 507–516

Johns H E, Bates L M, Watson T A 1952 1000 Curie units for radiation therapy. Br J Radiol 25: 296–302

Johnson E W, Dahlin D C 1959 Treatment of giant cell tumor of bone. J Bone Joint Surg 41A: 895–904

Johnson J T H 1978 Reconstruction of the pelvic ring following tumor resection. J Bone Joint Surg 60A: 747–751

Johnston J 1987 A modular prosthetic knee system for tumor surgeons. In: Enneking W F (ed) Limb Salvage in Musculoskeletal Oncology. Churchill Livingstone, New York, pp 234–237

Julien P, Ledermann F, Touwaide A 1993 Cosma e Damiano. Antea, Milan

Kardinal G C, Tarbro J W 1979 A conceptual history of cancer. Sem Oncol 6: 396–408

Kienbock R 1900 Die einwirkung des rontgenlichtes auf die haut. Med Wschr 47: 1581–1582

Kolodny A 1927 Bone Sarcoma: The Primary Malignant Tumors of Bone and the Giant Cell Tumor. Surgical Publishing Co., Chicago

Kotz R, Salzer M 1982 Rotation-plasty for childhood osteosarcoma of the distal part of the femur. J Bone Joint Surg 64A: 959–969

Langenbeck B 1850 Grossses enchondrom (gallertknorpel-geschwulst) des Schulterblattes: Extirpation des ganzen Schulterblattes mit Ausnahme des process coracoides. Dtsch Klin-Berl 2: 302–319

Langer F, Gross A E, West M, Urovitz E P 1978 The immuno-genicity of allograft knee joint transplants. Clin Orthop 132: 155–162

Lebert H 1845 Physiologie Pathologique, 2 vols. Paris J B Ballière

Lederman M 1981 The early history of radiotherapy: 1895–1939. Int J Rad Oncol Biol Phys 7: 639–648

Lederman M, Greatorex C A 1953 A cobalt 60 telecurie unit. Br J Radiol 26: 525–532

Lewis M M, Spires Jr W P, Bloom N 1987 Extendable pros-thesis: an alternative to amputation. In: Enneking W F (ed) Limb Salvage in Musculoskeletal Oncology. Churchill Livingstone, New York, pp 606–610

Lexer E 1908 Die Verwendung der freien Knochenplastik nebst Versuchen uber Gelenkversteifung und Gelenktrans-plantation. Arch Klin Chir 86: 939–954

Lexer E 1925 Joint transplantation and arthroplasty. Surg Gynec Obstet 40: 782–809

Lichtenstein L 1956 Benign osteoblastoma. Cancer 9: 1044–1052

Lichtenstein L 1959 Bone Tumors, 2nd edn. C V Mosby, St Louis

Linberg C F 1928 Interscapulothoracic resection for malignant tumors of the shoulder with preservation of a functional extremity. J Bone Joint Surg 1: 344–349

Lord C F, Gebhardt M C, Tomford W W, Mankin H J 1988 The incidence, nature and treatment of allograft infections. J Bone Joint Surg 70A: 369–376

Loty B, Courpied J P, Tomeno B, Postel M, Forest M, Abelanet R 1990 Bone allografts sterilized by irradiation. Biological

properties, procurement and results of 150 massive allo-grafts. Int Orthop 14: 237–242

Lyon T G 1896 The rontgen rays as cure for disease. Lancet i: 326

Lysholm E 1923 Apparatus for the production of a narrow beam of rays in treatment by radium at a distance. Acta Radiol 2: 516–519

Lytton D G, Resuhr L M 1978 Galen on abnormal swellings. J Hist Med Allied Sci 33, 531–49

Macewen W 1881 Observations concerning transplantation of bones: illustrated by a case of inter-human osseous trans-plantation, whereby over two-thirds of the shaft of the humerus was restored. Proc Roy Soc London 32: 232–234

Makley J T 1985 The use of allografts to reconstruct intercalary defects of long bones. Clin Orthop 197: 58–75

Malawer M M, Dunham B K, Zaleski T, Cielinski C J 1987 Management of aggressive benign and low-grade malignant bone tumors by cryosurgery: analysis of 40 cases. In: Enneking W F (ed) Limb Salvage in Musculoskeletal Oncology. Churchill Livingstone, New York, pp 498–510

Malawer M M, McHale K 1989 A limb sparing surgery for high grade malignant tumors of the proximal tibia. Surgical technique and a method of extensor mechanism recon-struction. Clin Orthop 239: 231–248

Malmud L S, Charkes N D 1975 Bone scanning. Principles, techniques and interpretation. Clin Orthop 107: 112–122

Mankin H J 1983 Complications of allograft surgery. In: Friedlaender G E, Mankin H J, Sell K W (eds) Osteochondral Allografts. Little, Brown, Boston, pp 259–274

Mankin H J, Doppelt S H, Sullivan T R, Tomford W W 1982 Osteoarticular and intercalary allograft transplantation in the management of malignant tumors of bone. Cancer 50: 613–630

Mankin H J, Gebhardt M C, Jennings L C, Springfield D S, Tomford W W 1996 Long-term results of allograft replacement in the management of bone tumors. Clin Orthop 324: 86–87

Mankin H J, Gebhardt M C, Tomford W W 1987 The use of frozen cadaveric allografts in the management of patients with bone tumors of the extremities. Orthop Clin N Am 18: 275–289

Mankin H J, Lange T A, Spanier S S 1982 Hazards of biopsy in patients with malignant primary bone and soft tissue tumors. J Bone Joint Surg 64A: 1121–1127

Marcove R, Lewis M, Huvos A G 1977 En bloc upper humeral interscapulo-thoracic resection. The Tikhoff–Linberg procedure. Clin Orthop 124: 219–228

Marcove R, Lewis M, Rosen G, Huvos A 1977 Total femur and total knee replacement. Clin Orthop 126: 147–152

Marcove R, Martini N, Rosen G 1975 The treatment of pulmonary metastasis in osteogenic sarcoma. Clin Orthop 111: 65–69

Marcove R C, Mike V, Hajek J V, Levin A G, Hunter R V P 1970 Osteogenic sarcoma under the age of 27. A review of 145 operative cases. J Bone Joint Surg 52A: 411–423

Marcove R C, Weis L D, Vaghaiwalla M R, Pearson R 1978 Cryosurgery in the treatment of giant cell tumors of bone. Clin Orthop 134: 275–279

Martland H F, Conlon P, Knet J P 1925 Some unrecognized dangers in the use and handling of radioactive substances. J Am Med Assoc 85: 1769–1776

McCarthy E F 1980 Giant cell tumor of bone: an historical perspective. Clin Orthop 153: 14–25

McGoveran B M, Davis A M, Gross A E, Bell R S 1986 Evaluation of the allograft-prosthesis composite technique for proximal femoral reconstruction after resection of a primary bone tumour. Cancer Surg 42: 37–45

Miller H 1950 A 2 MeV X-ray generator for therapy. Br J Radiol 23: 731–739

Mnaymneh W, Malinin T 1989 Massive allografts in surgery of bone tumors. Orthop Clin N Am 20: 455–467

Mnaymneh W, Malinin T I, Makley J T, Dick H M 1986 Massive osteoarticular allografts in the reconstruction of extremities following resection of tumors not requiring chemotherapy and radiation. Clin Orthop 227: 666–677

Moore A T, Bohlman H R 1943 Metal hip joint. A case report. J Bone Joint Surg 25A: 688–692

Morris H 1876 Conservative surgery. Lancet i: 440

Mott V 1828 An account of a case of osteosarcoma of the left clavicle in exsection of that bone was successfully performed. Am J Med Sci 3: 100–108

Muhm J R, Brown L R, Crowe J K 1977 Detection of pulmonary nodules by computed tomography. Am J Radiol 128: 267–280

Muscolo D L, Ayerza M A, Calabrese M E, Redal M A, Araujo E S 1996 Human leukocyte antigen matching, radiographic score and histologic findings in massive frozen bone allografts. Clin Orthop 326: 115–126

Olson J S 1989 The History of Cancer: An Annotated Bibliography. Greenwood, New York

Ortiz-Cruz E, Gebhardt M C, Jennings L C, Springfield D S, Mankin H J 1997 The result of transplantation of intercalary allografts after resection of tumors. A long term follow-up study. J Bone Joint Surg 79A: 97–106

Otis J C, Lane J M 1987 Nonmodular segmental knee replacements: design and performance. In: Enneking W F (ed) Limb Salvage in Musculoskeletal Oncology. Churchill Livingstone, New York, pp 22–24

Ottolenghi C E 1955 Diagnosis of orthopaedic lesions by aspiration biopsy. J Bone Joint Surg 37A: 443–464

Ottolenghi C E 1966 Massive osteoarticular bone grafts. J Bone Joint Surg 48B: 646–659

Pack G T, Ariel I M 1958 Tumors of the Soft Somatic Tissues. A Clinical Treatise. Hoeber-Harper, New York

Paget J 1853 Lectures in Surgical Pathology, 2 vols. Longman, Brown, Green & Longmans, London

Parrish F F 1966 Treatment of bone tumors by total excision and replacement with massive autologous and homologous grafts. J Bone Joint Surg 48A: 968–990

Parrish F F 1973 Allograft replacement of part of the end of a long bone following excision of a tumor: report of twenty-one cases. J Bone Joint Surg 55A: 1–22

Peltier L F 1961 The use of plaster of Paris to fill defects in bone. Clin Orthop 21: 1–31

Phemister B 1945 Rapid repair of defect of femur by massive bone grafts after resection for tumors. Surg Gynec Obstet 80: 120–127

Phemister D B 1930 Chondrosarcoma of bone. Surg Gynec Obstet 50: 216–233

Phemister D B 1940 Conservative surgery in the treatment of bone tumors. Surg Gynec Obstet 70: 355–364

Poretta C A, Dahlin D C, Janes J M 1957 Sarcoma in Paget's disease of bone. J Bone Joint Surg 39A: 1314–1329

Pringle J H 1916 The interpelvi-abdominal amputation with notes on two cases. Br J Surg 4: 283–287

Quimby E 1941 The specification of dosage in radium therapy. Am J Rontgenol 45: 1–16

Ramach W, Sigmund R, Sekera J, Salzer-Kuntschik M, Kotz R, Knahr K, Salzer M 1987 Functional results of customized prosthetic devices for the knee region after resection of bone and joints. In: Enneking W F (ed) Limb Salvage in Musculoskeletal Oncology. Churchill Livingstone, New York, pp 215–220

Rinaldi E 1987 The first homoplastic limb transplant according to the legend of Saint Cosmas and Saint Damian. Ital J Orthop Traumatol 13: 394–406

Ritschl P, Braun O, Pongracz D, Eyb R, Ramach W, Kotz R 1987 Modular reconstruction system for the lower extremity. In: Enneking W F (ed) Limb Salvage in Musculoskeletal Oncology. Churchill Livingstone, New York, pp 237–243

Röntgen W C 1895 Ueber eine neue Art von Strahlen. Sitzungsberichte der physikalisch-medicinischen Gesellschaft zu Wurzburg. Sitzung 30: 132–141

Rosen G 1987 Neoadjuvant chemotherapy for osteogenic sarcoma. In: Enneking W F (ed) Limb Salvage in Musculoskeletal Oncology. Churchill Livingstone, New York, pp 260–267

Rosen G, Caparros B, Huvos A G, Kosloff C, Nirenburg A, Cacavio A, Marcove R C, Lane J M, Metta B, Urban C 1982 Preoperative chemotherapy for osteogenic sarcoma: selection of postoperative adjuvant chemotherapy based on the response of the primary tumor to preoperative chemotherapy. Cancer 49: 1221–1230

Rosen G, Suwansirikul S, Kwon C, Tan C, Wu S J, Beattie E J, Murphy M L 1974 High dose methotrexate with citrovorum factor rescue and adriamycin in childhood osteosarcoma. Cancer 33: 1151–1163

Rosenthal D I, Hornicek F J, Wolfe M W, Jennings L C, Gebhardt M C, Mann N H J 1998 Percutaneous radiofrequency coagulation of osteoid osteoma compared with operative treatment. J Bone Joint Surg 80A: 815–821

Salzer M, Knahr K, Kotz R, Ramach W 1987 Cementless prosthetic implants for limb salvage of malignant bone tumors the knee joint: clinical results of three modes of anchorage. In: Enneking W F (ed) Limb Salvage in Musculoskeletal Oncology. Churchill Livingstone, New York, pp 26–29

Sauerbruch F 1922 Die Extirpation des Femur mit Umkipp-Plastik des Unterschenkels. Dtsch Zeit Chir 169: 1–12

Scales J T, Wait M, Wright K W J 1984 Intramedullary fixation of 'custom-made' major endoprostheses with special reference to the bone response. Engl Med 13: 185

Schachar N S, Cucheran D J, McGann L E, Novak K A, Frank C B 1994 Metabolic activity of bovine articular cartilage during refrigerated storage. J Orthop Res 12: 15–20

Schachar N S, McGann L E 1991 Cryopreservation of articular cartilage. In: Friedlaender G E, Goldberg V M (eds) Bone and Cartilage Allografts. American Academy of Orthopaedic Surgeons, Park Ridge, pp 211–230

Schajowicz F 1942 La degeneracion sarcomatosa de la osteitis deformante de Paget. Rev Orthop Traumatol 12: 131–148

Schajowicz F 1981 Tumors and Tumor-like Lesions of Bones and Joints. Springer, New York

Sim F H, Beauchamp C P, Chao E Y 1987 Reconstruction of musculoskeletal defects about the knee for tumor. Clin Orthop 221: 188–201

Sim F H, Chao E Y 1979 Prosthetic replacement of the knee and a large segment of the femur or tibia. J Bone Joint Surg 61A: 887

Simon M A, Aschliman M A, Thomas N, Mankin H J 1986 Limb salvage treatment versus amputation for osteosarcoma of the distal end of the femur. J Bone Joint Surg 68A: 1331–1337

Simon M A, Enneking W F 1976 Management of soft tissue sarcomas of the extremities. J Bone Joint Surg 58A: 312–327

Sinks L F, Mindell E R 1975 Chemotherapy of osteosarcoma. Clin Orthop 111: 101–104

Spanos P K, Payne W S, Ivins J C, Pritchard D J 1976 Pulmonary resection for metastatic osteogenic sarcoma. J Bone Joint Surg 58A: 624–628

Stauffer R N 1991 Problems with using metallic implants for replacement of bony defects. In: Friedlaender G E, Goldberg V M (eds) Bone and Cartilage Allografts. American Academy of Orthopaedic Surgeons, Park Ridge, pp 295–299

Steiner G C 1965 Post radiation sarcoma of bone. Cancer 18: 603–612

Stewart F W 1933 The diagnosis of tumours by aspiration. Am J Pathol 9: 801–811

Stewart F W 1954 James Ewing MD. Arch Pathol 36: 325–340

Stout A P 1953 Tumors of the Soft Tissues. Fascicle 5, Section 2. In: Ferminger H I (ed) Atlas of Tumor Pathology. Armed Forces Institute of Pathology, Washington DC

Strong D M, Friedlaender G E, Tomford W W, Springfield D S, Burchardt H C, Enneking W F, Mankin H J 1996 Immunological responses in human recipients of osseous and osteochondral allografts. Clin Orthop 326: 107–114

Strong D M, Sayers M H, Conrad III E U 1991 Screening tissue donors for infectious markers. In: Friedlaender G E, Goldberg V M (eds) Bone and Cartilage Allografts. American Academy of Orthopaedic Surgeons, Park Ridge, pp 193–209

Struhal E 1976 Tumors in the remains of ancient Egyptians. Am J Physical Anthropol 45: 613–619

Subramanian G, McAfee J G 1971 A new complex of ^{99m}Tc for skeletal imaging. Radiology 99: 192–196

Suit H D 1975 Radiotherapy in osteosarcoma. Clin Orthop 111: 71–75

Suit H D, Proppe K H, Mankin H J, Wood W C 1981 Preoperative radiation therapy for sarcoma of soft tissue. Cancer 47: 2269–2274

Suit H D, Russell W O 1975 Radiation therapy of soft tissue sarcomas. Cancer 36: 759–764

Suit H D, Russell W O, Martin R G 1973 Management of patients with sarcoma of soft tissue in an extremity. Cancer 31: 1247–1255

Suit H D, Russell W O, Martin R G 1975 Sarcoma of soft tissue: clinical and histopathologic parameters and response to treatment. Cancer 35: 1478–1483

Suit H D, Tepper J E, Mankin H J, Truman J T, Wood W C, Harmon D C, Schiller A L, Rosenberg A 1988 Sarcomas of soft tissue and bone. In: Wang C C (ed) Clinical Radiation Oncology, PSG Publishing, Littleton, MA, USA pp 331–349

Sullivan M P, Sutow W W, Taylor G 1963 L-phenylalanine mustard as a treatment for metastatic osteogenic sarcoma in children. J Pediat 63: 227–237

Sutow W W, Gehan E A, Vietti T J, Frias A E, Dyment P G 1976 Multidrug chemotherapy in primary treatment of osteosarcoma. J Bone Joint Surg 58A: 629–633

Sweetnam R 1973 Amputation on osteosarcoma. Disarticulation of the hip or high thigh amputation for lower femoral growths? J Bone Joint Surg 55B: 179–182

Sweetnam R 1975 The surgical management of osteosarcoma. Clin Orthop 111: 57–64

Tan M H, Mankin H J 1997 Blood transfusion and bone allografts. Effect on infection and outcome. Clin Orthop 340: 207–214

Tomford W W 1983 Cryopreservation of articular cartilage. In: Friedlaender G E, Mankin H J, Sell K W (eds) Osteochondral Allografts. Little, Brown, Boston, pp 215–218

Tomford W W, Doppelt S H, Mankin H J 1989 Organization, legal aspects and problems of bone banking in a large orthopaedic center. In: Aebi M, Regazzoni P (eds) Bone Transplantation. Springer, Berlin, pp 145–150

Tomford W W, Mankin H J 1999 Bone banking: update on methods and materials. Orthopedic Clin N Am 30: 553–565

Tomford W W, Thongphasuk J, Mankin H J, Ferraro M J 1990 Frozen musculoskeletal allografts. A study of the clinical incidence and causes of infection associated with their use. J Bone Joint Surg 72A: 1137–1143

Van Nes C P 1950 Rotation-plasty for congenital defects of the femur. J Bone Joint Surg 32B: 12–16

Vesalius A 1543 De Humani Corporis Fabrici. Basle

Virchow R 1863–67 Die Krankhaften Gewulste. Hirschwald, Berlin

Volkov M 1970 Allotransplantation of joints. J Bone Joint Surg 52B: 49–53

Von Recklinghausen F D 1882 Uber die multiplen Fibroma der haut und ihere Beziehungen zu die Neuromen. A Hirschwald, Berlin

Von Recklinghausen F D 1891 Die fibrose oder deformierende Ostitis, die osteomalazie und die osteoplastiishe Carcinose in ihren gegenseitigen Beziehungen. Fortsch R. Virchow, Berlin

Weis L, Hellan R L, Watson R C 1978 Computed tomography of orthopedic tumors of the pelvis and lower extremities. Clin Orthop 130: 254–259

Wilson J N 1971 Prosthetic replacement of long bone for tumour (two cases). Proc Roy Soc Med 64: 716–717

Wilson J W 1947 Virchow's contribution to the cell theory. J Hist Med 2: 163–178

Wilson P D, Lance E M 1965 Surgical reconstruction of the skeleton following segmental resection for bone tumors. J Bone Joint Surg 47A: 1629–1656

Wright J R Jr 1985 The development of the frozen section technique, the evolution of surgical biopsy, and the origins of surgical pathology. Bull Hist Med 59: 295–326

15

Orthopaedic product technology during the second half of the twentieth century

Dane Miller

The significance of implants and the biotechnology surrounding them are frequently underestimated by the lay observer. For example, it is currently estimated that between 8 and 10% of Americans have a permanent implant of some kind. It is further estimated that one in four Americans over sixty years of age has an implant, and that nearly five million total joints are currently in use in the USA. While it was difficult to find similar statistics outside of America, most would probably agree that similar percentages exist in the entire Western world.

Much of the advances in biomaterials, biomechanics and surgical instrumentation technology have occurred during the past fifty years. Therefore, this chapter concentrates on the steps forward and backward during this time leading to the very successful and gratifying experience most patients have with their total hip and total knee replacements today.

While many orthopaedic implants are used in procedures other than the replacement of arthritic joints, this chapter is principally oriented toward total joint replacement, which represents nearly half of the revenue generated by the orthopaedic industry today. It will also be heavily oriented toward the US experience due to the fact that the author's primary experience is within the American orthopaedic industry.

During the early decades of the twentieth century only a few meaningful steps in treating orthopaedic problems with implants were significant. However, the rate of the introduction of new technology increased substantially over time, especially during the last decade or two.

PRE-1950S

The earliest identified foreign material implanted to treat arthritic disease was reported in 1902 and involved gold foil as an interposition material by Robert Jones (Jones & Lovett 1929). In the early twentieth century, materials such as zinc, magnesium, celluloid, silver, rubber and decalcified bone were also used in a similar fashion. Unfortunately, neither the surgical approach nor the foreign materials used were successful, and such uses were only reported anecdotally well into the twentieth century.

By the 1920s several surgeons were using glass interposition arthroplasty cups with some level of success, but unfortunately the implants carried with them a continuous risk of catastrophic fracture. In hip arthroplasty, probably the most important advance in biomaterials of the early twentieth century was the fabrication by Marius Smith-Petersen of cup arthroplasties made of a cobalt–chromium–molybdenum alloy, trade-named Vitallium® (Fig. 15.1). Two years after the death of Smith-Petersen, Otto AuFranc, his assistant, published the results of a series of one thousand Vitallium® cup arthroplasties performed at Massachusetts General Hospital with 82% of results being good to satisfactory (Aufranc 1957). This publication and the results of the study formed the true foundation for the treatment of hip arthritis with engineered foreign implants.

The early positive experiences by Smith-Petersen encouraged Willis Campbell to use a similar interposition plate for hemi-arthroplasty of the knee in 1938 (Campbell 1940). He used a Vitallium® plate formed to the contour of the distal femur and attached it using hooks (Fig. 15.2). Little success occurred with this early mould arthroplasty of the knee until some of the surgeons at Massachusetts General Hospital, including W. N. Jones, AuFranc and W. L. Kermond attached a medullary stem (Jones et al 1967). Unfortunately, none of these early hemi-arthroplasty approaches, whether resurfacing the tibia or femur, provided clinical satisfaction in more than a small fraction of the patients.

Unlike Smith-Petersen's experience in the hip, neither distal femoral nor proximal tibial hemi-arthroplasty

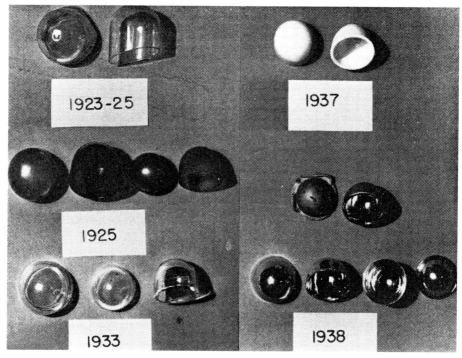

Fig. 15.1 Evolution of Smith-Petersen's mould: 1923, glass; 1925, Viscaloid; 1933, glass (Pyrex); 1937, Bakelite; 1938, Vitallium (Smith-Petersen 1939)

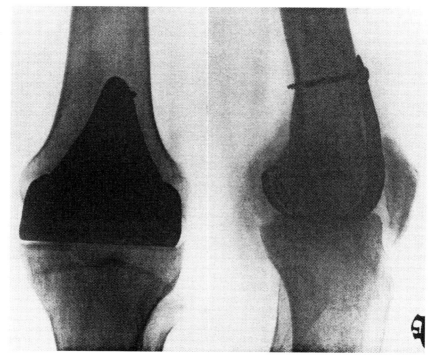

Fig. 15.2 (A) Anteroposterior and (B) lateral radiographs of the knee following arthroplasty showing a Vitallium plate in position (Campbell 1940)

proved to provide significant long-term pain relief in the knees of most patients. Most of the designs showed early and painful loosening, and these early attempts at hemi-arthroplasty of the knee were completely abandoned during the 1950s.

The preceding paragraphs were not meant to be an all-encompassing review of what happened during the first half of the twentieth century. They were to identify a few high points in the establishment of a technology base that would lead into the exciting events that were to occur during the second half of the twentieth century.

THE 1950S: 'FITS AND STARTS'

I have named this section 'Fits and Starts' because in my opinion it reflects a decade of real progress in implant design, the philosophy of fixation and materials, but on several occasions throughout the decade there were disappointing steps backward. In the area of both hip and knee replacement it was recognised during the 1950s that under the right set of circumstances stemmed intramedullary fixation of implants at both

ends of the femur and in the upper tibia showed some elements of success. Among the steps backward, as the term 'fits' suggests, were the use of various polymers, especially polymethylmethacrylate, which led to early wear problems and loosening.

In 1951 Frederick Thompson, Austin Moore and R. K. Lippman began performing hemi-arthroplasty surgery using intramedullary endoprostheses. The Thompson and Moore designs were similar with tapered stems and collars designed to wedge tightly into the medullary canal and rest on the proximal calcar (Fig. 15.3). Prostheses by Thompson and Moore continue to be used today in nearly unmodified form. The Lippman device was significantly different and relied on a technology called 'transfixation' (Fig. 15.4). Despite some early clinical success with the prosthesis, it was eventually abandoned in preference for single-piece, stemmed, intramedullary, hemi-arthroplasty prostheses.

Before these successful applications of cobalt and stainless steel alloys in hemi-arthroplasty fabrication, the Judet brothers in France began using an acrylic,

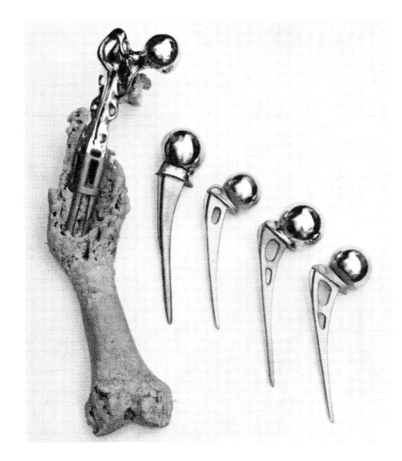

Fig. 15.3 Original Moore–Bohlman prosthesis and early models of the Moore prosthesis

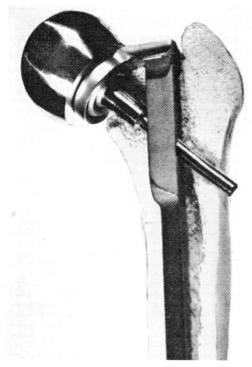

Fig. 15.4 Lippman's transfixion prosthesis in a femoral specimen (Lippman 1957)

short-stemmed, mushroom-shaped 'resection-reconstruction' design (Judet & Judet 1950). The stem on the Judet prosthesis was not designed to pass distally into the femoral medullary canal, but instead to pass transversely through to the lateral cortex of the femur (Fig. 15.5).

A variety of other surgeons developed similar prostheses to the Judet during the late 1940s and early 1950s showing, along with the Judet, positive short- and medium-term results. Unfortunately, medium- to long-term loosening, wear of the acrylic femoral head and resorption of the femoral neck became significant complications.

It is important to remember that during the 1950s more than fifty different types of hemi-arthroplasty prostheses were introduced. By the end of the decade the trend moved away from short-stem Judet prostheses to the Moore and Thompson type of intramedullary long stems. There was also significant movement away from polymeric components to implants made from either stainless steel or cobalt–chrome–molybdenum alloys. Running parallel with the work described above in hemi-arthroplasty of the hip was a series of efforts aimed at developing total hip replacements.

McKee and Watson-Farrar began implanting a metal-on-metal stainless steel design in 1951 with limited

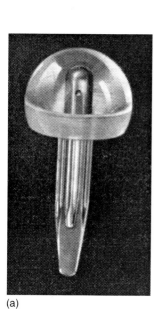

(a)

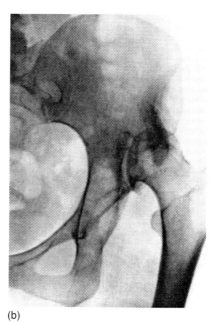

(b)

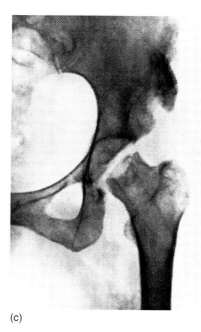

(c)

Fig. 15.5 (A) Original Judet acrylic prosthesis. (B) Radiograph of twenty-six-year-old female with congenital dislocation of left hip. The patient had an unsuccessful shelf operation with marked upward displacement of the femoral head. (C) New acetabulum formed in a normal position; the head was excised and replaced with an acrylic Judet prosthesis, which is radio lucent (Judet & Judet 1950)

success (McKee 1970). In 1953 McKee modified his femoral component to add a stem similar to the Thompson prostheses, and made both components out of cobalt–chrome–molybdenum alloy and began to see a success rate similar to that of cup arthroplasties (McKee & Watson-Farrar 1966).

In 1958 John Charnley reported his clinical experience using a stainless steel femoral component and a polytetrafluoroethylene acetabular component combined with a cementing or grouting technique using self-curing polymethylmethacrylate (PMMA) bone cement (Charnley 1961). Attempts had been previously made to use PMMA as a grouting agent but they met with limited success. Charnley would later report the failure of this total hip system due to rapid wear and tissue response to the polytetrafluoroethylene. The experience with this first acrylic fixed metal/polymer total hip was Charnley's both greatest accomplishment and greatest disappointment. It is noteworthy that by the late 1950s to early 1960s McKee and Watson-Farrar would be using PMMA to cement their implants.

We will now turn toward prosthetic knee surgery during the 1950s. It is interesting to note that prosthetic knee arthroplasty was following a parallel pathway to hip arthroplasty during this decade. Because of the relative success of cup or mould arthroplasty in the hip, several surgeons applied similar approaches to the knee. Early attempts in both the 1940s and 1950s to use free-moving mould arthroplasty implants in the knee met with little success (Campbell 1940, Jones et al 1967, Platt & Pepler 1969). The addition of a medullary stem to such a free-floating device for fixation in the femur provided minimal improvement in the clinical results. At the same time several authors, most notably MacIntosh and McKeever, were using a metallic tibial prosthesis fixed to the tibia in the hope of avoiding the reported clinical problems with fixation to the femur (MacIntosh 1958, McKeever 1960). McKeever's design is given in Fig. 15.6.

By the late 1950s it became apparent that neither femoral nor tibial hemi-arthroplasty provided significant medium- to long-term relief of pain of the knee. In a literature review published in 1957, Professor Walldius discusses the reported 896 hemi-arthroplasty procedures with the knee, showing only a long-term success rate of 46% (see Chapter 3). This review supported Walldius's conclusion that total knee replacement, not hemi-arthroplasty, was required for successful implant arthroplasty treatment of the knee.

As with many other prosthetic implants during the 1950s, the initial Walldius design was produced in a polymethylmethacrylate material. This early design was changed several times to increase strength and provide

metallic reinforcing inserts and ultimately the material was abandoned altogether. In the late 1950s the Walldius prosthesis was briefly made of stainless steel with a polytetrafluoroethylene bearing. By the end of the decade it was manufactured from cobalt–chrome–molybdenum alloy and began to show some positive clinical results (Fig. 15.7).

While there were other hinged total-knee implants produced, the early work by Walldius and the evolution to the stemmed cobalt alloy design of the late 1950s became the foundation from which future knees would be designed.

THE 1960S: REAL BREAKTHROUGHS

The 1960s were to experience the most significant event affecting the orthopaedic industry, profession and patient of the entire century. Interestingly enough, it would be at least ten if not fifteen years before the significance of this event was understood by the constituency involved. After the disappointments in 1958 experienced with John Charnley's selection of polytetrafluoroethylene, he changed his acetabular cup material to high-density polyethylene. The introduction of this ultrahigh molecular weight version of linear polyethylene combined with a metallic stem and cement fixation of both components became the gold standard for future developments in total hip replacement.

To understand the slowness by which the orthopaedic profession and industry responded requires an understanding of the historical environment in which this breakthrough in materials was achieved. The early part of the century had involved the application of various polymeric materials including celluloid, phenolics and especially acrylics with highly disappointing, maybe even disastrous, results. Even Charnley had had a disappointing experience with polytetrafluoroethylene. Many clinicians and material scientists were not sure that orthopaedics needed another polymer disappointment. In the environment of the 1960s, it would take at least five years of clinical results to awaken the field of orthopaedics to the significance of this development.

Many other clinicians and manufacturers began developing total hip systems with modification of the Charnley concept. Still, much of the orthopaedic research community remained sceptical of polyethylene's long-term clinical success and therefore new metal-on-metal articulations were also beginning to surface. The most significant new concepts involved a system developed by Peter Ring in Britain involving a Moore-style uncemented femoral component with a screw-in acetabular component fixed with a long central

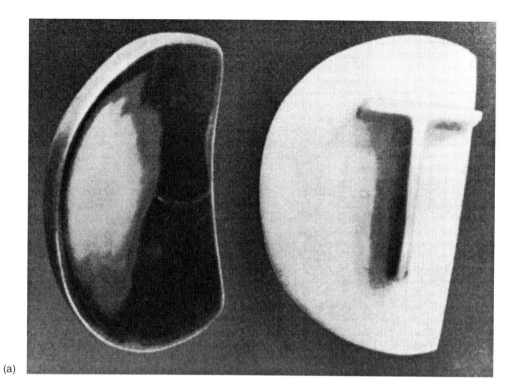

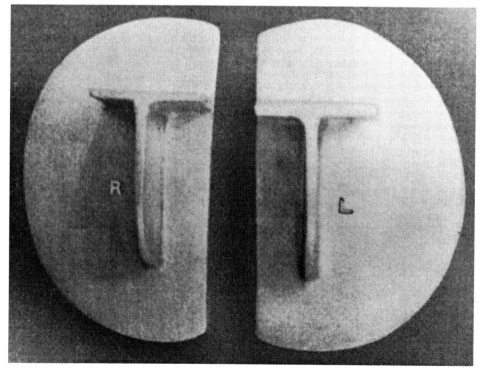

Fig. 15.6 (A) Tibial plateau prosthesis with the articulating surface (left) and undersurface and stem (right). (B) Undersurface and stem of both the left and right prostheses for a knee (McKeever 1960)

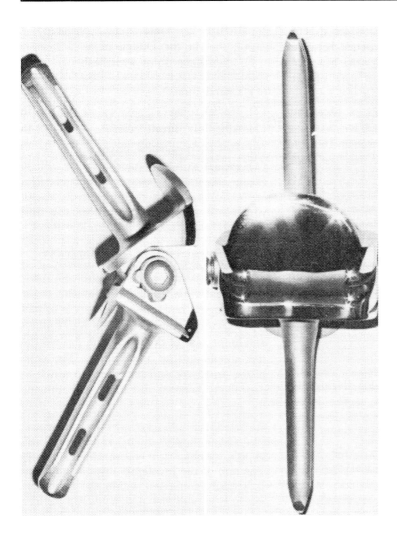

Fig. 15.7 Two views of the Walldius prosthesis (Jones 1973)

screw (Ring 1968) (Fig. 15.8). Professor Maurice Müller of Bern had developed a total hip system involving a polyethylene acetabular component and Thompson-like femoral component with a 32 mm head. This system, often termed the Charnley–Müller Hip, was fixed to the bone using methyl methacrylate bone cement. Charnley argued that his 22 mm low-friction total hip arthroplasty created lower friction and less wear debris, while Müller proposed that the larger femoral head diameter provided better stability against dislocation and a more forgiving system with regard to positioning of components. This argument still exists today with many compromising femoral head diameters in the 25–28 mm range.

The field of total knee replacement surgery experienced significantly less excitement during the 1960s than the field of total hip replacement. Several simple hinged knee prostheses were developed and implanted either with or without bone cement (Shiers 1954, Hungerford et al 1984). One of the most important examples of such an implant was the Stanmore hinged knee prostheses developed by Professor John Scales at the Royal National Orthopaedic Hospital in Stanmore, Middlesex (Lettin et al 1978).

Toward the end of the decade manufacturers and the clinical community began looking at ways to apply Charnley's developments of materials to total knee replacement. The first of these, the polycentric prosthesis, reached the clinic in 1968 and resulted from a development between Frank Gunston working with Charnley in Wrightington, England (Fig. 15.9). By the end of the 1960s it had become apparent that we would enter the next decade in orthopaedics with a new total joint paradigm which had been developed by Charnley.

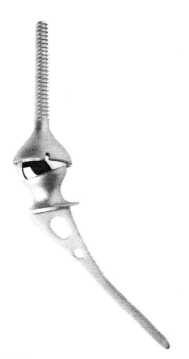

Fig. 15.8 Metal-on-metal prosthesis developed by Peter Ring

THE 1970S: 'WEAR – IS POLY TOO GOOD TO BE TRUE?'

The 1970s were characterised by many new total hip designs that can be characterised retrospectively as spin-offs of the basic concepts popularised in earlier decades by John Charnley and Maurice Müller. The orthopaedic industry in America identified an 'opinion leading' surgeon champion and introduced hip designs such as the Harris Hip developed by William Harris of Boston, the AuFranc–Turner Hip developed by Rod Turner of Boston, the Bechtol Hip from Charlie Bechtol of Los Angeles, the T-28 developed by Harlan Amstutz of Los Angeles, along with a variety of other lesser known total hip systems. With hindsight we can now look back at this early 1970s' total hip development and imagine that it was a little like preparing a Mexican meal. A Mexican meal consists of about six or eight basic ingredients combined to create a large number of individual menu items. For example, in the total hip developments taking place in the early 1970s the combination of 'ingredients' included: (1) femoral head diameter: between 22 and 32 mm; (2) femoral component metal: cobalt alloy or stainless steel; (3) femoral fabrication technique: casting, forging or machining; (4) stem shape: straight or curved; (5) stem cross-section: tapered or constant; and (6) acetabular OD design: groove or dimples. About

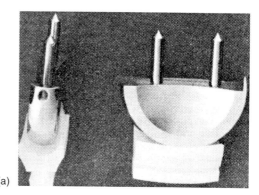

(a)

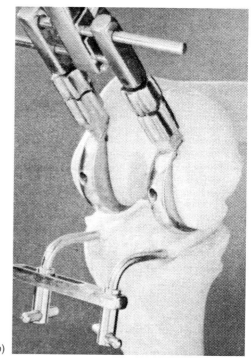

(b)

Fig. 15.9 (A) Polycentric prosthesis. (B) The jig used during installation of the prosthesis (Gunston 1973)

the only constant in these early designs was high-density or ultrahigh molecular weight polyethylene.

Throughout the 1970s the real goal in total hip design as the outstanding clinical results of the Charnley and Charnley–Müller designs were becoming better recognised was to improve upon these gold standards. Unfortunately, there were a few miscues along the way. It was assumed that any metal processed in any fashion would have adequate strength for long-term success of the joint. It was learned that with a growing number of fractured stems, solution annealing of the cobalt alloy and investment casting of the stainless steel alloy did not produce stems of adequate strength for long-term durability. The manufacturers using these techniques would abandon them by the end of the decade.

There was also another interesting process taking place in America's orthopaedic research laboratories. This was the study of the wear of polyethylene against various metallic surfaces. This effort took place despite the fact that growing clinical experience with polyethylene as a bearing material was not generally demonstrating a significant long-term clinical problem with polyethylene wear. There were anecdotal pieces of worn acetabular components requiring revision, but frequently these could be traced to the use of lower molecular weight high-density polyethylene instead of the now proven ultrahigh molecular weight polyethylene. The disparity between clinical experience and university and industrial research during this decade regarding wear is difficult to explain. It is the author's opinion that this led to misguided efforts to 'solve the wear problem' by introducing new materials such as polyesters, polyacetels, carbon-fibre reinforced polyethylene and ceramic on ceramic bearings. Fortunately these 'solutions to the wear problem' were relatively short-lived and, for the most part, were not broadly commercialised. During the last half of the 1970s a new problem now truly connected to clinical results had surfaced and had become known as the 'cement disease problem'. It was a growing opinion in most orthopaedic circles by the end of the decade that bone cement was the biggest problem in total hip replacement and sooner or later its use would have to cease.

It is interesting to note that much of the early research on 'living fixation' or porous ingrowth fixation had begun in the late 1960s and early 1970s. Much of this work was discussed at the early 'Clemson Meetings', which later became the International Society for Biomaterials. By the mid-1970s, chemical and mechanical problems with bone cement and their solutions with porous ingrowth fixation became a popular subject at the Orthopedic Research Society meetings.

The move toward commercialisation of these technologies took place relatively slowly for a variety of reasons. First, the orthopaedic industry was slow to recognise the significance of fixation in the long-term success of total joint replacement. Second, difficulties in the processing of femoral and acetabular components and the compromise in certain mechanical properties were a barrier to bringing a product to market. And finally, there was great concern on the part of both clinician and manufacturer of the complications that might exist if revision surgery was necessary with such well-fixed porous ingrowth prostheses.

By the mid-1970s, however, the first of these systems, the Madreporique hip replacement developed

by Gerald Lord of France, was introduced (Lord et al 1979, Lord & Bancel 1983) (Fig. 15.10). At the same time, Robert Judet, also of France, introduced the Judet macro-ingrowth stem and acetabular component (Judet et al 1978).

Similar work was underway in the USA with the AML Prosthesis developed with the input of Charles Engh of Baltimore (Engh et al 1981, 1984). The prosthesis, manufactured by DePuy of Warsaw, Indiana, was fully coated with sintered beads and had no collar. Later versions of the AML prosthesis with partial stem coating were introduced and are still clinically and commercially successful today. A little side note to the AML name may be appropriate. Readers familiar with orthopaedic products may know that the AML trademark stands for Anatomic Medullary Locking, as trademarked by DePuy. It is rumoured, although unconfirmed, in orthopaedic circles that AML really stood for Austin Moore Lundsford. The leading surgeon in this development with DePuy was Emmit Lundsford who had previously studied under Moore. However, due to Lundsford's untimely death in an aeroplane accident in the late 1970s, the manufacturer decided to look for an alternative definition for the trademark AML. Whether this story is true is academic, but at least it offers an additional opportunity to recognise a true pioneer in orthopaedic research – Emmit Lundsford.

The final development in total hip technology from the 1970s involved the development of a variety of surface replacement or 'conservative' total hip implant systems. These were systems developed to avoid replacing large segments of bone, especially in the upper femur, and allow reloading of the calcar in a more anatomically correct biomechanical fashion. The theory was that if the upper femur including the neck of the natural femur could be loaded under more natural conditions without a stem to offload the stresses distally,

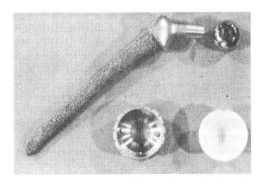

Fig. 15.10 Lord's Universal Madreporic prosthesis with a porous coated stem, threaded acetabular shell and modular polyethylene liner (Lord & Bancel 1983)

the disuse of the proximal femur that led to resorption and osteolysis might be eliminated. Such systems were the THARIES (Total Hip Articular Replacement with Internal Eccentric Shells) developed by Harlan Amstutz of Los Angeles and the Indiana Conservative developed by William Capello of Indianapolis (Fig. 15.11). The lesson to be learned from this experience is that a seemingly elegant biomechanical solution often leads to biological disappointment (Matthews et al 1973, Amstutz et al 1986). Early loosening and revisions were

characteristic with these systems. While some clinical attention was paid to this concept well into the 1980s, no further discussion will occur throughout the remainder of this chapter.

The story for total knee replacement in the 1970s is considerably different than that for total hip replacement. The total knees achieving any kind of clinical and commercial success during the first part of this decade can be divided into two categories. First were the surface replacement types as described above,

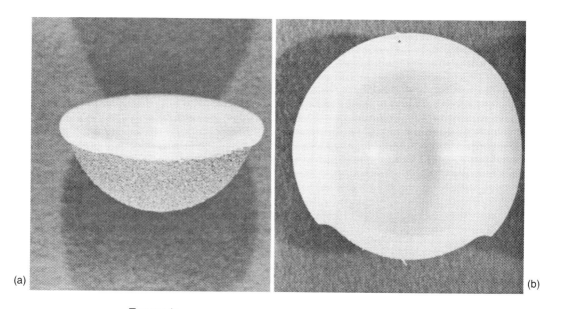

(a)

(b)

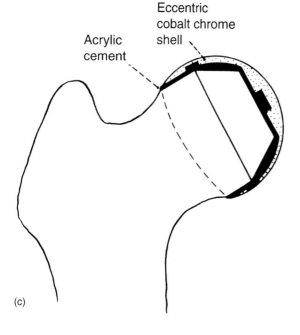

Eccentric
cobalt chrome
shell

Acrylic
cement

(c)

Fig. 15.11   (A) THARIES low-profile metal-backed socket, introduced in 1984 with cobalt–chrome plasma spray beads. (B) Trimmable polyethylene rim. (C) Conceptualised THARIES arthroplasty c.1975 (Amstutz et al 1986)

such as the Geometric, Polycentric and later Marmor modular designs that dealt principally with arthritic disease of the femoral/tibia joints. Second were the various intrinsically stable hinged or modified hinged designs such as the Guepar and Stanmore Knees.

The surface replacement designs generally failed for one of two reasons. First, patello-femoral disease could not be dealt with when using a surface replacement design and thus complete pain relief was not often obtained. Second, and the primary reason for failure of these early designs, was inadequate understanding of and attention to soft tissue balancing which led to ultimate instability and component loosening.

The intrinsically stable designs developed to address many of these problems failed for different reasons. These posted- or hinged-type of knees failed due to loosening and it soon became known that the soft tissue function could not be absorbed in the implant design itself. Other designs of this type, such as the Herbert, developed by J. J. Herbert, failed to a great extent through component fracture (Fig. 15.12) (Herbert & Herbert 1973). The Attenborough Total Knee (Fig. 15.13), which was a constrained design allowing for some translation and rotation, failed primarily through the polyethylene tibial component (Attenborough 1978). Later, the Spherocentric Knee was developed at the University of Michigan by Larry Matthews and Herbert Coffer (Matthews et al 1973). While achieving some level of commercial success, it also proved to be a disappointing design due to loosening and component fracture.

Generally, by the end of the 1970s, total hip replacement was considered to be a glowing success on a short- to medium-term basis, and many early designs were showing long-term clinical success. Throughout both the USA and Europe, however, total knee replacement was falling into disfavour. About 250,000 total hips were being replaced with a high level of confidence annually, while total knee replacement had probably peaked at less than 100,000 joints per year and was declining from that into the 1980s.

THE 1980S: 'BONE CEMENT – FRIEND OR FOE?'

As we leave the 1970s, much of the clinical community and orthopaedic industry was moving rapidly to cure the greatly overstated 'bone cement disease'. There was a rapid move toward sintered bead designs, ceramic coatings and diffusion-bonded wire mesh pads by various manufacturers. During the 1980s the sintered bead designs by DePuy called the AML Hip saw the sintered beads begin to move up the stem to prevent stress shielding from distal stem fixation. Howmedica

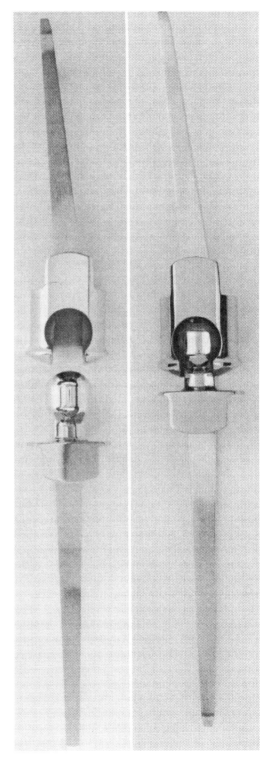

Fig. 15.12 Herbert total knee prosthesis (Herbert & Herbert 1973)

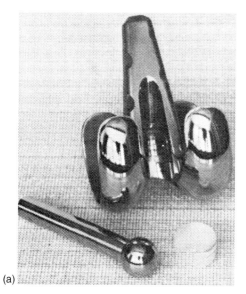

(a)

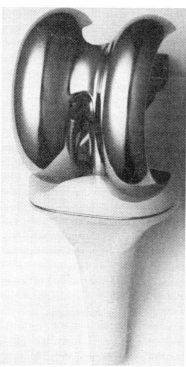

(b)

Fig. 15.13 Attenborough total knee. (A) Femoral component, stabilising rod and polyethylene circlip. (B) Entire prosthesis shown in flexion (Attenborough 1978)

was introducing the PCA design, first in the knee and then in the hip, with primary clinical leadership from John Hungerford. Various types of smooth press-fit hydroxyapatite coated stems were introduced by a

number of manufacturers with leadership coming from the Osteonics Division of Stryker and the Furlong Hip developed by Ronald Furlong and commercialised by Joint Replacement Instrumentation of England. The most widely used titanium wire mesh system was developed through the cooperation of William Harris of Boston and Jorge Galante of Chicago. These designs involved the diffusion bonding of mesh pads to strategic areas of the proximal implant surface and, along with the PCA Hip, gained a significant market share in the non-cemented total joint field.

Early clinical results with most of these designs were characterised by thigh pain, rationalised away as 'short-term pain for long-term gain'. In other words, it was expected that as the ingrowth process took place, femoral pain was a way of life but would be replaced by better long-term fixation of the stem. Unfortunately, this did not turn out to be the case and many systems experienced high levels of permanent thigh pain and ultimately premature revision due to proximal osteolysis.

Similar things were happening on the acetabular side of the joint. After several decades of simple all-polyethylene cemented acetabular components, several developments began to take place in the reinforcement and modified fixation of the socket side of the hip. Long-term clinical results with a metal-backed and replaceable acetabular component developed by William Harris and produced by Howmedica in the 1970s suggested that such designs led to lower rates of long-term loosening of the acetabular component. This, combined with several biomechanical studies of the acetabulum, encouraged the reinforcement of polyethylene-lined acetabular components with metal shells. Such early designs were the Bioclad, introduced by Biomet, and several porous-coated metal-backed systems by both Howmedica and Zimmer. Many of these early reinforced and non-cemented acetabular components were abandoned early due to premature loosening, osteolysis and revision. By the end of the decade only two cementless technologies seemed to survive in commercial application: titanium plasma spray-coated components, both acetabular and femoral, whose technology had been led earlier in the decade by Biomet; and the AML partially coated beaded stems introduced in the 1970s by DePuy. With these two exceptions, the rapid clinical and commercial migration away from bone cement was now equally rapid back toward the use of bone cement in fixation of implants.

As much as the 1970s showed significant progress in total hip replacement and relative disappointment in total knee replacement, the 1980s were to show great progress in successful total knee surgery improvement and a general 'progress stumble' in total hip replacement. By the beginning of the 1980s the general conclusion was that total knee designs to date were not working well. Considerable attention needed to be invested into design and fixation before total knee replacement would ever compare in popularity with total hip replacements. The Total Condylar design was initially developed by Insall and Walker in New York and commercialised by Johnson and Johnson Orthopedics and Howmedica. Combined with an expanding understanding of the soft and hard tissue biomechanics of the knee, the Total Condylar design gradually led to significant improvement in total knee replacement success. While there were other improvements that helped in the success of total knee replacement in the area of design and materials, the principal factor in the extraordinary improvements in long-term clinical results came not from the implant itself, but from instrumentation and surgical techniques.

Much of the early work in developing instrumentation was begun by M. A. R. Freeman in London with his early concept for soft tissue balancing during surgery. Many of these concepts for soft tissue balancing were further developed by both Howmedica with their advanced instrumentation system used with the PCA knee and by Biomet, which ultimately developed a calibrated ligament balancing instrument set. By the mid-1980s the American market for total knee replacement was expanding rapidly as longer clinical results were being reported with success rates approaching, if not exceeding, that in total hip replacement.

As with total hip replacement, the elimination of bone cement and introduction of porous or press-fit fixation systems also took place. However, by the end of the decade it became apparent that soft tissue was probably more important than the fixation method for long-term clinical success with total knee replacement.

There was another interesting clinical research dynamic taking place at this time. While much research attention was being paid to, and clinical results reporting on, a new disease called 'polyethylene wear debris disease', we had nearly forgotten the bone cement disease of the 1970s. This subject will receive further attention below.

THE 1990S: 'ONLY THE FIXED SURVIVE'

The 1990s can most accurately be termed a decade of regrouping. By the early 1990s, large studies with medium-term results were beginning to report relatively high revision rates with most cementless and/or press-fit systems introduced in the 1980s. It soon became apparent that 'short-term pain for long-term gain' was gradually turning into long-term pain for little or no gain. Attempts to eliminate bone cement disease in the

1980s had resulted in a new reported disease entity now called 'polyethylene wear disease'.

The author believes that history will demonstrate that the bone cement disease of the 1980s and polyethylene wear disease of the 1990s in fact are the same entity. Even the press-fit ceramic on ceramic hips marketed by Smith and Nephew Orthopaedics (then Richards Manufacturing) was showing similar problems of osteolysis at the interface. When we look back from 2010 I believe these osteolysis problems will be proven to be associated with the pumping of synovial fluid, with or without particulate contaminate into the interface within the joint capsule. The effect of the synovial fluid is to create creeping osteolysis at the interface until gross loosening of one or more components occurs and revision becomes necessary.

In the field of total hip replacement, the two most popular cementless designs of the 1980s were Howmedica's PCA and Zimmer's Harris–Galante Hips. Many other cementless systems were introduced, but these two were the most prevalently used, certainly in the American market. Relatively high rates of revision were being reported within five years following implantation, and as rapidly as we moved away from cement in the 1980s users of these systems were moving back to cemented systems.

There was, however, good news on the cementless fixation front. DePuy's AML and several titanium alloy plasma-sprayed coated systems produced by Biomet were showing good medium- to long-term clinical results. It is suggested that these two stems set themselves apart because they were coated with an ingrowth surface in a fully circumferential fashion. This allowed for a complete seal at the porous coating to bone interface, thus preventing the pumping of synovial fluid into the interface as described above.

If we now turn to the acetabular side of the hip, similar revelations were being reported. Certain of the porous beaded and wire mesh systems were showing reasonable fixation and relatively low acetabular revision rates. There had also been a move toward threaded acetabular components in the 1980s following the design of the Autophor ceramic acetabular cup. Unacceptable revision rates were also being reported with these threaded acetabular systems.

The experiences with threaded acetabular components, porous-coated, screw-fixed acetabular components, and stems with different surface ingrowth technology created a debate over the definition of a hybrid hip. Some clinicians thought that an appropriate hybrid hip included a cemented stem and cementless acetabular component, while others considered just the opposite to be the ideal hybrid system.

By the end of the 1990s there had been a complete move away from partially coated stems and acetabular components and a growing popularity with circumferentially coated bead systems such as the AML and plasma-spray systems produced by Biomet and now several other manufacturers. During the same period many manufacturers were dusting off old cemented designs and reintroducing them into the marketplace.

A different revelation was occurring in the area of total knee replacement. By the early 1990s it had become apparent that the Total Condylar-type design was very reliable long term when proper attention was paid to soft tissue or ligament balance. Much work within the industry was done in the 1990s to introduce systems with improved reinforced tibial bearing configurations and significantly improved instrumentation. Proper attention to the joint line positioning and medial and lateral soft tissue balance were beginning to show nearly flawless results in the two- to ten-year clinical use period. By the end of the 1990s the appropriate knee design appeared to be a Total Condylar femoral component, either cemented or cementless, and cemented tibial and patellar components. There had been a brief period during the late 1980s when reinforced patellar components became popular, but by the 1990s premature failure of such designs had led to their complete abandonment.

Also, unicompartmental knee replacement became popular during the 1990s. After several decades of popularity in Northern Europe, especially Scandinavia, unicompartmental knee replacement was replacing high tibial osteotomies or premature total knee replacement when only one compartment was affected by arthritic disease.

The popularity of unicompartmental knee replacement was further enhanced by improving the techniques for arthroscopically assisted, minimally invasive procedures. Unicompartmental knee replacement by the end of the 1990s was becoming the procedure of choice for conservative early intervention in unicompartmental osteoarthritis. Rapid recovery periods and high patient satisfaction were driving this segment of the market very rapidly by the year 2000.

In both hip and knee surgery it had become apparent that those systems showing good long-term fixation of all components had survived the test of time, whether cemented or cementless. As we enter the next millennium, it is expected that many new technologies will find their way into total joint replacement. However, mass-market success will only be preceded by a minimum of ten-year clinical studies. The overreaction to bone cement disease and polyethylene disease and the subsequent problems resulting

therefrom will lead to a much more cautious market in the years to come.

CONCLUSIONS

If we look back fifty years at the orthopaedic industry and practice of orthopaedic medicine, dramatic changes have taken place. Until nearly 1970, orthopaedic surgery was principally a field of trauma and the treatment of deformities. During the last thirty years, total joint replacement has become the single largest component of the orthopaedic industry and as well the most exciting and clinically satisfying segment of orthopaedic medicine. As the world's health care systems begin to reassess its reimbursement priorities into the next century, a high priority should be assigned to total joint replacement and similar medical technologies. The social payback and economic return on total joint replacement has been demonstrated to be among the highest of any treatment modality. Total hip and total knee replacement have probably improved the quality and quantity of life in the Western world, more than any other single medical technology in the history of mankind.

ACKNOWLEDGEMENTS

The author would like to thank Phillip M Gibbs, Development Engineer with Biomet, Inc. for his efforts in editing and obtaining illustrations and references for use in this chapter.

REFERENCES

Amstutz H C, Dorey F, O'Carroll, P F 1986 Tharies resurfacing arthroplasty evolution and long-term results. Clin Orthop 213: 92–114

Attenborough C G 1978 The Attenborough total knee replacement. J Bone Joint Surg 60B: 320

Aufranc O E 1957 Constructive hip surgery with Vitallium mold. A report on 1000 cases of arthroplasty of the hip over a 15 year period. J Bone Joint Surg 39A: 237–248

Calandruccio R A 1980 Campbell's Operative Orthopaedics, 6th edn. C V Mosby, St Louis

Campbell W C 1940 Interposition of Vitallium plates in arthroplasties of the knee. Am J Surg 47: 639

Charnley J 1961 Arthroplasty of the hip. A new operation. Lancet i: 129

Engh C A, Bobyn J D, Gorski J M 1984 Biological fixation of a modified Moore prosthesis. Orthopedics 7: 285

Engh C A, Brooker A F, Kenmore P I, Chandler H P, Lunceford E M 1981 Porous-coated hip replacement: a three-year follow-up study. Paper presented at the AAOS meeting, Las Vegas

Gunston F H 1973 Polycentric knee arthroplasty. Clin Orthop 94: 130

Herbert J J, Herbert A 1973 A new total knee prosthesis. Clin Orthop 94: 202

Hungerford D S, Krackow K A, Kenna R V 1984 Total Knee Arthroplasty: A Comprehensive Approach. Williams & Wilkins, Baltimore

Jones G B 1973 Total knee replacement – the Walldius Hinge. Clin Orthop 94: 50–57

Jones R, Lovett R W 1929 Orthopaedic Surgery. Wood, Baltimore

Jones W N, Aufranc O E, Kermond W L 1967 Mold arthroplasty of the knee. J Bone Joint Surg 49: 1022

Judet J, Judet R 1950 The use of an artificial femoral head for arthroplasty of the hip joint. J Bone Joint Surg 32B: 166–173

Judet R, Siguier M, Brumpt B, Judet T 1978 A noncemented total hip replacement. Clin Orthop Rel Res 137: 77–84

Lettin A W F, Deliss L J, Blackburne J S, Scales J T 1978 The Stanmore hinged knee arthroplasty. J Bone Joint Surg 60B: 327

Lippman R K 1957 The transfixion hip prosthesis. J Bone Joint Surg 39A: 759–785

Lord G, Bancel P 1983 The Madreporic cementless total hip arthroplasty. Clin Orthop Rel Res 176: 67–76

Lord G A, Hardy J R, Kummer F J 1979 An uncemented total hip replacement. Clin Orthop Rel Res 141: 2–16

MacIntosh D L 1958 Hemiarthroplasty of the knee using a space occupying prosthesis for painful varus and valgus deformities. J Bone Joint Surg 40: 1431

Mai M T, Schmalzried T P, Dorey F J, Campbell P A, Amstutz H C 1996 The contribution of frictional torque to loosening at the cement–bone interface in THARIES hip replacements. J Bone Joint Surg 78A: 505–511

Matthews L S, Sonstegard D A, Kaufer H 1973 The spherocentric knee. Clin Orthop 94: 234

McKee G K 1970 Development of total prosthetic replacement of the hip. Clin Orthop Rel Res 72: 85–103

McKee G K, Watson-Farrar J 1966 Replacement of arthritic hips by the McKee–Farrar prosthesis. J Bone Joint Surg 48B: 245–259

McKeever D C 1960 Tibial plateau prosthesis. Clin Orthop 18: 86

Moore A T 1960 The self-locking metal hip prosthesis. J Bone Joint Surg 39A: 811–827

Platt G, Pepler A 1969 Mould arthroplasty of the knee: a ten-year follow-up study. J Bone Joint Surg 51B: 76

Ring P A 1968 Complete replacement arthroplasty of the hip by the ring prosthesis. J Bone Joint Surg 50B: 720–731

Shiers L G P 1954 Arthroplasty of the knee. J Bone Joint Surg 36B: 553

Smith-Petersen M N 1939 Arthroplasty of the hip, a new method. J Bone Joint Surg 21: 269–288

Walldius B 1957 Arthroplasty of the knee using an endoprosthesis. Acta Orthop Scand 24 (suppl.): 19

SECTION 4:

The Future

16

Orthopaedics in 2050: a look at the future

Henry J. Mankin

One of the advantages of growing old is that it may not be necessary to live with your mistakes. Thus asking a person of my age to predict the way things will be in orthopaedics fifty years from now is fairly safe for me! Nevertheless it is a difficult and in fact in many ways an impossible task. For instance, those of us who were growing up in the early 1930s could never have predicted the way things have happened in the last seventy years. We could not have possibly guessed at wonderful things like air and now space travel, communication systems, television, the computer and, more specifically, the Internet. In medicine, we now view as commonplace undreamed of capabilities and events such as antibiotics, life-support systems, radiographic imaging, surgical technology, the disappearance of smallpox and polio, a vast array of drugs for control of many diseases, gene alteration and the like. On the less happy side of our naivety, none of us in our country at least would have thought that we would have had to deal with three additional wars (after the War to end all wars!), the A-bomb, the Holocaust, the Berlin Wall, the increased use of hallucinogenic drugs and dangerous weapons, AIDS and most recently the return of tuberculosis as a worldwide epidemic.

It is still possible based on the knowledge of the past, present and indications as to directions currently in progress to hazard some guesses as to the way things will be. It is important to point out a simple caveat, however. The Otis Company developed the first elevators before the end of the nineteenth century and even then could make them go much faster than they did or still do. The limiting feature of that system is not the technical capability of the equipment, but the brains of the human passengers, which in fact limit how rapidly the rise and descent can be. So it is with orthopaedic surgery in the next fifty years. The technological advances may be virtually unlimited in scope and extent, but the limiting feature may be the capacity of the human mind to understand and utilise these advances in caring for patients, in educating students and in performing quality research.

Let us now look into the crystal ball and see what the future may hold for the specialty of orthopaedic surgery. It seems logical to do this in terms of subject-matter and we should start with research and science, then education and finally clinical care.

SCIENCE

Engineering

In consideration of science and research in the orthopaedic specialty area, it is possible to predict that there will be some startling discoveries. I still firmly believe as I wrote in my Presidential Address for the American Orthopaedic Association in 1983 that mechanical engineering is near the end of its possible improvements and additions to our caretaking systems. Nevertheless the engineers continue to provide us with new devices and new approaches to our problems. It can be predicted that in the next fifty years our patients will fare better and our surgeons will find it easier based on competent engineering research. It may be predicted that we will see better systems for internal fixation of fractures, improved designs for joint implants and even robotic systems to correct the human errors in implantation and many more. The ankle and elbow that have resisted competent design of implants will surely be solved in these intervening years and the new devices although clearly similar in structure to those currently in use will be easier to implant, have fewer complications, last longer and function better. Engineers can now predict the likelihood of a fracture with bone malalignment or anatomical structural weakness but the technology is still experimental. In fifty years the equipment will be so sophisticated that they will be able to predict not only if the bone is in danger of breaking, but also what the fracture will consist of and when it will occur.

The future of engineering however is probably not really in the design of devices but in a new world of *tissue engineering*, which combines the specialties of engineering, mechanics and biology. It should be possible using the expanded technology and capacity to overcome immune responses, to transplant stem cells with cytokine elements in a medium which will allow virtually complete reconstitution of bony, cartilaginous or ligamentous components of the skeletal system. Thus, one will be able to repair a fracture, or replace a diseased or resected portion of the skeleton, or replace a tendon or a ligament, or heal a defect in cartilage with systems which start out quite differently in design and structure but ultimately become identical to the parent tissue, not only in histological appearance, but also in mechanical capabilities. It is even possible that one can reconstruct a metacarpal or even a major joint if the components have been destroyed. Of considerable importance to this system is the likelihood that autogenous cells may not be necessary and indeed allogeneic cell structures, for instance from the newborn's umbilicus can suffice. Of even greater potential value is the possibility that some form of xenogeneic tissue may be the material implanted. For the latter two possible sources of cells it is reasonable to assume that safe immunosuppressive agents may be developed but even more remarkable is the possibility that some form of immune modification may be directed at the implanted tissue such that the recipient accepts it as native material.

Biology

As one might expect in terms of advances in science, biological research will be explosive over the next half century. Knowledge will advance in terms of the biology and biochemistry of normal bone, cartilage, tendon and ligament and the mysteries of the anatomical structure and variations which occur from the time of conception until old age will be fully established. Epiphyseal growth will be well defined; intramembranous ossification will be now fully understood; the pattern of trabecular architecture will now be predictable; and Wolfe's law will be further exploded into a multiplicity of mechanical and chemical variables, which ultimately change the structure of the bone. The true effect of electricity and magnetism will be fully defined (for better or worse) and the role of osteocalcin, osteopontin, TGF-β, angiogenic factors, degradative enzymes, prostaglandins and growth factors will be daily reading matter in our orthopaedic literature package (surely by then on a sophisticated website rather than in a book!). It seems

logical that the bone morphogenic protein (BMP) family will be further expanded and that the true action of the array of materials included in this important group will not only be defined, but also available to the treating physician to solve problems such as disordered growth of bone or cartilage or non-union of fractures. The true action of the newest generation of bis-phosphonates (presumably much more potent and easier to use than the current ones) will be fully explored so that bone loss seen in fibrous dysplasia, metastatic cancer, Paget's disease and even senile or postmenopausal osteoporosis will be easier to treat.

Many of the mysteries of the articular cartilages and their diseases will be solved. We should be able to define the variation in structure in the different parts of the joint and in different joints; the materials which allow chondrocytes to proliferate and resist destruction; the role of the interleukins and dermatan sulphate proteoglycans in joint disease; and the actions and controlling elements for the matrix metalloproteases which are responsible for the degradative cascade, so critical to the arthritic process. Transport of materials across the matrix barrier will be carefully evaluated and scientists will clarify whether agents which are effective in controlling synovial disease are harmful to the aneural, avascular cartilage. The rheumatologists have been searching for a cause for rheumatoid arthritis and the other inflammatory arthritides for over two centuries – one would hope that they will be successful in the next fifty, but I am not sure we can count on that. The secrets seem to be too deeply buried.

Molecular biology

No field in all of medicine shows more promise of vast achievement than molecular biology. From the original identification of the structure of the chromosomes by Watson and Crick in 1953, we have progressed to the point where we are well on our way to discovering the structure of the entire human genome and, more importantly perhaps for clinicians, we have identified the gene error in many disorders. Especially striking amongst these are those diseases which in the past presented to orthopaedic surgeons with skeletal deformities many of which were genetic in origin and were eponymically identified, but were impossible to define in terms of causation and more importantly could not be treated other than in some cases by difficult or complex surgery. Many of these have now been 'solved' in terms of genetic error so that we can look at a case of achondroplasia and identify not only the clinical syndrome, but also more importantly that the gene locus for the error is at 4p16.3; or at a case of Morquio's disease and know that the locus of 16q24.3

is defective and that that is the cause of the child's difficulty. A partial listing of these errors is shown in Table 16.1. That is one of the great accomplishments of the last twenty years of the twentieth century, but it is only half done. Finding the gene error is important but of even greater importance is discovering the abnormal or absent proteinaceous and often enzymatic material made by the cell which is the cause of the clinical syndrome. One of the best examples is that of Gaucher disease where the gene error has been recognised but of greater importance is that evident fact that the defect causes a failure of production of glucosylceramide hydrolase, which results in the accumulation of intracellular lysosomal bound microtubular glucosylceramide. The presence of this material in the cells of the liver, spleen and bone marrow is the cause of this rare disease (Barton et al 1991) and patients who have been receiving modified β-glucosidase are clinically much improved. Of importance is the fact that some of these patients are now being treated with gene modification in an attempt to eliminate the error in the cells and thus hopefully eliminate the disease in them and the need for treatment. Similar studies are occurring with many other genetic disorders, only some of which are identified in Table 16.1, but in fact this work has only begun. It is predictable with the knowledge and capabilities of today's scientists that in the next half decade many of these disorders will be solved, not just as to genetic cause or protein error, but in terms of very competent and well-directed treatment. Thus patients with Tay-Sachs disease, or Hurler's syndrome, or osteogenesis imperfecta or hereditary multiple osteocartilaginous exostoses will be treated at birth or even while still in the uterus (after the defect is identified by amniocentesis or some other more sophisticated technique), their defective gene modified, and not only will they never show any clinical manifestation of these terrible disorders, but also they will never pass it on to their progeny – thus in time eliminating the disease. What an accomplishment for the science of tomorrow … what a great joy for the human race … what a delight for the treating orthopaedic surgeon … and what a relief to the anguished parents!

EDUCATION

Education in orthopaedics has been a major activity for many orthopaedic surgeons. The teachers teach the students and the students teach the teachers. Everybody wins! In recent years there have been some problems associated with this chiefly in terms of the impact of healthcare administrative and funding agencies, which consider education as less than a necessary function (Mankin 1999). Education in the last decade of the twentieth century is clearly less directed and less well conducted as it was in the prior decades, despite the fact that there is more to teach and the students are more capable and avid for knowledge than ever before.

Table 16.1 Gene loci for some orthopaedic diseases (partial listing)	
1. Achondroplasia	4p16.3
2. Charcot–Marie–Tooth Disease	17p11.2
3. Cleidocranial dysplasia	6p21
4. Diastrophic dysplasia	5q31-q34
5. Duchenne muscular dystrophy	Xp21.2
6. Hereditary multiple osteocartilaginous exostoses	8q21.11-q24.13
7. Facioscapulomuscular dystrophy	4q35
8. Fibrodysplasia ossificans congenita	20p12
9. Gardner's syndrome	5q21-q22
10. Klippel–Feil syndrome	5q11.2
11. Marfan's syndrome	15q21.1
12. Polyostotic fibrous dysplasia	20q13.2
13. Metaphyseal dysostosis (Type Schmid)	6q21-q22.3
14. Mucopolysaccharidosis (Hurler)	4p16.3
15. Mucopolysaccharidosis (Morquio)	16q24.3
16. Nail patella syndrome	9q34.1
17. Neurofibromatosis Type 1	17q11.2
18. Osteogenesis imperfecta	17q21.31-q22.05
19. Osteopetrosis	1p21-p13
20. Pseudohypoparathyroidism	20q13.2
21. Vitamin D-resistant rickets	12q12-q14
22. Spondyloepiphyseal dysplasia	Xp21.2-p22.1
23. Turner's syndrome	Xq13.1

If we are to maintain the quality of our orthopaedic care and research, we must make a very strong effort over the next few years to maintain and enlarge our educational commitment to medical students, residents, registrars, fellows and of course each other. Without research in one generation, the specialty will not grow ... without education in one generation there will be no specialty!

Education will be different. The books and journals will remain the way we learn, but they are now already at least in part delivered in a different way and in the future will be infinitely easier to access. The computer already can provide us with electronic full-text journals and books through the Internet and all of that is available on every computer (desktop, laptop, hand held and soon a virtual reality visual system). Accessing information will be spectacularly easy, rapid and inexpensive and should be possible to do in any setting about any subject. Learning will be programmed and directed and delivered everywhere via telesystems and it should be possible to call up imaging studies, lab data, clinical photographs and outcome data on any patient or group of patients, both as direct information or as rapidly performed regression statistics. Equally exciting is the possibility that one can learn anatomy, patient examination for physical findings and surgical technique by virtual reality systems.

But what will happen to the teacher and the lecturer? And equally important, what will happen to books and libraries? Will they be extinct in 2050? I think not. The human mind seems to need a 'book' or a 'journal' to look at or to read when it wishes and the library will remain, the 'wings' of medical education. Having said that, it is apparent that the library will be different in terms of structure and accessing systems to conform with the computer dependence we are already discovering is critical. As to the teacher, humans seem to learn and respond best to good interactive communication; and the lecture (albeit with better visual aids than currently available) and especially the question and answer period that follows will remain a major part of medical education. In fact the oldest form of such education, teaching at the clinic, bedside or operating table, will still serve our students and our teachers well. Both groups will learn from such Hippocratean encounters.

National organisations are already into computer communication. Currently one can submit abstracts for presentations at meetings, provide data for multicentre studies, apply for residency positions, etc. by computer. It is likely that meetings may be held at least in part through telecommunication systems, so that one need not travel to attend a national or international orthopaedic meeting. Having said that, it should be carefully noted that the social and communicative aspects of these meetings are also important; and although it will be possible to have interactive one-on-one direct verbal and visual communication with colleagues (and patients!) via computer, the warmth of a handshake or a friendly touch on a shoulder remain as important human requirements. Having dinner with friends is still an important and often very educational part of any meeting.

CLINICAL CARE

There is absolutely no doubt that clinical care will change radically over the next fifty years in terms of diseases we treat, the way we treat them, and our systems for outcome assessment and analysis. We had best recognise these changes ... they are in fact on their way, admittedly in rudimentary fashion and form.

The diseases:

1. *Genetic diseases*: as indicated above there will be some major developments in terms of recognition of syndromes both in newborn child or actually *in utero* by amniocentesis; both by a soon to be available form of non-invasive magnetic resonance spectroscopic system. The gene error will be assessed on a first drop of blood, the protein defect identified on the second drop; and the gene modification system introduced safely and easily immediately afterwards. If all this occurs as I believe it will, paediatric orthopaedic surgeons will no longer be required to deal with the terrible curses of the mucopolysaccharidoses, epiphyseal dysplasias, osteogenesis imperfecta, osteopetrosis, Ollier's and Maffucci's syndromes, florid fibrous dysplasia and the like. They will still have developmental hip dysplasia, club foot, scoliosis and other disorders of unknown and presumably non-genetic cause but be spared the most difficult of this group of unfortunate maladies.

2. *Infections*: it is our fervent hope and prayer that AIDS will be solved in the next few years and that no other such viral scourge will arise to threaten the health of continents ... but one cannot be sure. The AIDS virus is presumably a mutation and that can occur again ... and again ... and again over these next fifty years. Let us hope that the next ones will be easier to diagnose and treat and will be caught early enough to save the world the difficulties encountered with this terrible disease. Just as anterior poliomyelitis has been eliminated for most of the world in the 1950s by the introduction of a vaccine, we should anticipate that the same can be done for AIDS, Lyme disease, babesiosis, echinococcus, histoplasmosis and an array of other rare infectious disorders which now

represent major health problems in some parts of our world. Bacterial infections are another matter, however. We now have potent antibiotics that do an excellent job of preventing and controlling wound infections and osteomyelitis and one presumes that they will continue to do so and do it better. There is a nagging concern however that the bacteria may be developing resistant strains more rapidly than the bacteriologists can develop appropriate antibiotics to kill them and that just as we have resistant strains now that they will increase in number and potency. This would be a disaster in terms of clinical infectious disease, particularly in terms of the return of haematogenous osteomyelitis and, perhaps even more devastating, an increase in postoperative wound infections.

A special circumstance should be considered for tuberculosis, which is still the most frequent cause of death in the world today and infects more people than any other disease. We thought we had gained control of the disease in the past five decades based on the development of streptomycin, isonicotinic acid hydrolase, rifampin and many other drugs, but the new strains of the mycobacterium are more resistant to these agents (Valway et al 1998) and the genetically resistant strains of human are disappearing or are no longer passing their gene on to their progeny in the same way. It may be that the next few decades will see the return of the sanatorium and the tuberculous infections of spine, joints and even such rarely seen disorders as scrofula, Pott's disease and spina ventosa. Not a happy thought!

3. *Trauma*: there is little doubt that orthopaedic surgeons will continue to see and treat patients with traumatic injuries to their extremities. The injuries will be less likely to change in nature, causation and extent and in fact because people will live longer and feel well enough to continue sports and a more active life there may be considerably greater numbers of injuries to the elderly. The mean life span in 2050 may be as much as ninety-five or more, particularly if smoking is outlawed. The problem will lie only with the capacity of physicians to continue to treat patients in their nineties or older for injuries previously not treated because of the age and status of the patient. Some of these patients may be harder to care for than the younger group related in part to their mental status.

Furthermore, patients with multiple injuries who now die shortly after being seen in the emergency room setting will in the future have life support systems that far exceed the capacity of the current ones. Orthopaedic surgeons may then be faced with the management of multiple sites of extensive injury that will require the efforts of teams to restore the patient to musculoskeletal health. Of some likelihood, neural injuries to the spinal cord now resulting in paralysis or limited function and sensory deficit may be treated with drugs and other agents to restore function, possibly even late in the course. The ability to deal with nerve and blood vessel injury will surely improve to the point where nerve grafts and vascular repairs of all sorts will be commonplace even for injuries which we now think of as impossible to restore. The devices used for management of bony trauma will likely be much the same in design but may be considerably easier to apply. Skin and muscle grafts, free or on a pedicle will be used for many cases that currently would be doomed to fail because of poor healing, thus improving the outcome of some of the extensive trauma cases.

4. *Early osteoarthritis*: although there is current excitement about some of the cyclo-oxygenase inhibitors, chondroitin sulphate, glucosamine and hyaluronin injections it seems likely that the future holds a much larger step than these. Of greater interest is the possibility that osteoarthritic disease can be detected very early (perhaps by a high Tesla magnetic resonance imaging or spectroscopy system) and treated with appropriate medicinal agents to decrease the rate at which the disease progresses and indeed in some cases correct the process. The chemical materials may be administered orally or by injection and may over several months alter the process of the disease. There are some evidences in current research protocols that the success of this programme will lie in research areas which seek to enhance cartilage growth with some combination of cytokine factors such as fibroblast growth factor, insulin-like growth factor and TGF-β; and/or decrease the rate of degradation by interfering with interleukin 1, plasminogen-activator or some of the matrix metalloproteases such as collagenase or stromelysin.

5. *Localised cartilage defects*: currently there is a storm of interest in the treatment of localised cartilage damage of traumatic or osteonecrotic origin. The current systems are interesting and several of these such as cartilage cell replacement, periosteal flaps, mosaicplasty, stem cell and cytokine introduction have been tried and have stood up reasonably well through the early phase. There are doubts that they will continue to do so and it is evident to the 'chondrophilosophers' that more needs to be done. Whether this will include tissue engineering (see above), allograft implantation or improved 'cytokine cocktail' treatment is not clear but it would seem likely that in the next fifty years there will be a series of new systems that will put some of the athletes back on the playing field, despite defects in their cartilages.

6. *Late phase osteoarthritis*: when the entire joint has been destroyed by osteoarthritis, there remains little more to do than to insert a prosthetic implant. It is unlikely that 2050 will see many changes in the current excellent systems in use, except to enhance the longevity and functional capacity of the systems for hip, knee and shoulder by improved design of the device, a better and longer-lasting polyethylene or other plastic which will not disintegrate with time, and newer cements and methods of cementation (or non-cemented technique). It is hoped that by using the technology of tissue engineering, the method of fixation to bone will be firmer and longer lasting based on a bone bonding system. The areas of greater interest and potential improvement are prosthetic implants for the ankle, elbow and wrist, which currently have systems which are less than optimal.

7. *Metabolic bone disease*: there is little doubt that the most prevalent orthopaedic disorder in the elderly is osteopenia. Currently it is believed that the majority of this problem is caused by senile or post-menopausal osteoporosis and/or a little suspected osteomalacia, all of which destroy the strength and integrity of the bones and lead to wrist, hip and spine fractures and the multiple consequences thereof. It is clearly recognised that the percentage of the world-wide population over the age of seventy in 2050 will be much higher than presently and because of retirement systems and the sense of well-being associated with good general care, these patients will be at great risk for multiple injuries. As indicated above, these injuries will not be easy to treat and just as occurs today the fractures, particularly of the lower extremity, may lead to a deterioration of the patient's functional capacity and mentation and possibly an earlier demise. The answer does not really lie in improved methods of fixing fractures but in some preventative measures. Improving the brain's balance systems by better blood flow will certainly help but it seems logical and likely that biological treatment of bone strength is the key to reducing this unfortunate disorder, so prevalent now and soon to be over-whelming in extent.

What can do that? For women it seems logical that a 'safe' form of oestrogen replacement at menopause will help enormously. The currently used agents are implicated in carcinogenesis for breast and uterine tumours and it has been demonstrated that many connective tissue tumours have oestrogen and progesterone receptors. There must be some way of altering the structure of bone with hormones without increasing the likelihood of developing such neoplasms. Calcium and vitamin D supplements have been shown to be an important addition to the anti-osteopenia regimen and these should start early in life. A balanced diet is also essential. Anorexia should be avoided, particularly in their teen years. Adult humans are for the most part optional carnivores except for children who in their early years are pretty much obligate carnivores. An exercise programme maintained throughout life should be an essential of maintaining the strength of the skeleton. It is likely however that the new agents such as the bis-phosphonates which interfere with osteoclastic activity will be major forces in the fight against osteo-porosis in the elderly. It is possible that new drugs will be necessary to enhance the response and avoid complications, but it is likely that they will keep our bones stronger as we age and improve our lifestyle. It is also critical to keep track of the bone densitometry and although some systems are now available, newer more accurate and easier to access programmes will surely be available in the next fifty years.

8. *Bone and soft tissue tumours*: there is little doubt that great strides were made in the care of patients with bone and soft tissue tumours, either metastatic or primary in the last half of the twentieth century (see Chapter 14). As stated there, in the early 1960s, a patient with an osteosarcoma had only a 10% chance at survival and usually lost their leg; while almost all of those with Ewing's sarcoma died. Because of better staging, competent chemotherapy, well-ordered radiation and limb-sparing surgery, both for these two entities and other high-grade tumours including the soft tissue tumours we can now expect a prognosis of in some cases well over 60% survival. Most patients now have limb-sparing surgery. Similarly, metastatic disease can be controlled by radiation, chemotherapy and in some cases resection, and many patients with breast, renal or prostatic carcinoma have a long survival. Metallic implants and allografts have been developed to the point where insertion of the device after resection will leave the patient functional and ambulatory.

But what can we expect in the next fifty years? It is clear that a number of new approaches will be made and in fact some are in trial. The angiostatic agents, newer chemotherapeutic regimens, marrow replacement, laser treatment, interoperative radi-ation, proton beam therapy, immunological agents and even gene modification all are currently under consideration and will be expanded in scope and ease of administration, tested in animal systems and then applied to the bony or soft tissue lesions. We presume that they will be successful in eradicating or limiting many of the neoplastic diseases and improving the status of the patient.

There are, however, some things that will be required if that is to be effective. We need to establish a series of markers that will help to define the optimal course for the patient. The markers include:

- A definitive diagnostic marker possibly based on genetic sampling.
- A prognostic marker that will help to define the risk of metastasis for that particular tumour of that size at that anatomical site in the patient of that age, sex and health status.
- A marker that provides us with some clues as to the optimal treatment protocol, be it radiation, chemotherapy, surgery or some combination.
- A marker that defines the sensitivity of that tumour to the array of treatment modalities, especially chemotherapeutic agents. Is it sensitive to adriamycin, ifosfamide, methotrexate, vinblastine, *cis*-platinum or all the other new agents to be introduced over the next fifty years or some combination of them?
- A marker that defines the success of the treatment protocol during or immediately after administration. Currently some centres have started to use positron emission tomography (PET) for this purpose but it is just the beginning of a very exciting world of discovery.
- A marker that can define with certainty the presence of metastatic deposits in the lungs and other sites. We are currently dependent on computed tomography, magnetic resonance imaging, bone and gallium scans, and other less-specific forms of imaging, but surely when we fully define the tumour with a specific marker we should be able to scan for that marker and know if it is in another site.

Another issue is improvement in surgical systems for the treatment of these diseases. Clearly better imaging and defining the extent of the surgery will make resective surgery less disabling or deforming. The metallic implants that are now frequently modular rather than custom designed need to borrow from the page of the total joint people (see above) if they are to last longer. Devices that can be made to grow with the young child will be an essential system and hopefully these will be designed with a system such as magnetism so that the expansion can be performed without surgical intervention. Similarly allo-implants that now last longer than the metallic devices and are more anatomically competent are regrettably fraught with complications which occur in over 20% of the patients. These are surely related to the immune response. If matching can be done particularly in the Class 2 antigens or some system of immunosuppression introduced which does not diminish the patient's immune

system's control of the tumour, it should be possible to introduce not only the bone, but also soft tissues and possible vascular components.

Based on all this it is highly likely that patient's bone and soft tissue tumours and even metastatic disease in 2050 will have an earlier diagnosis, an easier course and a far better prognosis.

SURGICAL PROCEDURES

It is difficult to predict how surgery will change in the next fifty years, but it is quite clear that some things will be different. In the section on disease above there are a number of discussions of the changes seen in trauma, joint replacement, arthritis surgery, tumour treatment, etc. which provide some definition of the anticipated changes in the operative procedures. There are some issues and questions.

Will we have a lower complication rate? Will infection, bleeding, postoperative oedema, vascular injury, damage to nerve or spinal cord, postoperative deep venous thrombosis, and pulmonary embolism and other such current issues be reduced in frequency? Will the current debates about pedicle screws and spinal arthrodesis systems lead to improved systems? Will the complication rates for allo-implants be diminished? Will the arthroscopic systems be sufficiently improved so that the treatment of internal derangements of the knee and rotator cuff injuries to the shoulder will be easier to treat?

The answer to all of these questions is a guarded 'yes'. Surgery will be safer, easier and more effective for the patient. It is difficult to predict the way these things will happen, but it seems likely that minimally invasive surgical systems for the joints and spine will play a role, as will robotics and the improved design of implants. It is highly likely that tissue engineering will play a crucial role in surgery for hand injuries, joint disease, trauma and especially the necessary bonding of metallic implants to bone. Better drugs than are currently available will control postoperative deep vein thrombosis. Postoperative pain may disappear completely and infection will be partly controlled by a germ-free system and the liberal use of appropriate antibiotics.

Although I would like to predict that instruments will be sharper and always available, that operating room lighting will be much improved and that cases will always start on time, I think that may have been the same thing that I would have said about the year 2000 if I had been asked to write this chapter in 1950. There may be an important lesson there!

A final statement must be added to this collection of information, some of which is based on current information, some on speculation and some on what all of us hope to have available for our patients, our students and ourselves. It should be clear however that orthopaedic surgery has come a long way in the last two centuries. We started with learning we had a skeleton and that it sometimes did not work the way we wanted it to; and in the year 2000 we know more about all of it than I or any of the readers of this volume who are over sixty years of age ever dreamed we could. Few of these advances occurred by chance. They represent the effort and intellectual commitment and dedication of a group of wonderful people ... the orthopaedic surgeons and their colleagues. It is now a better world because of them and it is entirely predictable that their progeny will make it an even better world fifty years from now.

REFERENCES

Barton N W, Brady R O, Dambrosia J M, DiBisceglie A M, Doppelt S H, Hill S C, Mankin H J 1991 Replacement therapy for inherited enzyme deficiency macrophage targeted glucocerebrosidase for Gaucher's disease. N Engl J Med 324: 1464–1470

Mankin H J 1983 Orthopaedics in 2013: a prospection. J Bone Joint Surg 65A: 1183–1189

Mankin H J 1999 A managed care world: can academic activities survive? Clin Orthop 362: 256–260

Valway S E, Sanchez M P C, Shinnick T F, Orme I, Agerton T, Hay D, Jones J S, Westmorland H, Onorato M 1998 An outbreak involving extensive transmission of a virulent strain of mycobacterium tuberculosis. N Engl J Med 338: 633–639

Watson J D, Crick F H C 1953 Genetical implications of the structure of deoxyribonucleic acid. Nature 171: 964–967

Index